Occupational Therapy: Work-Related Programs and Assessments

Occupational Therapy: Work-Related Programs and Assessments
Second Edition

Karen Jacobs, M.S., OTR/L, FAOTA
Assistant Professor, Boston University
Sargent College of Allied Health Professions,
Department of Occupational Therapy
Boston

Foreword by
Florence S. Cromwell, M.A., OTR, FAOTA

Little, Brown and Company
Boston/Toronto/London

Contents

To Florence S. Cromwell, mentor and expert in work-related programming

Contributing Authors

Carl Bettencourt, OTR/L
Coordinator, WORK P.R.E.P., New England Rehabilitation Hospital
Ambulatory Care Center, Billerica, Massachusetts
Chapter 7

Theresa L. Breen
Occupational Therapy Student, Boston University, Boston
Chapter 10

KimAnn Clark
Occupational Therapy Student, Boston University, Boston
Chapter 10

Nancy Feldman, M.S., CCC Sp.
Speech Pathologist, Devereux Foundation—Center for Head Trauma, Devon,
Pennsylvania
Chapter 7

Sherlyn L. Fenton, OTR/L
Occupational Therapist, Liberty Mutual Rehabilitation Medical Service Center,
Boston
Chapter 7

Maria Foschi, M.Ed.
Cognitive Remediation Specialist, Devereux Foundation—Center for Head
Trauma, Devon, Pennsylvania
Chapter 7

Patricia Gagnon-Stryke, OTR/L
Senior Occupational Therapist, Liberty Mutual Rehabilitation Medical Service
Center, Boston
Chapter 7

Thelma Wellerson Hook, M.A., OTR
Director, Hand Therapy and Rehabilitation Associates, Los Gatos, California
Chapter 7

Glenda Jeong, M.A., OTR
Director, Keystone Vocational Services, San Francisco
Chapter 6

Valerie Shaw Jones, OTR/L
Occupational Therapist, Liberty Mutual Rehabilitation Medical Service Center,
Boston
Chapter 7

C. Shana Krell, OTR/L
Consultant, Occupational Therapy, United Cerebral Palsy Association of
MetroBoston, Inc., Watertown, Massachusetts
Chapter 7

Nancy MacRae, M.S., OTR
Assistant Professor, University of New England, Biddeford, Maine
Chapter 8

Deborah L. Maloney, OTR/L
Occupational Therapist, Devereux Foundation—Center for Head Trauma,
Devon, Pennsylvania
Chapter 7

Patricia A. McGauley, OTR/L
Occupational Therapist, Liberty Mutual Rehabilitation Medical Service Center,
Boston
Chapter 7

Michelle Moran
Occupational Therapy Student, Boston University, Boston
Chapter 10

Kathleen Murphy, B.A., B.Sc.OT(C)
Chief Occupational Therapist, CPRI, London, Ontario, Canada
Chapter 5

Jack Rabin, M.S., LCSW
Assistant Clinical Director, Division of Mental Health, Substance Abuse, and
Forensic Services, San Francisco
Chapter 6

Richard Schwartz, M.S., OTR
Director and Associate Professor, Occupational Therapy Program, and Director, Industrial Accident/Industry Prevention Lab, University of Texas Health
Science Center at San Antonio, San Antonio, Texas
Chapter 9

Foreword

Five years have passed since the initial publication of this text, which provided the first contemporary statement about and collection of models for occupational therapy in work-related programs. It undoubtedly led many therapists to think about how to include this philosophy in their programs. Now, however, it is time for an update on what has been happening in work-related treatment in our profession.

The public is increasingly aware of how health issues, prevention activities, and general fitness affect daily function at home and work. Smart CEOs, in their pursuit of cost-effective measures to increase U.S. competitiveness in the world market, constantly seek ways to ensure an able and healthy work force. For these reasons alone, the training of all workers for safe performance on the job and the timely rehabilitation of sick or injured workers have become paramount concerns in many businesses. Ordinary medical care no longer suffices. In addition, in the climate of worker shortages, employers have learned that hiring disabled, handicapped, and elderly workers is smart. Fitted to jobs within their capabilities and interests, these persons become productive and dependable workers.

In all of these facets of work and worker performance, occupational therapists have become increasingly involved. This second edition of *Occupational Therapy: Work-Related Programs and Assessments* brings some new perspectives on such roles.

The author has wisely augmented the original content to reflect the broadened arena of worker health for occupational therapist concern and participation. In addition, the original text has been updated but still provides the fundamental principles and activities that anyone new to this field of practice needs. Importantly, the philosophy of the book still centers on core beliefs of the profession—the uses of activity as the mediator for healing and adaptation.

For those already experienced in work-related treatment, here is a welcome injection of fresh thinking about programming. For the occupational therapist who wishes to get involved in this area of practice, you will not find such a rich resource elsewhere. We all thank the author for her continued efforts in bringing this field of occupational therapy into sharp focus.

Florence S. Cromwell, M.A., OTR, FAOTA

Preface

Work is at the heart of the philosophy and practice of occupational therapy. In its broadest sense, work, as productive activity, is the concern in almost all therapy.

Occupational Therapy: Work-Related Programs and Assessments comprehensively examines the topic of work: Historically, conceptually, and programmatically, throughout the life span, across various disabilities and facilities. In its first edition, this book was designed to fill a void in the occupational therapy literature. In its second edition, some of the original information has been retained and some updated.

Chapter 1 traces the historical perspective of occupational therapy's role in work practice from our founding years, outlining the way the foundations were laid for present programs.

Chapter 2 formulates a conceptual framework with which the occupational therapist can develop work assessments and programs. Uniform terminology is presented and its use is stressed.

Chapter 3 offers an overview of the "state of the art" of work assessment and evaluation.

Chapter 4 is devoted to an in-depth presentation of the Jacobs Prevocational Skills Assessment (JPSA), which was developed to evaluate a learning-disabled adolescent population. Although a standard evaluation, it is viable as a useful screening tool because it can be adapted to the individual client's needs. The JPSA is presented in its entirety, including graphic illustrations. It is hoped that therapists will find this a practical instrument and reproduce it in photocopies for their personal clinical use. Please note that some of the graphic illustrations must be enlarged for ease of use and for conformity to the standard feature of the assessment materials (for complete size listings, refer to the "shopping list" section of Chapter 4).

To facilitate a better understanding of the JPSA, the chapter is arranged in five sections.

The section on the development of the JPSA describes the way the JPSA evolved, as a guide for other therapists, who may some day find themselves faced with the task of developing their own assessment. The rationale for selecting specific work skill areas, tasks, and recording media is explored.

The next section of Chapter 4 describes the test elements. The recording medium, a single-page checklist-style profile sheet, was devised to facilitate recording data and to make the raw data accessible for further analysis, as was the JPSA manual, which includes for each of

15 tasks its purpose, materials, set-up of materials, and instructions for the therapist or client student or both. Numerous photographs and graphic illustrations facilitate comprehension.

The next section of Chapter 4 consists of a "shopping list" of all the items needed to construct your own JPSA. All graphic illustrations, including the profile sheet itself, are provided throughout the chapter. Please carefully refer to this "shopping list" when constructing your own assessment to be sure the materials are kept in a standard form.

The penultimate section of Chapter 4 contains three case studies to exemplify the ease of assessment implementation, data recording, and write-up of results. One of these case study sample evaluation reports is followed in greater depth in Chapter 5. The third case study illustrates the usefulness of the JPSA to complement other work evaluations, in this case, the Skills Assessment Module (SAM). Individual client case studies, which add clarity to the textbook content, are interwoven throughout Chapters 5, 6, and 7.

The final section of Chapter 4 is the chapter appendix, containing the complete JPSA manual ready for photocopying. (It is recommended that the photocopied manual later be spiralbound for ease of use.) However, no reproduction of the material can be used for commercial or educational purposes without the express written approval of the publisher.

I invite therapists who use the JPSA to share their experience with me. I am particularly interested in adaptations you may make for the needs of your individual clients. I envision that eventually a network can be established to allow users a forum for exchange.

Chapters 5 through 10 describe work practice throughout the life span; from childhood and adolescence to adulthood. I have endeavored to provide comprehensive coverage of this topic by presenting case studies of programs by experts in this area throughout the United States and, to a limited extent, in Canada and Australia.

Chapter 5 begins with an overview of the need for work programming for children. It stresses that programming for the child with special needs begins at an early age to facilitate incorporation of these occupational performance components into their behavioral repertoire.

Four facilities are described regarding their care of children and adolescents with various disabilities. The Little People's and Learning Prep School has been examined in particular detail. Although I am no longer affiliated with the school and programming has changed since this description was written for the first edition, I believe the school remains a superlative example of the range of possibilities available for creative work program development. For current information about the Learning Prep School, the reader is advised to contact the school. In this chapter, the use of community as a resource for program development and maintenance is a recurring theme. Finally, the sample evaluation report on "Stacey" continues to reflect the results of the JPSA and the implementation of those results in therapy.

Chapter 6 has been divided into two sections. The first section, written by Rabin and Jeong, provides an in-depth perspective of work programming for psychiatric clients. The second section continues this theme by providing descriptions of five programs, including case studies. Special attention has been given to describing correctional institutions, because the field of corrections appears to be one that offers increasing opportunity to therapists.

Chapter 7 is divided into two sections. The first section, written by Bettencourt, describes chronic pain, disability, and rehabilitation of the injured worker. The second part provides examples of innovative work practice for adults with neurophysiologic problems. Seven programs incorporate individual case studies.

Chapter 8 completes the life span continuum for work practice. It has been written by MacRae, a leader in the field of gerontology.

The subject of prevention is described in depth in Chapter 9 by Schwartz.

Home-based employment is explored in Chapter 10 as a viable environment for the disabled worker. This chapter was written by three occupational therapy students from Boston University: Breen, Clark, and Moran.

Chapter 11 proposes that occupational therapy educational curricula include a course on work practice. Content areas and requirements for a course on work are explored.

Chapter 12 asks "What is the future outlook for occupational therapists in work practice?" I believe we should be quite optimistic; however, success will require a proactive stance on the part of individual therapists and the profession itself.

The text provides the therapist with a detailed set of guidelines and program models for developing and implementing work assessments and programs. The book is intended to serve as a resource and reference whenever any work program is being planned or refined and/or the subject is being addressed in the classroom.

The task of concluding this text was a difficult one, due to the dynamic nature of this area of practice. Since work practice is expanding so quickly, I urge therapists who read this book to be in touch with me about their programs, so that we can exchange material and have an ongoing dialogue.

—K.J.

Acknowledgments

Appreciation is due to everyone who helped in the preparation of this textbook. I would like to express my gratitude to all by listing them by specific chapters.

Chapter 1 was developed in part from information originally provided by Florence S. Cromwell and Edwinna M. Marshall.

The following occupational therapists have worked at The Little People's and Learning Prep School and contributed to the metamorphosis of the Jacobs Prevocational Skills Assessment: Kathy Pepicelli, Irene Noble, Nancy Mazonson, Wynne Leekoff, Debra Viens, Sara Sicilano, Stacey Schrope-Szklut, Linda Gow, and Joan Schiff. Special thanks to Walter Loan, who posed for photographs, and to Nancy Mazonson, who posed for photographs and also contributed case studies to Chapters 4 and 5. Full acknowledgment must be given to graphic artist Roger Tirrell for his tireless efforts in preparing the illustrations for the Jacobs Prevocational Skills Assessment.

I thank the following individuals for their assistance in Chapter 5 on the Little People's and Learning Prep School: the director of the school, Nancy Rosoff; the administrators; the staff; and the students who participated via photographs and the exchange of information. Much of what I have learned about work programming with children and adolescents came from direct work with all these people. Appreciation is due to others involved in Chapter 5: Sherry Olin and Mary Haldy for their contribution on the Margaret Walters School; Terry Lyons, who shared information on the Handicapped Employment Training Assistance Unit in Australia; and Kathleen Murphy, both for her description of CPRI and for being my Canadian connection on work practice with children and adolescents.

For the first section of Chapter 6, I would like to express my gratitude to Jack Rabin and Glenda Jeong for writing a superb manuscript on work programming and the psychiatric client; and to Susan Lang, for her support in their endeavor. The following individuals kindly shared information on their programs: Lauren Kirson for the New York Veterans Administration Medical Center program; both Donna Gatti and Francis Palmer for information about McLean Hospital's Thrift Shop; Robin Klein for information on the Clifton T. Perkins Hospital; Robert Schneider for the Calgary General Hospital section, including the photographs; and Sandra Palmer, who provided information on Washington State Special Offenders Center.

To my friend Carl Bettencourt, many thanks for writing the first section of Chapter 7. For the second section of this chapter, I would like to thank Deborah Maloney, Maria Foschi, and Nancy Feldman for writing about GROWS. In addition, I would like to acknowledge the assistance of the following individuals: Ralph Colangelo, Karen Haggarty-Weake, and Holly T. Ehle, for the information and photographs on Braintree Hospital's Comprehensive Driver Education Program; Sherlyn L. Fenton, Patricia Gagnon-Stryke, Valerie Shaw Jones, and Patricia McGauley for the photographs, information, and case studies for Liberty Mutual Rehabilitation Medical Center; Rhonda Auricht, Pam Dean, and Robert Cox, for their information on the Western Dominiliary Care and Rehabilitation Service of Queen Elizabeth Hospital–Alfreda Rehabilitation Unit; Dorie Milner, who kindly shared both information and photographs on the Institute of Rehabilitation Medicine, New York University Medical Center; Karen Schultz, for both photographs and information on Downey Community Hospital; Thelma Hook, for writing the section on Hand Therapy and Rehabilitation Associates; Carolyn Austin and John Basile, who provided information on Walter E. Fernald State School; and friend Shana Krell, for sharing her work at United Cerebral Palsy Association of MetroBoston, Inc.

I thank my dear friend Nancy MacRae for writing the chapter on the older worker. I hope this chapter provides the catalyst for others to enter into this area of practice.

Grateful acknowledgment is extended to Richard Schwartz for his definitive chapter on prevention.

I am proud to include the chapter on home-based employment, which was written by occupational therapy students Theresa Breen, KimAnn Clark, and Michelle Moran. Thank you all for accepting the challenge of writing!

My publisher, Little, Brown and Company, has my appreciation for their assistance.

Finally, my love and appreciation are extended to my family and friends, who have endured my absenteeism during this writing endeavor!

Occupational Therapy: Work-Related Programs and Assessments

History of Work Practice in Occupational Therapy

The 1980s were a banner decade for renewed interest in work practice, and this trend is predicted to continue into the 21st century. In particular, interest was established in the area of work hardening.

Environmental trends have provided the climate for occupational therapists to become more involved in work practice. Some of these trends include:

1. Increased number of industrial injury cases
2. Lack of adequate comprehensive services
3. Escalating, prohibitive costs of supporting injured workers
4. Regulatory agency guidelines
5. Workers' Compensation and Public Laws (e.g., PL 88–210 and 99–142).

For example, in 1989 the Commission on Accreditation of Rehabilitation Facilities (CARF) established its "Work Hardening Guidelines," which are predicted to have a significant impact on work practice (Appendix 1–1) [13]. At present, Kentucky, Florida, and Ohio have incorporated these guidelines as mandatory for reimbursement in their Worker Compensation system [63]. It is predicted that many other states will follow. Since the release of these guidelines, 130 facilities have become accredited by CARF and approximately 200 should be accredited by the end of 1991 [9a].

The membership of the American Occupational Therapy Association (AOTA) confirmed their commitment to work practice in 1986 through the establishment of the Work Programs Special Interest Section (WPSIS). In 1990, there were approximately 2,900 members [2]. As part of the WPSIS membership, individuals receive a quarterly newsletter, which provides short articles on work practice topics such as ergonomics, educational curricula, prevention, and the burn client. An additional aspect of the WPSIS is an appointed state liaison network to exchange current and emerging information on statewide work practice. The *Working Papers* is the quarterly exchange vehicle for this network. In 1990, the 1987–1990 WPSIS Standing Committee completed its first demographic survey of work hardening programs and an outcome study of over 40 programs, which included 400 individuals. Results from both the survey and the study are planned to be disseminated through articles submitted to the *American Journal of Occupational Therapy* [67].

The interest in work practice has been evidenced through an increase in the number of textbooks, professional articles/papers, conferences, and workshops on this subject.

TEXTBOOKS

In 1990, AOTA published a comprehensive textbook on work practice entitled *Work in Progress*. This edited textbook includes chapters on work hardening, ergonomics, supported employment and prevention [34].

Ogden-Niemeyer and Jacobs published in 1989 the first comprehensive textbook on work hardening, appropriately titled *Work Hardening: State of the Art*. The text includes definition and history of work hardening, program models for work hardening, the issue of abnormal illness behavior, work hardening in the health care system, and over 20 descriptions of current programs [55].

The seventh edition of *Willard and Spackman's Occupational Therapy*, published in 1989, contains an updated chapter called "Occupational Therapy for the Workplace" [39].

In 1988, two texts were published on work practice. *Work Injury: Management and Prevention* is an edited text by Susan Isernhagen, a physical therapist [40]. *Physical Capacity Assessment and Work Hardening Therapy: Procedures and Applications* is an edited text by a rehabilitation counselor [32].

In 1985, the first edition of *Occupational Therapy: Work-Related Programs and Assessments* was published as one of the first comprehensive textbooks on work practice for occupational therapists [41].

PROFESSIONAL ARTICLES

In 1990, a new journal devoted solely to work practice was published. *Work, a Journal of Prevention, Assessment and Rehabilitation*, a quarterly journal targeted for occupational and physical therapists and other professionals in work practice, provides thematic articles on work. Topics include "Industrial Rehabilitation," "The Psychiatrically Challenged," "Work Assessments," and "Back Injury" [43].

Occupational Therapy Practice entitled its second issue, "Work: Occupational Therapy Interventions" [42]. Articles included "The Effectiveness of Work Programming with an Alzheimer Population" [9], "Overview of Standardized Worksamples and Norms for Injured Workers" [8], and "An Accident/Injury Prevention Program for Occupational Therapy Employees" [5].

The majority of articles in the September, 1987, *Journal of Hand Surgery* were on work practice. Examples of articles were "Work Capacity Evaluation for Occupational Hand Injuries" [33] and "Tool Design for Preventing Hand and Wrist Injuries" [49].

The Winter 85/86 issue of *Occupational Therapy in Health Care*, entitled "Work-Related Programs in Occupational Therapy," included articles such as "The Expanding Role of Occupational Therapy in the Treatment of Industrial Hand Injuries" and "A Private Practice Work Evaluation Unit" [20].

The May 1985, issue of *American Journal of Occupational Therapy (AJOT)* was devoted to work evaluation. Prior to that time, *AJOT* included periodic articles on work practice, such as "The School Therapist and Vocational Education" [14], "The Role of Occupational Therapy in Vocational Evaluation" [35, 36], "To Market, To Market" [37], and "Factors Affecting Return to Work After Hand Injury" [4]. In 1980, the American Occupational Therapy Association (AOTA) published an official position paper entitled "The Role of Occupational Therapy in the Vocational Rehabilitation Process" [1], and in 1986 they published "Work Hardening Guidelines." AOTA is reformulating a position statement on Work Practice that should be available sometime in 1992. The *Canadian Journal of Occupational Therapy* continues to have a steady flow of work practice articles [11, 31, 44, 51, 52].

CONFERENCES AND WORKSHOPS

Presentations on various areas of work practice have been on a steady increase since 1981. In 1982, AOTA initiated a three-year project, funded through the Office of Special Education and Rehabilitation Services, U.S. Department of Health and Human Services, called "Occupational Therapist's Role in Vocational Readiness for Handicapped Students." The project resulted in the development of a curriculum for occupational therapists working in the area of work practice for disabled students. Based on this project, in 1985 the five-day workshops entitled "Planning and Implementing Vocational Readiness in Occupational Therapy" (PIVOT) were made regionally available.

Workshops on selected work practice topics are offered periodically throughout the United States. Examples include "How to Market and Sell Work Hardening Services Successfully," "Consulting with Industry: Selling Services to Employers," and "Work Injury Management Advances in Evaluation, Treatment and Prevention of Injuries in Industry." In recent years, there has been an increase in the number of workshops devoted to refinement of present work programs and the development of marketing strategies.

PRECURSORS TO CURRENT WORK PRACTICE

Renewed interest in and enthusiasm for the area of work practice is not unusual for the profession. The following brief historical overview is presented so that the reader can appreciate more fully the scope and importance of current interest.

For the sake of brevity, this history will begin in the decade of the founding of the profession, 1910 to 1920. This was a time of "watchful . . . custodial conservative treatment and long-term caring for people"

[18]. It was a time of reactivation of moral treatment* for the mentally ill and of the use of reconstruction aides, who concerned themselves with the return to work of disabled Great War soldiers [66]. Eleanor Clarke Slagle, earlier a social worker, became one of the first known advocates of occupational therapy as a means of treating the wounded. By the close of the war, thousands of soldiers had received some form of "occupation therapy" [38].

The time was right for the emergence of the profession. As noted by Woodside [66], "The war, a severe polio epidemic in 1916, industrial accidents and the widening use of the automobile all contributed to the need for new methods of treating residual disabilities." The concept of employing crafts to reactivate the minds and motivation of these disabled persons paved the way for the entrance of the occupational therapy profession into vocational training and rehabilitation [54].

In Canada, the Military Hospitals' Commission established schools for vocational training in convalescent hospitals and offered instruction in activities that would aid patients to prepare for work [65].

In 1920 the Vocational Rehabilitation Act (Smith-Fess Act, Public Law 66-236) was passed. This landmark legislation defined rehabilitation as "return to remunerative employment," with the provision of funds on a matching basis to states for helping disabled persons. The Act allowed solely for "training in existing schools, industry and commercial establishments, or by a tutor." Medical service was covered only "if needed to determine eligibility for help." Since the training was carried out by state vocational education departments, there were many opportunities for occupational therapists in centers such as sheltered and curative workshops to participate in prevocational programming.† At this time former psychiatric patients were ineligible for benefits derived from the Act. The founders of the AOTA were instrumental in enlisting the assistance of veterans' groups and physicians' associations in campaigning for legislative changes. Public Law 236 gave the profession the ideal opportunity to introduce work-related programming tailored to disabled persons. At this point "our founders were quite committed to look at the total day and future of the individual, not just his current pathology" [18]. Concurrently, other important contributions were made by George Edward Barton, William Rush Dunton, Jr., and Eleanor Clarke Slagle.

Barton became the advocate of occupation therapy who, after suffering tuberculosis and stroke, organized Consolation House in Clifton Springs, New York, as a vocational bureau and community-based activity workshop for ill and disabled persons. "By means of occupations, people could be retrained or adjusted to gainful employment [the phi-

---

*Moral treatment came into existence in the early nineteenth century with the development of psychiatric programs such as that of McLean Hospital in Belmont, Massachusetts. According to Sanbourne Bockoven [7], "The history of moral treatment in America is not only synonymous with but is the history of occupational therapy before it acquired its twentieth-century name."

†The Rehabilitation Service Administration (U.S. Department of Health, Education and Welfare) evolved from this legislation. At present the agency serves the psychiatrically and developmentally disabled and, to a more limited degree, the physically disabled. As a result of 1978 amendments, a large proportion of clients served are severely disabled [35].

losophy of which was] to give that sort [of activity] which will be preliminary to and dovetailed with the real vocational education which is to begin as soon as the patient is able to go farther along" [38].

Dunton, "the Father of Occupational Therapy," was involved in the use of occupational therapy with psychiatric patients at Sheppard and Enoch Pratt Hospital, Baltimore. He insisted on total workday planning for patients and was primarily concerned in developing and maintaining work habits [19].

Slagle made "habit training" the centerpiece of her methods of treatment, which were based on the use of a wide sample of daily occupations. This type of rehabilitation program, which included preindustrial and vocational work, attempted to create a balance of work, rest, and play for psychiatric patients [38].

In Canada, another founder of AOTA, T. B. Kidner, who came from an industrial background, was concerned with returning the disabled to work through activity [18, 56].

According to Cromwell [18], the profession received a strong message from its founders "that the occupational therapy profession, small as it was at the time, was devoted to the belief that productivity was possible to prevent the breakdown of skills, habits and attitudes."

During the 1930s, therapists were still feeling the impact of World War I and the Vocational Rehabilitation Act. This was the time of "curative workshops," which were specifically aimed at the injured industrial worker and which utilized work-related activity as the treatment. Occupational therapists were instrumental in the organization and development of such workshops in Philadelphia, Milwaukee, and St. Louis. The Pre-vocational Unit at the Institute for the Crippled and Disabled (ICD), founded in New York City in 1936, may be viewed as the forerunner of present prevocational programs. For this program, the institute modified evaluation techniques used for applicants to industry and trade schools to evaluate and train the disabled [38].

Similar trends were apparent in Europe and Canada, also because of the need to reeducate the disabled. In 1938 the Occupational Therapy Workshop of the Canadian Workmen's Compensation Board was opened. Its goal was to shorten the convalescent period of injured workmen, thus cutting costs of compensation, through a concentrated program of occupational, recreational, and physical therapy. In this workshop tasks specifically related to the patient's former job were utilized as treatment. For example, patients built brick walls, painted building, laid railroad ties, and repaired plumbing [46, 59]. Numerous articles in the *Canadian Journal of Occupational Therapy* during the early 1940s also reflected local interest in this area [46, 59, 61, 65].

West [65] notes that during the world wars occupational therapy as a profession grew tremendously as a result of its role in work adjustment of soldiers. World War II allowed disabled soldiers and workers to emerge as a major force in the United States because of the scarcity of able-bodied workers in an expanding industrial economy. Many industries modified work environments to accommodate disabled workers.

Passage of the Vocational Rehabilitation Amendments (Barden-La Follette Act) of 1943 (Public Law 78-113), for which AOTA founders

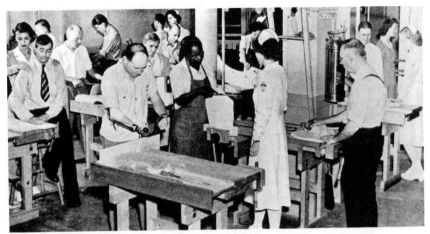

Figure 1-1.   The occupational therapy at the Liberty Mutual rehabilitation center, late 1940s. (Photo courtesy of Liberty Mutual Insurance Companies, Boston, Massachusetts.)

had actively campaigned in the 1920s, was another landmark. For the first time developmentally and psychiatrically disabled persons were made eligible for rehabilitation services. With this legislation, the need for vocational training for those who had *never* been employed was recognized.

Despite all the pioneering efforts that show continuing and active involvement in work-related treatment, the early postwar period saw a noticeable move by the occupational therapy profession away from prevocational rehabilitation activities. According to West [65], this trend may have resulted from heavy case loads, poor training of professional personnel, and the high cost of facilities. In addition, according to Cromwell [18], "Occupational therapists were looking for more scientific approaches and beginning to reject 'occupation' alone. Occupational therapists choose more often to be identified with the medical model than with a social or vocational model." This period, however, saw the rise of many military and veterans' hospitals. Therapists in these centers developed the army model of rehabilitation and used activities adapted from hospitals and industry as treatment. Occupational therapists also gradually turned from work related activities to the development of adaptive tools and devices for clients with various orthopedic and neurologic injuries [18].

During this same period Liberty Mutual became the first insurance company to establish rehabilitation workshops. These workshops, located in Boston and Chicago, provided rehabilitation services to disabled workers with the intent of returning them to their jobs as quickly as possible (Fig. 1–1). In San Francisco, Carlotta Wells and Signe Brunstrum established a program using intensive work-oriented treatment at the May T. Mornson Center, which served persons with many kinds of physical and psychological illnesses [18].

Declining professional interest in work-related programming was somewhat bolstered in 1954, with the adoption of amendments to the Vocational Rehabilitation Act. As a result of this legislation, prevocational units were established within rehabilitation facilities. Occupational therapists assumed a major responsibility in the development of principles of prevocational exploration [1,12]. The Department of Physical and Rehabilitation Medicine at New York University Medical Center established possibly the largest prevocational exploration unit in the world at the time [23].

In 1955 AOTA held an institute "to reassess professional education and practice as related to rehabilitation" [65]. In the following year the association held another institute with the specific purpose of addressing the concept, purposes, methods, values, and rationale of prevocational programming, as well as prevocational techniques and media [30, 56].

As noted by Reed and Sanderson [56], "Prevocational exploration and training became the glamor area of practice in the late fifties and early sixties." There even emerged within AOTA a prevocational specialty group. Interest in this group has come and gone through the years.

The content of the *American Journal of Occupational Therapy* between 1957 and 1961 reflects the increased interest in this area, with a total of 11 work-related articles [64, 65]. An example is Rosenburg and Wellerson's explanation of the differences between the prevocational and vocational evaluation programs at the Institute for the Crippled and Disabled [58]. Aims of prevocational programming for physically disabled populations at the ICD included the development of three aspects of the individual: work habits; work tolerance; and coordination, production, and speed. In the ICD program, clients were exposed to activities such as clerical and sales tasks, upholstery refinishing, power press operation, industrial leather manufacturing, and assembly and packaging tasks. Task selection was based on the client's interest and work history, and the average length of programming was between two weeks and six months [58]. The TOWER (Testing, Orientation, and Work Evaluation in Rehabilitation) system, an outgrowth of early programs developed at ICD, continues today to be a much-used evaluation instrument [38]. Many occupational therapists received training in the use of this instrument and were subsequently employed as vocational evaluators in rehabilitation centers serving patients with many kinds of disabilities.

One of the later leaders in the profession and a continued proponent of work-related programming is Florence Cromwell [15–21]. Her many articles, lectures, and research reports and her manual on prevocational evaluation continue to be valid references for today's therapist. Cromwell herself remains an inspirational role model and resource person for those committed to contributions by occupational therapy in work-related programs. In her 1962 presentation [16] to the Third International Congress of the World Federation of Occupational Therapists, she reiterated the profession's commitment: "Work adjustment is and has always been a function of occupational therapy."

The 1960 Iowa Conference on Prevocational Activities was another effort to clarify the role and structural framework of prevocational programs in occupational therapy [50]. The questions addressed in 1960 [53] are similar to those being asked today:

1. What progress has been made in more sharply defining the term pre-vocational?
2. Can we obtain agreement on working definitions for the following terms:
   a. work adjustment
   b. work conditioning
   c. pre-vocational unit
   d. job sampling
3. What are the characteristics of a good vocational evaluation system?

   I. What is the scope of pre-vocational activities?
   II. What contribution . . . [do] . . . the following personnel [make] to the pre-vocational process? . . .

According to West [65], despite the increase in publications on and interest in work-related programming, the literature was "extremely limited in terms of our total professional picture." Reed and Sanderson [56] note that "no specific issue diminished the interest in prevocational practice, but as health care swung toward acute and short term care there simply was not time to provide prevocational exploration and training." On the international scene, however, there remained a greater focus on work-related treatment [29], and, according to Cromwell [18], "Our colleagues in other countries really left us behind."

Curative workshops were beginning to turn from restoration and work-related treatment to straight vocational counseling. Much of the work performed by the occupational therapist was being passed by default to the emerging work evaluators. The University of Wisconsin–Stout, with strong federal support, established the Stout Vocational Rehabilitation Institute. A division of the institute, the Materials Development Center (MDC) [62], is presently "the national central source for the collection, development, and dissemination of information and materials in the areas of vocational evaluation, work adjustment, and rehabilitation facility management and operations. The goal of MDC is to improve the performance of rehabilitation facilities serving the handicapped, resulting in the increased economic independence for disabled persons."

In the early 1960s, Mary Reilly suggested the need for the profession to increase its knowledge of the work–play continuum as an appropriate base for occupational therapy. This continuum has subsequently been designated *occupational behavior*. Reilly's understanding of occupational behavior is built on the premise that "the play of childhood . . . contains a critical ability to transmit the adaptive skills necessary for complex work technology and urban living of today" [57]. She stresses the importance of "examining the various life roles of the population relative to community adaptation, to identify the various skills that support these roles, and to create an environment in treatment where the relevant behavior could be evoked and practiced" [57]. Much of what Reilly suggests is reminiscent of Slagle's habit training.

Articles published in the *American Journal of Occupational Therapy* after 1966 express concern about the sparsity of literature related to work-related programming, particularly in the treatment of psychiatric populations. Ethridge [26] noted that, over a period of years, literature discussing prevocational evaluation was totally concerned with the assessment of physically handicapped patients, with almost no mention of the psychiatrically disabled. Two notable exceptions were articles by Llorens and colleagues [45] and Fidler [27].

Beginning in the late 1960s and 1970s more interest in the psychiatrically disabled developed. Articles by Clark and Lerner [10], Ethridge [26], Diasio and Jones [24], Distefano and Pryer [25], Deacon and associates [22], and Solberg and Chueh [60] all relate to the psychiatric population and emphasize evaluation checklists. Theoretical articles by various therapists appeared at the same time. Bailey [3] identified work habits—attitudes toward work, punctuality, regular attendance, appearance, speed of work, manual dexterity, concentration, cleanliness, and social skills—and traced them to theories of childhood and vocational development. In Reed and Sanderson [56], Maurer defined skills important to vocational development: identifying with a worker, learning about work and its varieties, getting along with peers, developing basic habits of industry, developing a self-concept and translating it into occupational terms, and learning to work with and adjust to authority.

The impetus for establishing occupational therapy services in schools was provided by the enactment of Public Law 94-142, the Education of All Handicapped Children Act of 1975, which mandates the opportunity for appropriate education for every child. Public Law 93-112, Section 504, the Rehabilitation Act of 1973, also has played an important role in the provision of services to children [14]. Occupational therapy has been readily recognized as a valuable service within the educational system. The occupational therapist has become a vital member of teams developing and providing appropriate educational and health care programs for special needs students [14].

Gilfoyle and Hays [28] believe that occupational therapy will be important in student career development.

An increase in the number of handicapped children can be predicted for secondary schools and/or vocational training programs centers administered by public school programs as impact of Federal legislation will provide more appropriate education for the adolescent age group. Occupational therapy must play a vital role with educational programs of career development and prevocational training for handicapped students.

According to Cromwell [19], "Vocational educators in the school system who are beginning to get handicapped youngsters in labs and classes have indicated a real need for help. They need to know how to adapt settings, materials and methods, to manage these persons with different ways of functioning. What more perfect place for the occupational therapist to consult and aid in the development of these programs? Finally, great opportunities await occupational therapists with the passage of the Americans with Disabilities Act (ADA). If we take the initiative, we might become one of the primary players in its implementation. The future holds great promise for us!

REFERENCES

1. Ad Hoc Committee of the Commission on Practice. The role of occupational therapy in the vocational rehabilitation process: Official Position Paper. *Am.J.Occup.Ther.* 34:881, 1980.
2. AOTA Membership Files. Rockville, Maryland: AOTA, May 7, 1990.
3. Bailey, D. Vocational theories and work habits related to childhood development. *Am.J.Occup.Ther.* 25:298, 1971.
4. Bear-Lehman, J. Factors affecting return to work after hand injury. *Am.J.Occup.Ther.* 37:189, 1983.
5. Bettencourt, C. An accident/injury prevention program for occupational therapy employees. *Occupational Therapy Practice* 1:2, 1990.
6. Bing, R. K. Eleanor Clarke Slagle Lectureship—1981—Occupational therapy revisited: a paraphrastic journey. *Am.J.Occup.Ther.* 35:499, 1981.
7. Bockoven, J. S. Occupational therapy—a historical perspective: legacy of moral treatment—1800s to 1910. *Am.J.Occup.Ther.* 25:223, 1971.
8. Bryan, T. Overview of standardized worksamples and norms for injured workers. *Occupational Therapy Practice* 1:2, 1990.
9. Burns, T., and Buell, J. The effectiveness of work programming with an Alzheimer population. *Occupational Therapy Practice* 1:2, 1990.
9a. CARF. Personal communications, 1991.
10. Clark, B., and Lerner, G. E. Occupational therapists participate in prevocational screening. *Am.J.Occup.Ther.* 20:91, 1966.
11. Clements, L., and Dixon, M. A model of occupational therapy in back education. *Can.J.Occup.Ther.* 46:161, 1979.
12. Combs, M. H., Nadler, E. B., and Thomas, C. W. Vocational exploration—Methodological problems and a suggested approach. *Am.J.Occup.Ther.* 22:64, 1958.
13. Work hardening programs. In *Standards Manual for Organizations Serving People with Disabilities.* Tucson, Ariz.: Commission on Accreditation of Rehabilitation Facilities. 1989, pp 69–72.
14. Creighton, C. The school therapist and vocational education. *Am.J.Occup.Ther.* 33:373, 1979.
15. Cromwell, F. S. A procedure for prevocational evaluation. *Am.J.Occup.Ther.* 13:1, 1959.
16. Cromwell, F. S. Looking ahead in work evaluation: Work adjustment as a function of occupational therapy. In *Proceedings of the Third International Congress of the World Federation of Occupational Therapists,* Dubuque, Iowa: Wm. C. Brown, 1964. Vol. 5, p. 16.
17. Cromwell, F. S. *Occupational Therapist's Manual for Basic Assessment—Primary Prevocational Evaluation.* Altadena, Ca: Fair Oakes Printing Company, 1976.
18. Cromwell, F. S. The world of industry: arena for OT skills. Presented at the National Occupational Therapy Association Conference, Philadelphia, May 1982.
19. Cromwell, F. S. Personal communication, 1983.
20. Cromwell, F. Work-related programs in occupational therapy. *Occupational Therapy in Health Care,* Winter 85/86.
21. Cromwell, Florence S. Vocational readiness programming in occupational therapy: Its roots, course, and prognosis. In *Competency-Based Curriculum in Vocational Readiness.* Baltimore: American Occupational Therapy Association, 1984.

22. Deacon, S., Dunning, R. E., and Dease, R. Jobs: a job clinic for psychotic clients in remission. *Am.J.Occup.Ther.* 28:144, 1974.
23. Department of Physical Medicine and Rehabilitation. *Pre-Vocational Therapy Demonstration in a General Hospital and a Rehabilitation Center* (SP-234). Report to the National Advisory Council on Vocational Rehabilitation, U.S. Department of Health, Education, and Welfare. New York: New York University Medical Center, 1960.
24. Diasio, K., and Jones, M. S. Prevocational services for young adult psychiatric patients. *Hosp. Community Psychiatry* 21:217, 1970.
25. Distefano, M. K., and Pryer, M. W. Vocational evaluation and successful placement of psychiatric clients in a vocational rehabilitation program. *Am.J.Occup.Ther.* 24:205, 1970.
26. Ethridge, D. A. Prevocational assessment of rehabilitation potential of psychiatric patients. *Am.J.Occup.Ther.* 22:161, 1968.
27. Fidler, G. S. A second look at work as a primary force in rehabilitation and treatment. *Am.J.Occup.Ther.* 20:72, 1966.
28. Gilfoyle, E., and Hays, C. Occupational therapy roles and functions in the education of the school-based handicapped student. *Am.J.Occup.Ther.* 33:565, 1979.
29. Goode, D. G. The role of occupational therapy in work adjustment: Work adjustment as a function of occupational therapy. In *Proceedings of the Third International Congress of the World Federation of Occupational Therapists,* Dubuque, Iowa: Wm. C. Brown, 1964. Vol. 5, p. 99.
30. Granofsky, J. *A Manual for Occupational Therapists on Prevocational Exploration.* Dubuque, Iowa: Wm. C. Brown, 1959.
31. Green, A., Gould, L., Mailer, M., Otto, K., and Henderson, R. Task groups: how they work in one vocational assessment unit. *Can.J.Occup.Ther.* 45:61, 1978.
32. Havranek, J. (Ed.) *Physical Capacity Assessment and Work Hardening Therapy: Procedures & Applications.* Athens, Ga: Elliott & Fitzpatrick, Inc., 1988.
33. Herbin, M. Work capacity evaluation for occupational hand injuries. *Journal of Hand Surgery,* 12A(5), 1987.
34. Hertfelder, S., and Gwin, C. *Work in Progress.* Rockville, Md: AOTA, 1989.
35. Hightower-Vandamm, M. Nationally Speaking: The role of occupational therapy in vocational evaluation, Part 1. *Am.J.Occup.Ther.* 35:563, 1981.
36. Hightower-Vandamm, M. Nationally Speaking: The role of occupational therapy in vocational evaluation, Part 2. *Am.J.Occup.Ther.* 35:631, 1981.
37. Hightower-Vandamm, M. Nationally Speaking: To market, to market. *Am.J.Occup.Ther.* 36:293, 1982.
38. Hopkins, H. L., and Smith, H. D. (Eds.) *Willard and Spackman's Occupational Therapy* (6th ed.). Philadelphia: Lippincott, 1983.
39. Hopkins, H., and Smith, H. (Eds.) *Willard and Spackman's Occupational Therapy* (7th ed.). Philadelphia: Lippincott, 1989.
40. Isernhagen, S. (Ed.) *Work Injury: Management and Prevention.* Baltimore, Md: Aspen Publications, 1988.
41. Jacobs, K. *Occupational Therapy: Work-Related Programs and Assessment.* Boston: Little, Brown, 1985.
42. Jacobs, K. (Ed.) Work: occupational therapy interventions. *Occupational Therapy Practice* 1:2, 1990.
43. Jacobs, K. (Ed.) *Work: A Journal of Assessment, Prevention and Rehabilitation.* 1:1–77, 1990.
44. Lewchuk, S. The occupational therapist in industry—a developing challenge. *Can.J.Occup.Ther.* 47:159, 1980.
45. Llorens, L. S., Levy, R., and Rubin, E. Z. Work adjustment program—a pre-vocational experience, *Am.J.Occup.Ther.* 28:15, 1964.
46. Lomey, M. B. Rehabilitation under the workmen's compensation act. *Can.J.Occup.Ther.* 8:25, 1941.
47. Maurer, P. A. Prevocational activities and evaluation for the child and adolescent. *Phys. Ther.* 48:771, 1968.
48. Maurer, P. A. Antecedents of work behavior. *Am.J.Occup.Ther.* 25:295, 1971.

49. Meager, S. Tool design for prevention of hand and wrist injuries. *Journal of Hand Surgery*, 12A(5), 1987.
50. Moed, M. B. Procedures and practices in prevocational evaluation: a review of current programs. In J. E. Muthard (Ed.), *Proceedings of the Iowa Conference on Prevocational Activities*. Washington, D.C.: Office of Vocational Rehabilitation, U.S. Department of Health, Education and Welfare, 1960.
51. Monfette, L. Vocational counseling and the alienated worker. *Can.J.Occup.Ther.* 46:57, 1979.
52. Murphy, M. Developments in a rehabilitation service for psychiatric patients. *Can.J.Occup.Ther.* 47:15, 1980.
53. Muthard, J. E. (Ed.) *Proceedings of the Iowa Conference of Prevocational Activities*. Washington, D.C.: Office of Vocational Rehabilitation, U.S. Department of Health, Education and Welfare, 1960.
54. O'Donnell, D. T. A descriptive study of the frequency and nature of the application of pre-vocational activity in occupational therapy settings in the state of Maryland. University of Maryland Master's thesis, 1983.
55. Ogden-Niemeyer, L., and Jacobs, K. *Work Hardening: State of the Art*. Thorofare, NJ: Slack, Inc., 1989.
56. Reed, K., and Sanderson, S. R. *Concepts of Occupational Therapy* (2nd ed.) Baltimore: Williams & Wilkins, 1983.
57. Reilly, M. Occupational therapy can be one of the great ideas of 20th century medicine. *Am.J.Occup.Ther.* 16:1, 1962.
58. Rosenburg, B., and Wellerson, T. A structured prevocational program. *Am.J.Occup.Ther.* 14:57, 1960.
59. Smith, H. V. Workmen's compensation board, occupational therapy workshop. *Can.J.Occup.Ther.* 7:26, 1940.
60. Solberg, N. A., and Chueh, W. Performance in occupational therapy as a predictor of successful prevocational training. *Can.J.Occup.Ther.* 30:481, 1976.
61. Storms, H. D. Occupational therapy in the treatment of industrial casualties. *Can.J.Occup.Ther.* 10:40, 1943.
62. Stout Vocational Rehabilitation Institute Catalog, Menomonie, Wisconsin: University of Wisconsin, 1983.
63. Toppel, A. Work Programs Special Interest Section Annual Business Meeting. New Orleans, Louisiana: AOTA, April 29, 1990.
64. Wegg, L. S. Eleanor Clarke Slagle Lecture—The essentials of work evaluation. *Am.J.Occup.Ther.* 14:65, 1960.
65. West, W. L. The role of occupational therapy in work adjustment: Work adjustment as a function of occupational therapy. In *Proceedings of the Third International Congress of the World Federation of Occupational Therapists*. Dubuque, Iowa: Wm. C. Brown, 1964. Vol. 5, p. 1.
66. Woodside, H. H. Occupational therapy—a historical perspective: the development of occupational therapy—1910–1929. *Am.J.Occup.Ther.* 25:226, 1971.
67. Wyrick, J. Demographic Survey. Work Programs Special Interest Section Annual Business Meeting. New Orleans, Louisiana: AOTA, April 29, 1990.

Appendix 1-1. Guidelines for Work Hardening Programs*

Work hardening programs, which are interdisciplinary in nature, use conditioning tasks that are graded to progressively improve the biomechanical, neuromuscular, cardiovascular, metabolic, and psychosocial functions of the client in conjunction with real or simulated work activities. Work hardening provides a transition between acute care and return to work, while addressing the issues of productivity, safety, physical tolerances, and worker behaviors. Work hardening is a highly structured, goal-oriented, individualized treatment program designed to maximize the individual's ability to return to work.

1. Recognizing that attendance and workplace tolerance relevant to the competitive marketplace are integral parts of work hardening, the total work hardening program should make structured therapeutic activities available on a five-day-per-week basis.
2. Entrance/admission criteria should enable the program to admit:
   a. Persons who are likely to benefit from the program
   b. Persons whose current level of functioning due to illness or injury interferes with their ability to carry out specific tasks required in the work place, and
   c. Persons whose medical condition does not prohibit participation in the program
3. The initial steps in the process of entrance/admission should address:
   a. Questions to be answered
   b. Goals the achievement of which would enable the client to return to work
   c. Anticipated time frames for completion of program
4. Evaluation should include a personal interview to obtain work history, current reported functional status, lifestyle, and educational background.
5. Evidence of a recent evaluation of the individual's impairment must be obtained.
6. The evaluation process should take place within the context of the demands of competitive employment. The process should document a benchmark from which to establish the initial plan and/or the individual's functional/ vocational disposition and should include, but not be limited to, one or more of the following functional capacity evaluations:
   a. Baseline evaluation—a baseline assessment of functional ability to perform work activities, including the physical demand factors on which the *Dictionary of Occupational Titles* is based
   b. Job capacity evaluation—an assessment of the match between the individual's capabilities and critical demands of a specific job
   c. Occupational capacity evaluation—an assessment of the match between the individual's capabilities and the critical demands of an occupational group
   d. Work capacity evaluation—an assessment of the match between the individual's capabilities and the demands of competitive employment
7. Clinical reports as well as public information concerning evaluations should describe the content and state the time used.
8. Within the evaluation process, consideration should be given to attitudinal and behavioral factors that will affect the individual's ability to work or to benefit from further rehabilitation.
9. Services should be provided by a coordinated, interdisciplinary team.
   a. The team should be the major decision-making body in determining the goals, process, and time frames for completing the program.
   b. The team should meet on a formal basis as often as necessary to carry out its decision-making responsibilities. A team conference for each client should occur at least every other week. There should be interim informal conferences among the members of the team.

*Modified from the Standards Manual for Organizations Serving People with Disabilities.

    c. Assessment, coordinated program planning, and direct services should be provided on a regular and continuing basis by an interdisciplinary team. Team members should have special interest, training, experience, and expertise in work hardening programs. Depending upon the needs of those served and stated goals, the interdisciplinary team should include:
      (1) Occupational therapist
      (2) Physical therapist
      (3) Psychologist
      (4) Vocational specialist
    d. Depending upon the needs of the client and the goals, the program should provide for the services of:
      (1) Physician
      (2) Rehabilitation nurse
    e. The services of the following professionals should be available as necessary:
      (1) Alcohol and drug abuse treatment counselor
      (2) Dietitian
      (3) Exercise physiologist
      (4) Industrial engineer/rehabilitation engineer/ergonomist
      (5) Prosthetist/orthotist
      (6) Remedial educator
      (7) Social worker

10. Services in specific areas of expertise should be delivered by registered, certified, licensed, or degreed personnel or should be performed substantially in their presence.
11. The program should provide or arrange for, but not necessarily be limited to, the following services:
    a. Instruction, practice, and modification of work tasks
    b. Development of strength and endurance needed to perform work tasks
    c. Education to teach safe job performance to prevent reinjury
    d. Assessment of specific job requirements through work site evaluation and/or job analysis
    e. Education of the employer and/or union as to the implications of the individual's present status
    f. Involvement and education of the family or significant others regarding the implications of the individual's status
    g. Promotion of sense of responsibility and self-management by client
    h. Evaluation of client's productivity, safety in the workplace, and behavior on the job
    i. Identification of the client's transferable skills
12. The exit/discharge criteria for the client should include, but not be limited to:
    a. Ability to return to work.
    b. Achievement of program goals.
    c. Refusal of further services.
    d. Non-compliance with organizational policies.
    e. Limited potential to benefit from continuing the program
    f. Need for further health care.
13. For each client, the exit/discharge summary should include:
    a. Present functional status and potential.
    b. Functional status related to the targeted job, alternative occupations, or competitive labor market.
14. The exit/discharge summary should be prepared and disseminated within seven working days of the exit/discharge date.
15. An individual should be designated to administer and manage the work hardening program.
16. The organization should identify the desired knowledge, skills, and abilities of the director of the work hardening program, and ensure that the director meets these criteria. Examples of these skills include management and

supervisory skills, knowledge of organizational goals, and innovative methods of achieving these goals.

17. There should be a core designated area designed, organized, staffed, and equipped specifically for the work hardening program.
18. Space and equipment used in work simulation should approximate a relevant work environment.

Conceptual Framework

Lisa is a homemaker who provides care for her aged parent.
Erica attends first grade.
Bill is a vocational rehabilitation counselor.
Daniel is planning for retirement and is exploring avocational interests, such as gardening.

What these individuals have in common is that they are all workers. The occupational performance area of *work* (Figure 2-1) includes activities of home management, care of others, educational and vocational activities, and retirement planning [4].

TERMINOLOGY

Work includes all forms of productive activity, regardless of whether they are reimbursed. According to Gary Kielhofner [3],

> Productive activities are those that provide a service or commodity needed by another or that add new abilities, ideas, knowledge, artistic objects, or performances to the cultural tradition. The productive activity of work thus maintains and advances society. When an activity is considered to be one's work, it is generally organized into a major life role. Life roles are positions in life recognized by the social environment and by the role incumbent. Thus, activities engaged in to fulfill one's duties as a student, housewife, volunteer, serious hobbyist, or amateur, and that are part of one's identity, can be considered work.

According to this definition, work is not limited to adulthood but is relevant throughout the life span, from school age to retirement. In order to work, the individual needs specific performance components. Based on terminology found in *Uniform Terminology for Occupational Therapy,* Second Edition [4], the U.S. Department of Labor's *Dictionary of Occupational Titles* [5], and "Selected Characteristics of Occupations Defined in the *Dictionary of Occupational Titles*" [6], these performance components can be categorized as work behaviors, work skills, aptitudes, and physical capacities [2].

Work behaviors, commonly termed "prevocational or 'prevoc' readiness skills," are those behaviors that are necessary for successful participation in a job. They include but are not limited to grooming, interpersonal skills, punctuality, adherence to safety procedures, time management, coping skills, social conduct, self-control, termination of an activity, initiation of an activity, and attention span.

1. *Home Management*
   a. *Clothing Care*—Obtain and use supplies, launder, iron, store, and mend.
   b. *Cleaning*—Obtain and use supplies, pick up, vacuum, sweep, dust, scrub, mop, make bed, and remove trash.
   c. *Meal Preparation and Cleanup*—Plan nutritious meals and prepare food; open and close containers, cabinets, and drawers; use kitchen utensils and appliances; and clean up and store food.
   d. *Shopping*—Select and purchase items and perform money transactions.
   e. *Money Management*—Budget, pay bills, and use bank systems.
   f. *Household Maintenance*—Maintain home, yard, garden appliances, and household items, and/or obtain appropriate assistance.
   g. *Safety Procedures*—Know and perform prevention and emergency procedures to maintain a safe environment and prevent injuries.
2. *Care of Others*—Provide for children, spouse, parents, or others physical care, nurturance, communication, and use of age-appropriate activities.
3. *Educational Activities*—Participate in a school environment and school-sponsored activities (such as field trips, work-study, extracurricular activities).
4. *Vocational Activities*
   a. *Vocational Exploration*—Determine aptitudes, interests, skills, and appropriate vocational pursuits.
   b. *Job Acquisition*—Identify and select work opportunities and complete application and interview processes.
   c. *Work or Job Performance*—Perform job tasks in a timely and effective manner, incorporating necessary work behaviors such as grooming, interpersonal skills, punctuality, and adherence to safety procedures.
   d. *Retirement Planning*—Determine aptitudes, interests, skills, and identify appropriate avocational pursuits.

Figure 2-1.   Definition of the Occupational Performance Area of Work and its Occupational Performance Components as Defined in the *Uniform Terminology for Occupational Therapy*, Second Edition (Reprinted with permission from AOTA).

Work skills are the capabilities that an individual has learned or has the potential to learn (typing, cooking, sewing, welding, etc.). Work skills have been frequently called vocational skills.

Aptitudes are general capacities and abilities that are, to one degree or another, possessed by nearly all individuals. Examples are intelligence; verbal, numerical and spatial ability; form perception; clerical perception; motor coordination; finger dexterity; manual dexterity; eye–hand–foot coordination; and color discrimination.

Physical capabilities include lifting, carrying, pushing, pulling, climbing, balancing, stooping, kneeling, crouching, crawling, reaching, handling, fingering, feeling, talking, hearing, and seeing.

The Commission on Accreditation of Rehabilitation Facilities (CARF) has developed "Work Hardening Guidelines" that provide a basis for a uniform language, particularly important for work practice in industrial rehabilitation (see Appendix 1-1).

It is strongly suggested that uniform terminology be utilized in work practice. Not only will it facilitate ease in communicating information about your clients and/or program(s) to your various markets (e.g., insurance companies, physicians, educators); but it may be the key to receiving appropriate reimbursement and facilitating accurate recording of outcome information for efficacy studies. In addition, in those states that have embraced the CARF "Work Hardening Guidelines," uniform terminology becomes critical to both accreditation and reimbursement.

WORK PRACTICE

Work programming requires a holistic approach to the needs of the individual—social, psychological, physical, and educational—in his or her development of a work role, regardless of whether the person is "normal" or "disabled."

Traditionally, the occupational therapist has been faced with clients who are either unsuccessful at work or unable to work for a variety of reasons or who have never had the opportunity to acquire work-related skills. Such clients may include an upper-extremity amputee from a recent industrial accident; a stockboy with an acquired chronic back injury who now perceives himself as unable ever to return to work; a computer analyst who, after severe head trauma, has limited cognitive and physical functioning; a secretary who has become severely depressed and is unable to hold her office job; and an institutionalized developmentally delayed adolescent who has never been exposed to appropriate work behaviors and skills.

Functionally, these persons' disabilities can be put in two major categories: (1) a lack of work behaviors; and (2) neurophysiologic impairments. The importance of the first category is emphasized by the fact that most unemployed workers have lost their jobs because of problems with interpersonal relationships, that is, trouble getting along with co-workers and supervisors, rather than because of inadequate skills.

As therapists we can provide "the client with a series of learning experiences that will enable [him or her] to make appropriate vocational decisions and develop work habits necessary for eventual employment" [1].

In program development, I have found that many commonalities exist across the various client populations and clinical settings. When developing a work-related program for any population in any setting, the therapist must first obtain information on the clients for appropriate treatment planning. This can be done by performing a work-assessment. Historically, occupational therapists have often been involved in some type of assessment to measure work skills, aptitudes, and physical capacities. According to the 1980 official position paper by the American Occupational Therapy Association on the role of occupational therapy in vocational rehabilitation [1], the goal of work-related evaluation is

> . . . to assess and predict work behavior and vocational potential through the application of practical, reality-based assessment techniques. The objectives include: testing and evaluating work abilities related to a specific job task; assessing the client's learning abilities and retention of skills; evaluating physical, psychological, and social factors such as work tolerance, habits, and interpersonal qualities. Testing objectives are met through the use of

carefully selected media that stimulate or closely resemble actual job-related requirements.

From the information gathered in the assessment, the therapist can begin to plan an appropriate work-related program. Many factors must be taken into account: (1) What are the client's interests? (2) What are his or her aspirations and interests regarding future employment? (3) Are the client's job goals realistic? (4) What is the extent of the client's job experience? (5) What type of work is available to the client, particularly in his or her local community? Does the client have the necessary skills to do this kind of work? (6) What type of budget do you have in developing and operating the program? (7) Do you have access to equipment and supplies? (8) How much physical space will you have for the program? (9) Do you have the support of the administration and staff of your facility?

After these questions have been answered, the key word to keep in mind in setting up the program is *creativity*. Look to your own in-house resources for areas of simulated job experiences for your client. Check to see if you have access to a business office, food preparation area, or maintenance or laundry service; then make arrangements to use this area, equipment, or supplies. When appropriate, ascertain whether you can obtain support from the supervisors and workers for eventual work placement of your clients. In addition, contact your local community businesses—for example, copy shops, hardware stores, restaurants—for donations of supplies and equipment.

Programs should cater to the needs of the individual client, yet realistic expectations must be established. Many difficulties arise when a client returns to work or is first placed on a job site and finds that it is very different from the therapy milieu. Any problems should be brought back to the clinic, where the client can receive support and work on problem areas. A good example of this process comes from the Learning Prep School, a vocational work-study program for learning-disabled students. Eight students in the work-study program were placed in the student cafeteria at a local college. After a week on the serving line, the manager reviewed their performance and stated that, although the students were doing fine, they needed to increase their speed and accuracy. This area of difficulty was brought back to the treatment setting and addressed in simulated job experiences. In addition, the staff therapist devised a plan whereby these issues would be reinforced in both the students' vocational and academic classes.

Throughout this book you will read about work assessments and programs. I hope that this sampling will be a catalyst to you in your endeavor to develop programs and assessments suitable to your population.

REFERENCES

1. Ad Hoc Committee of the Commission on Practice. The role of occupational therapy in vocational rehabilitation process: Official position paper. *Am. J. Occup. Ther.* 34:881, 1980.
2. Jacobs, K. Work assessments and programming. In H.L. Hopkins and H.D.

Smith. (Eds.) *Willard and Spackman's Occupational Therapy* (7th ed.). Philadelphia: J.B. Lippincott, 1988.

3. Kielhofner, G. Occupation. In H.L. Hopkins and H. D. Smith. (Eds.) *Willard and Spackman's Occupational Therapy* (6th ed.). Philadelphia: J.B. Lippincott, 1983, p. 31.

4. Uniform Terminology for Occupational Therapy, Second Edition. *AJOT*, 43:808, 1989.

5. U.S. Department of Labor. *Dictionary of Occupational Titles* (4th ed.). Washington, D.C.: U.S. Government Printing Office, 1977.

6. U.S. Department of Labor. Selected Characteristics of Occupations Defined in the *Dictionary of Occupational Titles*. Washington, D.C.: U.S. Government Printing Office, 1981.

3

Work Assessments

Comprehensive client assessment provides the strategic foundation for the provision of rehabilitation services to persons with disabilities.

—Brian Bolton [3]

FCA, SAM, VCWS, JPSA, PCA, WEST, BTE, SAGE, TAP, JEVS, TOWER, WCED, and P-MAC are acroynoms used to describe some of the many work assessments and evaluations available to test persons with disabilities. The number of work assessments continues to expand. A combination of factors have precipitated this growth:

1. Reductions in rehabilitation funding have provided the incentive to improve accuracy and efficiency of assessments.
2. The Carl Perkins Act (PL 94-142) has mandated the assessment of all students with disabilities.
3. The number of injured workers is increasing, yet there has been a lack of adequate comprehensive evaluations.

Many standardized and nonstandardized assessment instruments have been developed, but at present there are no instruments applicable to all populations. This is not surprising, since a test developed for a blind, developmentally delayed client would probably not be valid for a cognitively normal right-upper-extremity amputee. For this reason, many occupational therapists have developed nonstandardized assessments to be used with their specific populations. Examples of these will be presented throughout the text. The formats differ, but the behaviors assessed remain fairly constant from assessment to assessment.

Available assessments and evaluations range in complexity from short to diagnostic. Many require special training to administer, and can be expensive and cumbersome to transport. Some lack optimal clinical utility because of these limitations.

Assessment is *not* synonymous with evaluation. Assessment is a much broader term and includes the intake interview, a general medical examination, and evaluation.

Occupational therapists use a variety of processes in assessment, including:

1. Review of medical, educational and vocational records
2. Interviews with the client, employer, family members, teachers, and significant others

3. Observation
4. Standardized and nonstandardized evaluations [11].

STANDARDIZED VERSUS NONSTANDARDIZED WORK EVALUATIONS

Standardized evaluation implies uniformity of procedure in administering and scoring the test, affords comparison of test results with a normative group, and assumes that validity and reliability have been established [1, 10].

With *nonstandardized evaluations*, a uniform procedure in administering and scoring the test may have been established, but normative data, validity, and reliability may not have been determined. In some instances, nonstandardized instruments are used as adjuncts to standardized assessments. As noted by Trombly and Scott [19], "Non-standardized tests are also used to observe work habits, physical capacities, and other areas of concern which may not be observed during standardized testing. When craft and shop activities are carefully analyzed, they allow for observation of many of the basic skills common to all work."

NORM-REFERENCED TESTS

A norm-referenced test compares an individual's performance to that of a standardized sample. For instance, a norm-referenced test asks, "How will Ariel perform on evaluation A compared to adult sheltered workshop employees?" It is assumed that the individual being evaluated is similar to the standardized sample. In the present scenario, Ariel is an adult with moderate development disabilities and was given evaluation A to ascertain job placement potential. In this case, a comparison to the norm group (sheltered workshop employees) would provide information relevant to successful job placement. However, if Ariel were an adult of normal intelligence who had sustained a back injury, and the question to be addressed was if she could return to her job as a supermarket cashier, comparison to the sheltered workshop norm group would be irrelevant.

CRITERION-REFERENCED TESTS

"Can Laela make change for $10.00?"

"Can Laela reach overhead and attach bolts to a board?"

These might be questions addressed in a criterion-referenced test. Hursh and Kerns remark, "Criterion-referenced tests provide information about the individual's ability to perform specific behaviors, skills or activities or to demonstrate mastery over a particular skill domain" [11].

Methods Time Measurement (MTM) is an example of a criterion-referenced procedure "which analyzes any manual operation or method into the basic motions required to perform it and assigns to each motion a predetermined time standard which is determined by the nature of the motion and the conditions under which it is made" [20].

MTM is based on 19 fundamental motions. A rating of 100% is considered entry level job readiness, and 150% represents a greater level of success. MTM is becoming more popular among the developers of work evaluations. Some work evaluations that include MTM are Valpar Component Work Samples # 1–19, 202, 203, 204, and 205, and the Skills Assessment Module (SAM).*

VALIDITY

A valid evaluation measures what it was designed to measure. *Validity* dictates the usefulness of an evaluation. There are four types of validity: content validity, construct validity, predictive validity, and face validity.

Hursh and Kerns stress that "the primary criterion for determining the usefulness of a test is its validity. The norming sample may be adequate and the test may demonstrate reliability over time, but unless it demonstrates acceptable validity, it is of little use to the evaluator" [10, p. 92].

RELIABILITY

Reliability assures that the results of an evaluation are consistent and stable from one measurement to another. That is, the client will receive the same or similar scores if the test should be repeated [10].

WORK EVALUATION GUIDELINES OF THE
COMMISSION ON ACCREDITATION OF REHABILITATION FACILITIES

The Commission on Accreditation of Rehabilitation Facilities (CARF) has prepared a list of components that should be included in work evaluations. These are:

Physical and psychomotor capacities
Intellectual capacities; emotional stability; interests, attitudes and knowledge of occupational information; personal, social, and work histories; aptitudes
Achievements (e.g., vocational, educational)
Work skills and work tolerances
Work habits (punctuality, attendance, concentration, organization, and interpersonal skills)
Work-related capabilities (e.g., mobility, communication skills, hygiene, homemaking, money management)
Job-seeking skills
Potential to benefit from further services that are specifically identified
Employment objectives, which may involve either competitive or non-competitive employment or programs in industry options

*To learn more about MTMs and becoming certified to perform them, contact the MTM Association for Standards and Research, 1411 Peterson Ave, Park Ridge, IL 60068.

Ability to learn through the evaluation experience

Assessment of the most effective modes of understanding and responding to various types of instruction

Identification of the need for tool and job site modification or adaptive equipment to enhance employability [6].

Many of the tests commonly used in occupational therapy practice to evaluate dexterity, strength, endurance, coordination, activities of daily living, and interpersonal skills can be considered appropriate for work evaluation. In Chapter 6, Rabin and Jeong will explore work assessments used with the psychiatric client. Therefore, the primary focus of the remainder of this chapter will be those work assessments used with individuals who have neurological and/or physical challenges, that is head injury, developmental delays, or physical injuries (carpal tunnel syndrome, back injury).

TYPES OF EVALUATIONS

Commonly used categories of work evaluation tools are:

1. On-the-job or job site evaluations
2. Situational assessments
3. Psychometric instruments
4. Work samples [4, 10, 11].

Using more than one evaluation category is often the most effective way to appraise an individual's work potential [11]. Not all categories are used by occupational therapists or are appropriate for every individual. For example, a middle-aged individual who has been fired from a series of jobs may be referred to determine the cause of job instability, whereas a school-aged person with no work history may be referred for assessment of occupational interests. In another example, an individual with a back injury may be referred for the purpose of identifying present physical capabilities.

On-the-Job or Job Site Evaluations

The purpose of on-the-job or "job site" evaluations is to evaluate the individual's ability to perform successfully in a competitive employment situation. Structured observation of the individual on the job and, ideally, in a variety of job-related environments (e.g., cafeteria, break room, using public transportation to travel to and from the job site) can be performed by the occupational therapist. The occupational therapist typically uses a job analysis form to categorize information about the job and the individual's ability to perform the job and its related activities. In cases of long-term assessment, observation might be performed by the employer or another employee(s). In these instances, the therapist must rely on information from these individuals in formulating recommendations.

Many types of job analysis exist. The U.S. Department of Labor has developed a Job Analysis Schedule, which is commonly used by vocational evaluators (Fig. 3-1). To some degree, most job analyses deal with the following information [14]:

Physical demands
Mental factors
Stress factors
Breakdown of the job
Tools and machines used
Description of the work environment
Hazards

As an example, Joshua sustained a back injury at work. He has completed six weeks of work hardening and appears ready to return to work. Prior to returning to his job, the occupational therapist observed Joshua perform some of his job tasks at the job site, noting the duration of static and dynamic postures and repetition of motions in lifting, bending, and reaching activities.

In contrast, evaluation of a developmentally delayed adult in a supported employment environment might focus more on determining the job-related abilities, interests, learning style, and needs of the individual. To accurately depict the job demands, the following additional information would be useful: direct observation of other workers in the area, an interview with the employer, and performance of the job tasks by the therapist. This additional information allows for a comparison of actual job demands relative to the individual worker's demonstrated abilities, interests, learning style, and needs. Spencer cautions,

> Isolated assessment of job related skills or the use of prevocational, developmentally referenced assessments have been found to be largely ineffective in developing on-the-job training strategies and in predicting supported employment needs and subsequent job success. Occupational therapy's reliance on these approaches is not recommended within a supported employment context. Situational observation of individual performance in relevant community and work environments, combined with job and environmental analysis, necessarily becomes the assessment method of choice [18, p. 78].

Situational Assessment

Situational assessment involves evaluating the individual in a realistic work situation. However, in contrast to on-the-job evaluation, variables such as supervision style or production demands can be systematically altered and the individual's performance under each circumstance can be observed. For example, with a learning-disabled adolescent in a mainstreamed high school setting, a realistic placement might be in the school's cafeteria or main office. If interpersonal skills were of concern, the therapist might arrange for the student to perform job tasks in a small group rather than alone. The therapist would then observe the individual's behaviors and job performance in reference to this change. Questions such as, Was the individual able to share job tools and materials? Was the individual able to wait his or her turn? could be answered to identify the factors that help promote or hinder work performance.

OMB 44-R0722

U.S. Department of Labor
Manpower Administration

Estab. & Sched. No. _____

Job Analysis Schedule

1. Estab. Job Title _____

2. Ind. Assign. _____

3. SIC Code(s) and Title(s) _____

_____

_____

4. Job Summary:

5. Work Performed Ratings:

Worker Functions	D Data	P People	T Things

Work Field _____

M.P.S.M.S. _____

6. Worker Traits Ratings:

GED	1	2	3	4	5	6					
SVP	1	2	3	4	5	6	7	8	9		

Aptitudes   G__ V__ N__ S__ P__ Q__ K__ F__ M__ E__ C__

Temperaments	D	F	I	J	M	P	R	S	T	V
Interests	1a	1b	2a	2b	3a	3b	4a	4b	5a	5b
Phys. Demands	S	L	M	H	V	2	3	4	5	6
Environ. Cond.	I	O	B	2	3	4	5	6	7	

(left margin labels: Code, WTA Group, DOT Title, Ind. Desig.)

MA 7-36

Figure 3-1.   A sample format for a job analysis from the U.S. Department of Labor. (From *Handbook for Analyzing Jobs* (pp. 33–36) by U.S. Department of Labor, Manpower Administration, 1972. Menomonie: University of Wisconsin-Stout, Stout Vocational Rehabilitation Institute, Materials Development Center.)

7. General Education

   a. Elementary _____ High School _____ Courses _____

   b. College _____ Courses _____

8. Vocational Preparation

   a. College _____ Courses _____

   _____

   b. Vocational Education _____ Courses _____

   _____

   c. Apprenticeship _____

   _____

   d. Inplant Training _____

   e. On-the-Job Training _____

   f. Performance on Other Jobs _____

9. Experience _____

10. Orientation _____

11. Licenses, etc. _____

12. Relation to Other Jobs and Workers _____

   Promotion: From _____ To _____

   Transfers: From _____ To _____

   Supervision Received _____

   Supervision Given _____

   _____

13. Machines, Tools, Equipment, and Work Aids

14. Materials and Products

Figure 3-1.   (continued)

15. Description of Tasks:

Figure 3-1. (continued)

16. Definition of Terms

17. General Comments

18. Analyst _____ Date _____ Editor _____ Date _____

    Reviewed By _____ Title, Org. _____

    National Office Reviewer _____

Figure 3-1. (continued)

Psychometric Instruments

Psychometric instruments include a wide variety of paper-and-pencil and apparatus tests that measure general intelligence, personality, achievement, abilities, and related characteristics, such as vocational aptitudes and interests.

Dougherty and Radomski developed an evaluation to assess work behaviors of brain-injured adults, which they stated can be used "to complement multidisciplinary evaluations findings" [7, p. 12]. The evaluation focuses on observing the following work behaviors [7, p. 11]:

1. Ability to follow written and verbal directions
2. Efficiency and accuracy of work
3. Vigilance
4. Response to feedback
5. Self-awareness

This is a *nonstandardized* evaluation and typically takes two one-hour sessions to complete. All the necessary forms and instructions to administer and score the evaluation can be found in *The Cognitive Rehabilitation Workbook* [7]. The evaluation is composed of six sections. They will be reviewed briefly:

1. *Computations*—The client uses a calculator to solve 26 arithmetic problems. The client is timed, required to record answers on the evaluation form, and must check his or her own work from an answer key.
2. *Use of the Yellow Pages*—This written test contains ten hypothetical situations that require the use of the yellow pages to determine the appropriate individual, service, or store to call [7, p. 26]. The client is provided with a yellow pages and a stopwatch, which the therapist shows the client how to use. The client is instructed to time him- or herself while completing the problems (Fig. 3-2).
3. *Reading Transportation Schedules*—The client must answer and then score responses to 10 questions based on a provided train schedule (e.g., "How long does it take the 9:18 A.M. train to get from Waconia to Garden Park?") [7, p. 17].
4. *Checking Accounts*—The client must carry out the necessary steps to manage a checking account, by following written instructions. This test is timed. The client is allowed to use a calculator. This section is divided into three steps. Step 1 instructs the client to write out seven checks to various people/parties for specified amounts. Step 2 asks the client to complete six deposit slips for specified amounts. Step 3 has the individual balance the checkbook using a checkbook register, based on information provided in Steps 1 and 2.
5. *Self Awareness* first part—The client is asked to list his or her responses to the question, "What personal characteristics or skills do you feel are your strengths at present?"
6. *Self Awareness*, second part—The individual is asked to list his or her responses to the following questions: "What problems re-

II. USE OF THE YELLOW PAGES

Instructions:
Take this form to the therapist. Request that the therapist tell you how to do the next
set of problems.

A. You are hungry for a steak dinner.

_____ Time: _____

B. You loosened a filling while eating taffy.

_____ Time: _____

C. You need to rent a car.

_____ Time: _____

D. You need to make photocopies of some important papers.

_____ Time: _____

E. Your cat is sick.

_____ Time: _____

F. You need to buy new custom draperies.

_____ Time: _____

G. You would like to purchase a baseball glove.

_____ Time: _____

H. You need to buy a new pair of eyeglasses.

_____ Time: _____

Figure 3-2.   Example of "Use of the Yellow Pages." (Reprinted from
The Cognitive Rehabilitation Handbook by P. Dougherty and M. Radomski (Eds.), p. 14, with permission of Aspen Publishers, Inc.,
© 1987.)

sulting from your injury continue to limit your ability to work optimally?" and "Are there specific techniques that you are able to use to compensate for your deficits? If so, list them."

Vocational Interest Inventories and Checklists

Occupational therapists use various checklists and inventories to gain insight into the client's interests, desires, and work objectives. Some of the more commonly used checklists and inventories are the Interest Checklist [14], the Activity Configuration [20], the Reading-Free Vocational Interest Inventory—Revised [2], and the Occupational Role History. There are many other interest inventories and checklists that are used more frequently by vocational rehabilitation counselors and other professionals, but that can be used by occupational therapists as well. The following are appropriate for use with the severely challenged:

Wide Range Interest and Opinion Test (WRIOT)
Gordon Occupational Checklist

A sixth-grade reading level is required for the following vocational interest inventories and checklists:

Self Directed Search [9]
Strong Vocational Interest Inventory
Career Assessment Inventory (CAI)
Kuder Vocational Interest Inventory
Ohio Vocational Interest Survey
Vocational Interest, Experience and Skill Assessment (VIESA)

The Self Directed Search (SDS) is composed of two booklets that guide the individual through a self-exploration and self-interpretation process [9]. The client selects from one booklet activities that he or she likes and dislikes, activities that he or she has the skill to perform, and interest or dislike for selected occupations (Fig. 3-3). In addition, the SDS requires the client to rate him- or herself on selected traits in comparison to persons of their own age. For example, in the section entitled "Occupational Daydreams," the client is instructed to list "occupations you have considered in thinking about your future. List the careers you have daydreamed about as well as those you have discussed with others" [9, p. 3]. A summary code, based on Holland's occupational category types, is obtained. Some of these codes are:

RSE = Realistic, Social, and Enterprising themes
AIR = Artistic, Investigative, and Realistic themes

Next, the individual uses the second booklet to locate appropriate jobs under this three-letter code.

Hursh and Kerns comment, "Although the SDS is useful for independent self-administration and exploration, the evaluator is encouraged to 'work' through the inventory with the student. This process

COMPETENCIES

Blacken under Y for "Yes" for those activities you can do well or competently. Blacken under N for "No" for those activities you have never performed or perform poorly.

R

	Y	N
I have used wood shop power tools such as power saw or lathe or sander	☐	☐
I know how to use a voltmeter	☐	☐
I can adjust a carburetor	☐	☐
I have operated power tools such as a drill press or grinder or sewing machine	☐	☐
I can refinish varnished or stained furniture or woodwork	☐	☐
I can read blueprints	☐	☐
I can make simple electrical repairs	☐	☐
I can repair furniture	☐	☐
I can make mechanical drawings	☐	☐
I can make simple repairs on a TV set	☐	☐
I can make simple plumbing repairs	☐	☐

Total No. of Y's ☐

I

	Y	N
I understand how a vacuum tube works	☐	☐
I can name three foods that are high in protein content	☐	☐
I understand the "half-life" of a radioactive element	☐	☐
I can use logarithmic tables	☐	☐
I can use a slide rule to multiply or divide	☐	☐
I can use a microscope	☐	☐
I can identify three constellations of the stars	☐	☐
I can describe the function of the white blood cells	☐	☐
I can interpret simple chemical formulae	☐	☐
I understand why man-made satellites do not fall to the earth	☐	☐
I have participated in a scientific fair or contest	☐	☐

Total No. of Y's ☐

A

	Y	N
I can play a musical instrument	☐	☐
I can participate in two- or four-part choral singing	☐	☐
I can perform as a musical soloist	☐	☐
I can act in a play	☐	☐
I can do interpretive reading	☐	☐
I can do modern interpretive or ballet dancing	☐	☐
I can sketch people so that they can be recognized	☐	☐
I can do a painting or sculpture	☐	☐
I can make pottery	☐	☐
I can design clothing, posters, or furniture	☐	☐
I write stories or poetry well	☐	☐

Total No. of Y's ☐

Figure 3-3. Competencies from the *Self-Directed Search* [9]. (Reproduced by permission of Consulting Psychologists Press, Inc., Palo Alto, California.)

S   Y   N

I am good at explaining things to others   ☐   ☐
I have participated in charity or benefit drives   ☐   ☐
I cooperate and work well with others   ☐   ☐
I am competent at entertaining people older than I   ☐   ☐
I can be a good host (hostess)   ☐   ☐
I can teach children easily   ☐   ☐
I can plan entertainment for a party   ☐   ☐
I am good at helping people who are upset or troubled   ☐   ☐
I have worked as a volunteer aide in a hospital, clinic,   ☐   ☐
    or home
I can plan school or church social affairs   ☐   ☐
I am a good judge of personality   ☐   ☐

Total No. of Y's ☐

E

I have been elected to an office in high school or college   ☐   ☐
I can supervise the work of others   ☐   ☐
I have unusual energy and enthusiasm   ☐   ☐
I am good at getting people to do things my way   ☐   ☐
I am a good salesperson   ☐   ☐
I have acted as leader for some group in presenting   ☐   ☐
    suggestions or complaints to a person in authority
I won an award for work as a salesperson or leader   ☐   ☐
I have organized a club, group, or gang   ☐   ☐
I have started my own business or service   ☐   ☐
I know how to be a successful leader   ☐   ☐
I am a good debater   ☐   ☐

Total No. of Y's ☐

C

I can type 40 words a minute   ☐   ☐
I can operate a duplicating or adding machine   ☐   ☐
I can take shorthand   ☐   ☐
I can file correspondence and other papers   ☐   ☐
I have held an office job   ☐   ☐
I can use a bookkeeping machine   ☐   ☐
I can do a lot of paper work in a short time   ☐   ☐
I can use a calculating machine   ☐   ☐
I can use simple data processing equipment such as   ☐   ☐
    a keypunch
I can post credits and debits   ☐   ☐
I can keep accurate records of payments or sales   ☐   ☐

Total No. of Y's ☐

Figure 3-3   (continued)

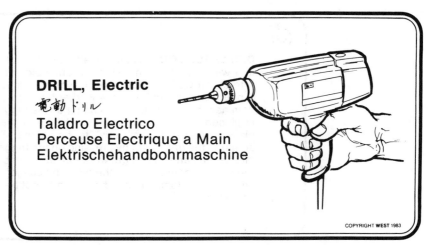

DRILL, Electric
電動ドリル
Taladro Electrico
Perceuse Electrique a Main
Elektrischehandbohrmaschine

COPYRIGHT WEST 1983

Figure 3-4.   Sample card from the WEST Tool-Sort. (Reprinted with permission.)

functions to further increase self-exploration and self-evaluation on the student's part" [10, p. 112].

WEST Tool-Sort

The WEST Tool-Sort has gained popularity in industrial rehabilitation as a useful interest inventory instrument.* It is composed of 80 cards, which depict 59 different tools (Fig. 3-4). The client is instructed to "look over each card and place it in one of five piles," according to his or her perceived ability to use the tool. The piles are divided into the following categories:

A. "I would have no change in the speed at which I work."
B. "I would have a decrease in the speed at which I work."
C. "I would be unable to continue work without an extra break."
D. "I would be unable to work."
DK. "I don't know whether or not I could use this tool."

The Tool-Sort assesses the client's performance on 26 work variables. It also may be used to identify Type 2 Malingerer Symptom Magnification Syndrome.

Aptitude and Achievement Tests

Some commonly used aptitude and achievement tests are:

Wide Range Achievement Test—Revised (WRAT)
General Aptitude Test Battery (GATB)
Peabody Individual Achievement Test
Peabody Picture Vocabulary Test
Minnesota Multiphasic Personality Inventory
Draw-a-Person Test

*WEST Tool-Sort. Work Evaluation Systems Technology. 1950 Freeman Ave., Long Beach, CA 90804.

(60)

DRILL, ELECTRIC - A unilateral/bilateral implement used in a wide variety of industries to drill holes and install or retract screws. This tool ranges in weight from 12 ounces to 6 pounds. In typical use, the worker holds this tool in the dominant hand with the index finger on the trigger. A drill bit is placed within the drill chuck. The tip of the drill bit is placed against the material to be drilled. The worker actuates the drill motor by pressing on the trigger while the middle, ring and little finger work with the thumb to stabilize the tool. Depending upon the type and size of the electric dirll, the non-dominant hand may or may not be involved as an assist.

Figure 3-4. (continued)

Performance Tests

These hands-on evaluations measure dexterity, coordination, and use of tools. The most commonly used performance tests are the Crawford Small Parts Dexterity Test, the Bennett Hand-Tool Dexterity Test, and the Purdue Pegboard.

Crawford Small Parts Dexterity Test
The Crawford Small Parts Dexterity Test is a timed test that measures fine motor and eye-hand coordination. It is composed of two sections. The first part involves using tweezers to (1) pick up a pin and place it in a hole and (2) pick up a collar and place it over the pin. The second section requires bilateral hand use of a blade-head screwdriver to turn a threaded screw in a hole. Normative data are based on a small sample size for students, employed workers, adults in a vocational training program, and mentally challenged adults (See Fig. 7-25).

Bennett Hand-Tool Dexterity Test
This timed test measures gross motor ability, coordination, and use of basic hand tools. Normative data are outdated and poorly documented. Available norms are based on job applicants, mechanics, and welders.

Purdue Pegboard
The Purdue Pegboard measures fine finger dexterity and upper extremity coordination (Fig. 3-5). The test, which takes 10–15 minutes to perform and can be administered to groups, involves placing pins, collars, and washers into holes on the test board. The test manual, which contains dated normative data, presents low reliability and validity coefficients. However, recent normative data for the Purdue Pegboard have been established for injured industrial workers by the Occupational Therapy Department at the J. Leonard Camera Industrial Rehabilitation Center [5, p. 7].

Hursh and Kerns noted the following about the use of psychometric tests in vocational evaluation of severely challenged students: "Major limitations of psychometric tests are inadequate norm groups, restrictive

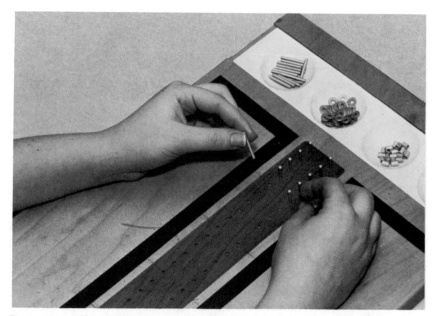

Figure 3-5. The Purdue Pegboard measures fine finger dexterity and upper extremity coordination. (Photographer Lucia Grochowska Little-field.)

standardized administration procedures, inappropriate test content, and limited ability to modify testing procedures. In addition, paper and pencil tests are familiar experiences for special needs students and have historically represented failure" [10, p. 47].

Some work evaluations can be categorized as psychometric instruments or work samples or interest inventories and checklists. For example, the Purdue Pegboard and Crawford Small Parts Dexterity Test have been categorized in the literature as single trait work samples instead of as psychometric performance tests.

When used with other work evaluations, psychometric instruments can supplement or complement a comprehensive work assessment [10].

Work Samples

Work samples are the primary technique of work evaluation. A work sample is "a well-defined work activity involving tasks, materials, and tools which are identical or similar to those in an actual job or cluster of jobs. It is used to assess an individual's vocational aptitude, worker characteristics, and vocational interests" [10, p. 119].

There are four categories of work samples: Single trait, cluster trait, simulated job, and actual job work samples [4].

Single Trait Work Samples

Single trait work samples measure a single worker trait or characteristic, such as finger dexterity. Hursh and Kerns noted "that in measuring only a single or isolated trait, we do not have a work sample, but only a psychometric test" [10, p. 121]. However, Roberts noted that the single trait work sample has a greater "degree or element of reality" than a psychometric test [11].

Cluster Trait Work Samples

Cluster trait work samples measure a group of traits, such as strength, endurance, and range of motion, that are inherent to a job. Some of the more common cluster trait work samples used by occupational therapists, particularly in industrial rehabilitation, are:

WEST 2A, 3, 4A, and 7—Whole Body Range of Motion
VALPAR Component Work Samples 1, 4, 8, 9, 11
Baltimore Therapeutic Equipment Bolt Box

A cluster trait work sample that has had increasing popularity with therapists working in school systems is the Perceptual-Motor Assessment for Children (P-MAC).

WEST 2A—Whole Body Range of Motion Work Sample

The WEST 2A is a wall-mounted frame that can be used in a standard evaluation of functional tolerances to determine an individual's level of performance on the U.S. Department of Labor's Physical Demand Factors, which include stooping, kneeling, crouching, overhead reaching, and handling. Manufactured or custom evaluation equipment can be combined with the WEST 2A to assess ability to perform brief to prolonged light and/or resistive tool handling and assembly/disassembly tasks in various postures. The WEST 2A is easily adaptable to a wheelchair. The "Brief Tool Use Assembly" task of the WEST 2A was normed on healthly male adults from a manual arts vocational training program.

WEST 3—Comprehensive Weight System

The WEST 3 contains seven handles, 36 weights, and a weight container. When used with the WEST 2A, it can assess unilateral or bilateral lifting/carrying capacity and range of motion under load up to 105 lbs.

WEST 4A—Upper Extremity Strength and Fatigue Tolerance Work Sample

The WEST 4A measures upper extremity strength and fatigue tolerance in tool handling tasks requiring pronation/supination and wrist flexion/extension against resistance. The WEST 4A contains three torque units and an accurate torque indicator. The indicator range is 2–100 pounds. The torque units can be adapted to accept standard socket drive tools and accessories. It was normed for upper extremity strength on healthy male adults attending a manual arts vocational training program and on healthy females.

WEST 7—Bus Bench

The Bus Bench is a cognitive assessment tool designed to measure upper extremity dexterity and coordination. It can measure full range of motion from knuckle to shoulder level and can be performed in groups. The evaluation is a two-step disassembly/assembly procedure.

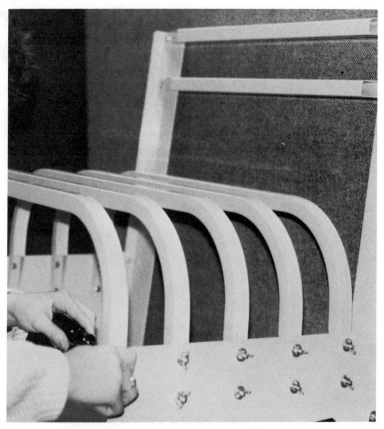

Figure 3-6.   Disassembly of the WEST 7—Bus Bench.

Disassembly (Phase I) measures finger dexterity and manual dexterity in the loosening and removal of bolts, washers, and wing nuts (Fig. 3-6). Assembly (Phase II) measures finger dexterity and manual dexterity in the rejoining of the structural components. Separate scores for both assembly and disassembly are obtained. The time required to complete the tasks becomes the score. Percentile norms are based on highly competitive non-disabled workers who have ongoing and recent experience with hand tools.

Valpar Component Work Sample (VCWS) #1—Small Tools: Mechanical

VCWS #1 measures an individual's understanding of and ability to work with small tools (Fig. 3-7). It is administered into two sections— assembly and disassembly—and the client can be seated or standing.

Valpar Component Work Sample (VCWS) #4—Upper Extremity Range of Motion

VCWS #4 measures an individual's upper extremity (shoulder, upper arm, forearm, elbow, wrist, and hand) range of motion (Fig. 3-8). The VCWS #4 is designed to provide an actuarial level of performance, including finger dexterity, tactile sense, and neck and back fatigue. The work sample is administered in two sections (assembly and disassem-

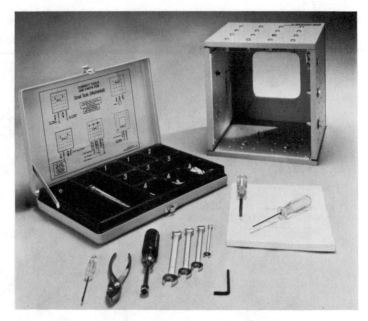

Figure 3-7.   Valpar Component Work Sample #1—Small Tools (Mechanical). (Photograph courtesy of Valpar International Corp., Tucson, Arizona.)

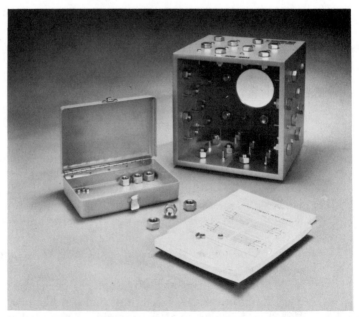

Figure 3-8.   Valpar Component Work Sample #4—Upper Extremity Range of Motion. (Photograph courtesy of Valpar International Corp., Tucson, Arizona.)

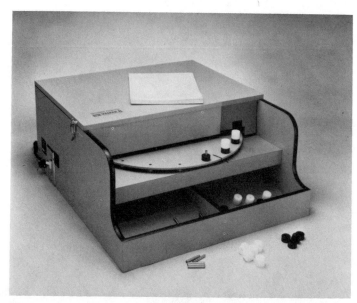

Figure 3-9.   Valpar Component Sample #8—Simulated Assembly.
(Photograph courtesy of Valpar International Corp., Tucson, Arizona.)

bly). Following the assembly section, the client is asked a series of questions to ascertain his or her physical reaction to the activity. The "Upper Extremity Body Position Chart" records the client's fatigue and/ or pain. The work sample is designed to be performed in a standing position; however, it can be done seated if noted on the scoring sheet.

Valpar Component Work Sample (VCWS) #8—Simulated Assembly
VCWS #8 measures an individual's ability to work at an assembly task requiring repetitive physical manipulation (Fig. 3-9). Scoring is based on the total number of units assembled correctly during a 20-minute period while the client is standing.

Valpar Component Work Sample (VCWS) #9—Whole Body Range of Motion
VCWS #9 measures an individual's gross motor movements as they relate to performing job tasks (Fig. 3-10). For example, the therapist is able to observe what effect kneeling for a period of time will have on the client's dexterity.

Valpar Component Work Sample (VCWS) #11—Eye-Hand-Foot Coordination
VCWS #11 measures an individual's eye-hand-foot coordination (Fig. 3-11). It is administered to a seated client and involves three sections.

Baltimore Therapeutic Equipment (BTE) Bolt Box
The BTE Bolt Box measures dexterity, manipulation skills with or without visual cues, eye-hand coordination, size discrimination, and work tolerance. It can be used for treatment or as an evaluation tool. The assembly and disassembly tasks are timed.

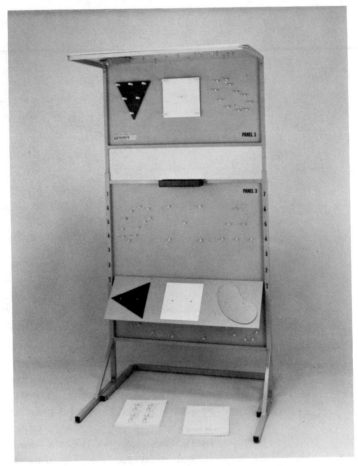

Figure 3-10.   Valpar Component Work Sample #9—Whole Body Range of Motion. (Photograph courtesy of Valpar International Corp., Tucson, Arizona.)

Perceptual-Motor Assessment for Children (P-MAC)

This is a computer-interpreted assessment designed for screening visual, auditory, and haptic (touch) perception, fine and gross motor abilities, and perceptual memory in children ages 4 years to 15 years, 11 months. P-MAC is portable (single suitcase), materials are nonconsumable, and no training is required. It is divided into three parts:

1. Two subtests from the McCarron-Dial System's Perceptual Motor Task are used:
    a. *Spatial Relations*—cubes are used to reconstruct printed cube patterns
    b. *Auditory—Visual Recognition and Sequencing*—colored blocks are used to match a sequence of orally presented colors, (Fig. 3-12).
2. Haptic Visual Discrimination Test: This test uses geometric and/ or textured objects that are obscured from the client's view and

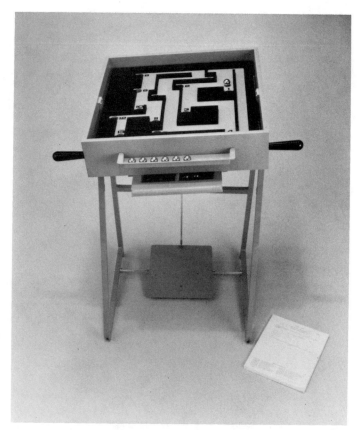

Figure 3-11.   Valpar Component Work Sample #11—Eye-Hand-Foot Coordination. (Photograph courtesy of Valpar International Corp., Tucson, Arizona.)

must be manipulated in one hand and then identified from draw-ings (Fig. 3-13).

3. McCarron Assessment of Neuromuscular Development (MAND):

Six of the MAND subtests are used:

a. *Beads in the box*—a 30-second test that requires the transfering of beads, one at a time, from one box to another (Fig. 3-14).

b. *Finger tapping*—a 10-second test of rapid continuous tapping of the index finger.

c. *Nut and bolt*—a test that requires the turning of a bolt into a nut. The test is timed and uses two sizes of nuts and bolts (Fig. 3-15).

d. *Hand strength*—a test that uses a dynamometer to measure strength of one hand and then the other.

e. *Standing on one foot*—requires standing on one foot (right, then left) with eyes open and then closed.

f. *Finger-nose-finger*—involves moving finger to nose using a specified movement. Performed first with eyes open and then closed for 10 seconds each.

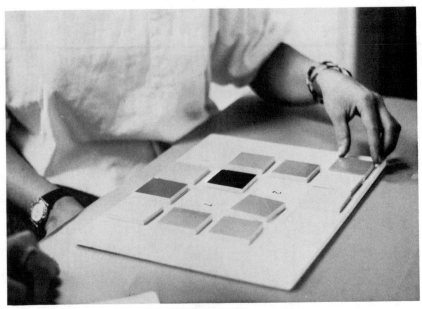

Figure 3-12. Auditory-Visual Recognition and Sequencing subtest from the Perceptual-Motor Assessment for Children.

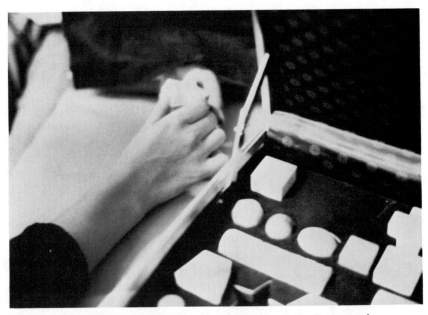

Figure 3-13. Haptic Visual Discrimination Test from the Perceptual-Motor Assessment for Children.

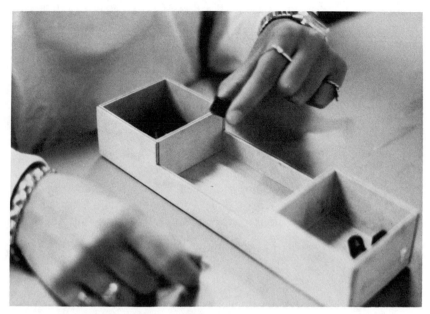

Figure 3-14. Beads in the Box, a subtest from the McCarron Assessment of Neuromuscular Development.

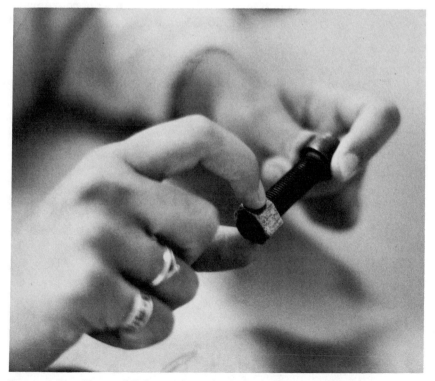

Figure 3-15. Nut and Bolt, a subtest from the McCarron Assessment of Neuromuscular Development.

Purchase of the P-MAC also includes a five-volume set of *Guides for Educational Management* (GEM). These are very useful in translating results from the assessment into appropriate activities for the classroom.

Simulated Job Work Samples

Simulated work samples replicate a *segment* of the essential work factors, materials, equipment, supplies, and tasks of one or more jobs. The VCWS #19 and the Skills Assessment Module (SAM) are two examples of simulated job samples.

Valpar Component Work Sample #19 (VCWS #19)

Twenty-three physical demand factors from the *Dictionary of Occupational Titles* (DOT) are measured with 28 exercises. The exercises require the client to read an invoice, locate a shipping carton, remove the carton from a shelf (climbing one step on a ladder), pack the carton correctly, weigh it, and put it in its proper place for shipping (Fig. 3-16).

Skills Assessment Module (SAM)

SAM evaluates an individual's affective, cognitive, and manipulative strengths and weaknesses in relation to vocational performance required in school-based training programs. The manual suggests that "the student can be evaluated before entering a training program to determine in which performances he or she demonstrates a deficiency or competency" [17]. SAM is directly correlated to the *Dictionary of Occupational Titles*.

The assessment is compact and nonconsumable, and it can be administered in 1.5–2.5 hours. It is computer based (IBM and Apple), with normative data established for average, mildly handicapped, and disadvantaged youths (14–21 years) and employed workers. MTMs have been developed. The technical manual presents encouraging reliability coefficients (.82–.95) on 11 of the 12 hands-on modules. Validity must be developed locally.

SAM is composed of three paper and pencil tests and 12 hands-on modules. The paper and pencil tests, which can be administered individually or in groups, are:

1. *Learning Styles Inventory*—This test helps to determine an individual's preference in the areas of information gathering, work conditions, and expression (Fig. 3-17)
2. *Revised Beta Examination*—This test ascertains a nonverbal measure of intellectual ability.
3. *Auditory Directions Screen* (ADS)—ADS assesses the individual's ability to follow oral directions.

The twelve hands-on modules can be administered in any order and include:

1. *Mail Sort*—sorting 100 preaddressed post cards in zip code order (Fig. 3-18)

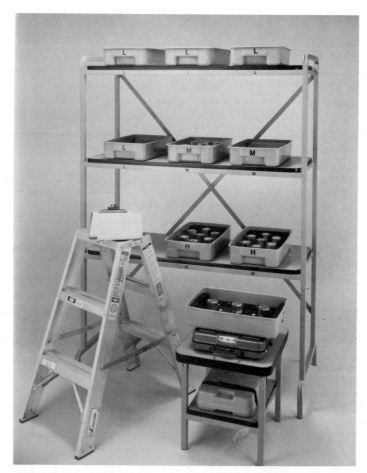

Figure 3-16.   Valpar Component Work Sample #19—Dynamic Physical Capacities. (Photograph courtesy of Valpar International Corp., Tucson, Arizona.)

2. *Alphabetizing Cards*—filing preaddressed postcards alphabetically
3. *Etch-A-Sketch Maze*—following a pattern by simultaneously turning the two dials on the Etch-A-Sketch (Fig. 3-19)
4. *Payroll Computation*—computing earnings with the aid of an adding machine
5. *Patient Information Memo*—involves reading, analyzing, and transcribing written material
6. *Small Parts*—manipulating small objects on a board using small tools (tweezer, screwdriver)
7. *Ruler Reading*—reading a ruler and measuring lines to the nearest 16th of an inch
8. *Pipe Assembly*—assembling a pipe and faucet with appropriate tools according to a printed diagram (Fig. 3-20)
9. *O-Rings*—sorting various rubber circles (O-rings) according to size
10. *Block Design*—constructing a design based on a printed diagram using a set of colored blocks diagram

		MOST LIKE ME			LEAST LIKE ME
1.	When I make things for my studies, I remember what I have learned better.	4	3	2	1
2.	Written assignments are easy for me to do.	4	3	2	1
3.	I learn better if someone reads a book to me than if I read silently to myself.	4	3	2	1
4.	I learn best when I study alone.	4	3	2	1
5.	Having assignment directions written on the board makes them easier to understand.	4	3	2	1
6.	It's harder for me to do a written assignment than an oral one.	4	3	2	1
7.	When I do math problems in my head, I say the numbers to myself.	4	3	2	1
8.	If I need help in the subject, I will ask a classmate for help.	4	3	2	1
9.	I understand a math problem that is written down better than one I hear.	4	3	2	1
10.	I don't mind doing written assignments.	4	3	2	1
11.	I remember things I hear better than things I read.	4	3	2	1
12.	I remember more of what I learn if I learn it when I am alone.	4	3	2	1
13.	I would rather read a story than listen to it read.	4	3	2	1
14.	I feel like I talk smarter than I write.	4	3	2	1
15.	If someone tells me three numbers to add, I can usually get the right answer without writing them down.	4	3	2	1
16.	I like to work in a group because I learn from the others in my group.	4	3	2	1
17.	Written math problems are easier for me to do than oral ones.	4	3	2	1
18.	Writing a spelling word several times helps me remember it better.	4	3	2	1
19.	I find it easier to remember what I have heard than what I have read.	4	3	2	1
20.	It is more fun to learn with classmates at first, but it is hard to study with them.	4	3	2	1
21.	I like written directions better than spoken ones.	4	3	2	1
22.	If homework were oral, I would do it all.	4	3	2	1
23.	When I hear a phone number, I can remember it without writing it down.	4	3	2	1
24.	I get more work done when I work with someone.	4	3	2	1

Figure 3-17.   Learning Styles Inventory from the Skills Assessment Module. (Reprinted with permission from Piney Mountain Press, Cleveland, Georgia.)

		MOST LIKE ME			LEAST LIKE ME
25.	Seeing a number makes more sense to me than hearing a number.	4	3	2	1
26.	I like to do things like simple repairs or crafts with my hands.	4	3	2	1
27.	The things I write on paper sound better than when I say them.	4	3	2	1
28.	I study best when no one is around to talk or listen to.	4	3	2	1
29.	I would rather read things in a book than have the teacher tell me about them.	4	3	2	1
30.	Speaking is a better way than writing if you want someone to understand what you really mean.	4	3	2	1
31.	When I have a written math problem to do, I say it to myself to understand it better.	4	3	2	1
32.	I can learn more about a subject if I am with a small group of students.	4	3	2	1
33.	Seeing the price of something written down is easier for me to understand than having someone tell me the price.	4	3	2	1
34.	I like to make things with my hands.	4	3	2	1
35.	I like tests that call for sentence completion or written answers.	4	3	2	1
36.	I understand more from a class discussion, than from reading about a subject.	4	3	2	1
37.	I remember the spelling of a word better if I see it written down than if someone spells it out loud.	4	3	2	1
38.	Spelling and grammer rules make it hard for me to say what I want to in writing.	4	3	2	1
39.	It makes it easier when I say the number of a problem to myself as I work it out.	4	3	2	1
40.	I like to study with other people.	4	3	2	1
41.	When the teachers way a number, I really don't understand it until I see it written down.	4	3	2	1
42.	I understand what I have learned better when I am involved in making something for the subject.	4	3	2	1
43.	Sometimes I say dumb things, but writing gives me time to correct myself.	4	3	2	1
44.	I do well on tests if they are about things I hear in class.	4	3	2	1
45.	I can't think as well when I work with someone else as when I work alone.	4	3	2	1

Figure 3-17. (continued)

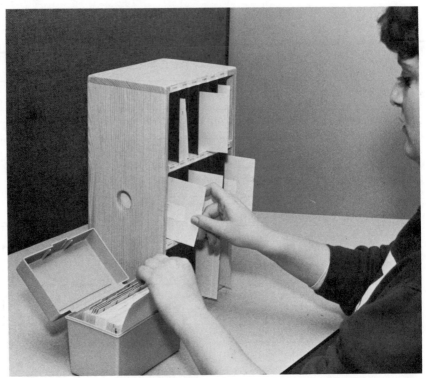

Figure 3-18. Mail Sort, from the Skills Assessment Module. (Photographer Lucia Grochowska Littlefield.)

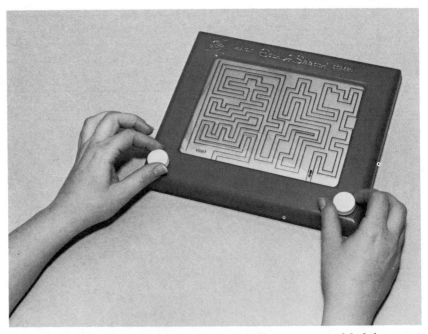

Figure 3-19. Etch-A-Sketch Maze, from the Skills Assessment Module. (Photographer Lucia Grochowska Littlefield.)

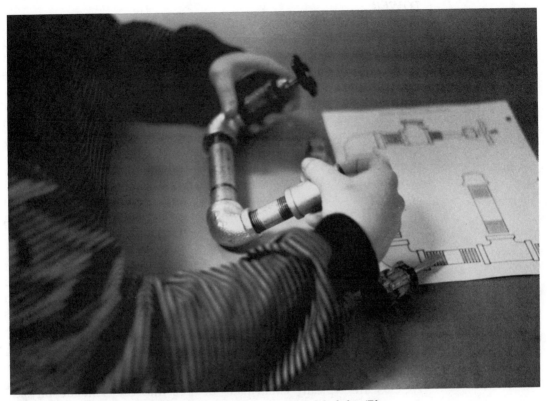

Figure 3-20.   Pipe Assembly, from the Skills Assessment Module. (Photographer Lucia Grochowska Littlefield.)

11. *Color Sort*—sorting seven different colors by identifying the center color in a pattern
12. *Circuit Board*—following a color coded pattern to wire a circuit board

During testing, the individual is rated by the evaluator on work behaviors, e.g., appearance, endurance, initiative, following rules, safety consciousness.

The Prevocational Assessment Screen (PAS) is a shorter version of the SAM. It takes 50 minutes to administer and is composed of eight of the twelve hands-on modules.

Actual Work Samples

Although similar to a simulated work sample, an actual work sample measures a client's performance on only *one* job. The most commonly used actual work samples are commercially produced, and are used by occupational therapists and other professionals, such as vocational evaluators. The best resource on commercially produced work samples is a monograph by Botterbusch [4]. TOWER and Singer Career Systems are two examples of actual work samples that are commercially made.

TOWER

TOWER is an acronym for "Testing, Orientation, and Work Evaluation in Rehabilitation." Work sampling began with the development of TOWER in 1936 by the New York Institute for Crippled and Disabled (now called the International Center for the Disabled, or ICD).* It was originally developed for persons with physical challenges, but it is now used with all types of disabled individuals.

TOWER contains 110 work samples arranged in 14 occupational areas: clerical, drafting, drawing, electronics assembly, jewelry manufacturing, leather goods, machine shop, lettering, mail clerk, optical mechanics, pantograph engraving, sewing machine operating, welding, and workshop assembly. Within each occupational area, the work samples are arranged in order of complexity. For example, the work sample "mail clerk" is composed of the following tasks: opening mail, date-stamping mail, sorting mail, delivering mail, collecting mail, folding and inserting, sealing mail, classifying mail, using a scale, and calculating postage. Selection of areas is at the therapist's discretion; not all samples are usually administered to each individual, because completion of the entire TOWER would take three weeks. Each facility constructs its own TOWER from the manual purchased from ICD. The manual includes work sample directions, response sheets, and scoring criteria. No hardware or materials are included.

Work Capacity Evaluation Devices (WCEDs)

WCEDs are typically clinic-made devices that can simulate physical demands and can be structured to gradually increase the demands made upon the individual, to assess a wide range of physical capabilities. Some familiar WCEDs are Matheson's bird cage, Blankenship's boxes, and sled and pipe tree assembly. Baltimore Therapeutic Equipment (BTE) designed "Assembly Tree," which may be categorized as a WCED.

Electronic/Computerized Work Simulators

These are essentially high-tech versions of WCEDs. They can assess a variety of physical demands, such as standing, torquing, pushing, pulling, and cranking. The BTE Work Simulator, LIDO Workset, and ERGOS are the most familiar models (Fig. 3-21).

Therapist-Designed Evaluations

Susan Isernhagen, a physical therapist, designs and markets a line of work products. One of her products is the Isernhagen Functional Capacities Evaluation. This five-hour test was designed to be helpful in medical, legal, and workers' compensation cases. Table 3-1 lists the procedures included in this functional capacities evaluation.

Proprietary Work Evaluations

Some companies and individuals have developed evaluation systems that provide a complete package of equipment and/or training. In some

*Institute for the Crippled and Disabled (ICD) Rehabilitation and Research Center. Write to ICD, 340 East 24th St., New York, NY 10010.

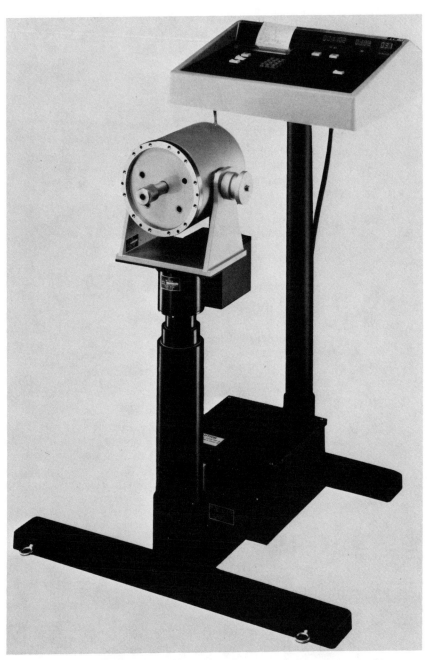

Figure 3-21.   Baltimore Therapeutic Equipment Work Simulator, used in both evaluation and treatment. (Photograph courtesy of Baltimore Therapeutic Equipment Co., Hanover, Maryland.)

Table 3-1.   Isernhagen Work Systems Functional Capacity Evaluation Procedures

---

History
Musculoskeletal Physical (brief)

Lifts
  Floor to waist
  Waist to overhead
  Horizontal

Push/Pull
  Static
  Dynamic

Carry
  Front
  Right or left-handed

Elevated Work

Forward-Bending Tolerance
  Sitting
  Standing

Unweighted Rotation Tolerance
  Sitting
  Standing

Low Activities
  Crawl
  Kneel
  Crouch
  Repetitive squat

Ambulation Activities
  Walking
  Stair climbing
  Stepladder climbing

Static Work
  Sitting
  Standing

Upper Extremity
  Hand grip
  Coordination

---

cases, with each use of the evaluation, an additional cost is incurred. Functional Capacities Assessment (Polinsky Medical Rehabilitation Center), and KEY Functional Assessment are two popular examples.

KEY Functional Assessment (KFA)

KFA is designed to measure a client's capabilities for a safe return to work. The KFA is composed of a Whole Body Assessment, which takes four hours to administer; the Special Purpose Assessment, which takes two hours and measures physical capabilities; and the Job Placement Assessment, which takes 25 minutes and evaluates a noninjured worker's capacity for jobs requiring weighted activities.

Use of the KFA requires three days of training, plus the purchase of equipment (including the ergonomically engineered Key Station and forms kits from Key Functional Assessments, Inc.). Company support is provided in the form of access to normative data on the injured worker, marketing, and continuing education.

SELECTION OF A WORK ASSESSMENT

Many variables, including the target population, cost, time, and labor need to be considered when selecting a work assessment. However, many tests have inadequate norms, inappropriate test content, unknown predictive capability, and procedures that are not adaptable to individual abilities and disabilities. The best tests are those most suited to the individual and the goals of intervention [10, p. 100].

The following list is provided as a guide in the selection of work evaluations [11, p. 290]:

1. Investigate the range and types of jobs available in the local catchment area; determine the relevance of the assessment/evaluation to local jobs and training programs.
2. Analyze your client population, considering their assets and deficits.
3. Review commercially available systems, either by visiting other facilities that have them or by borrowing them for a period of time. The Materials Development Center has many audiovisual materials on vocational assessment/evaluation that may aid in decision making.
4. Carefully review the assessment/evaluation manual, its answer sheet, and other materials. Answer the following questions: What is the purpose of this test? What is the reading level? Are the instructions and procedures clear? How much does it cost? How much time does it take to administer and score? Is training necessary? How much space is needed? For what population was the evaluation designed? Does the evaluation have reliability, validity, and established norms and/or MTMs? Are norm groups current, well described, and sufficient in size? [10] Read the review of the evaluation in the *Handbook of Measurement and Evaluation in Rehabilitation* [3] for a critical overview of this topic.

5. Investigate the resources you already have available at your facility or one nearby.
6. Consider whether you need to purchase an assessment/evaluation. Can you borrow it or develop your own from existing subcontract work, in-house jobs, or other sources?

CONCLUSION

The use of *a variety of* "low-tech" and "high-tech" work *assessment/evaluations* equipment and devices appears to be the most effective approach. This has been supported by a demographic survey performed in 1989–90 by the Standing Committee of AOTA's Work Programs Special Interest Section. This study, based on 192 work hardening and work adjustment programs in the United States, found that the most frequently used forms of work evaluations were "low-tech":

1. simulation of the physical demands of a job (87%)
2. realistic job simulations (76%)
3. aerobic training equipment, e.g., bicycle, treadmill (75%)

The "high-tech" work evaluations most frequently used were WEST (66%), BTE (65%), and VALPAR (57%) [22].

A word of caution for the future: The users of work assessments have the responsibility to become better educated in this arena. Knowledge can improve accuracy of assessment, influence the types of programming provided, and ultimately affect the quality of life of clients.

REFERENCES

1. Anastasi, A. *Psychological Testing* (3rd ed.). New York: Macmillan, 1968.
2. Becker, R.L. *Reading-Press Vocational Interest Inventory:* MF. Columbus, Ohio, Elbern Publications, 1981.
3. Bolton, B. *Handbook of Measurement and Evaluation in Rehabilitation.* Baltimore: Paul H. Brookes Publishing Co., 1987.
4. Botterbusch, K.F. *Vocational Assessment and Evaluation Systems: A Comparison.* Menomonie, Wis.: Materials Development Center, 1987.
5. Bryan, T.H. Overview of standardized worksamples and norms for injured workers. In K. Jacobs (Ed.). *Occupational Therapy Practice.* Rockville, Md.: Aspen Publishers, Inc., 1990. pp. 1–10.
6. Commission of Accreditation of Rehabilitation Facilities. Work hardening programs. In *Standards Manual for Organizations Serving People with Disabilities.* Tucson: Author, 1989, pp. 69–72.
7. Dougherty, P.M., and Radomski, M.V. *The Cognitive Rehabilitation Workbook.* Rockville, Md.: Aspen Publishers, Inc., 1987.
8. Gerber, P.J. Learning Disabilities and Vocational Education-Realities and Challenges. In K.P. Lynch, W.E. Kiernan, and J.A. Starks (Eds.). *Prevocational and Vocational Education for Special Needs Youth: A Blueprint for the 1980s.* Baltimore: Paul H. Brookes, 1982, pp. 185–197.
9. Holland, J.L. *The Self Directed Search: A Guide to Educational and Vocational Planning.* Palo Alto, Calif.: Consulting Psychologists Press, 1985.
10. Hursh, N.C., and Kerns, A.F. *Vocational Assessment and Evaluation Systems: A Comparison.* Boston: College-Hill Press, 1988.
11. Jacobs, K. Work Assessments and Programming. In H.L. Hopkins and H.D.

Smith. (Eds.). *Willard and Spackman's Occupational Therapy* (7th ed). Philadelphia: J.B. Lippincott, 1989.

12. Kester, D.L. Prevocational and Vocational Assessment, In H.L. Hopkins and H.D. Smith. (Eds.). *Willard and Spackman's Occupational Therapy* (6th edition). Philadelphia: J.B. Lippincott, 1983.

13. Lynch, K.P., Kiernan, W.E., and Stark, J.A. (Eds.). *Prevocational and Vocational Education for Special Needs Youth: A Blueprint for the 1980s.* Baltimore: Paul H. Brookes, 1982.

14. Matsutsuyu, J. The interest checklist. *Am. J. Occup. Ther.* 23:323, 1969.

15. Reynolds-Lynch, K. Job analysis. In M. Kirkland and S.C. Robertson (Eds.). Planning and Implementing Vocational Readiness in Occupational Therapy (PIVOT). Rockville, MD.: American Occupational Therapy Association, 1985, pp. 155–157.

16. Roberts, C. Definitions, objectives and goals in work evaluation. *Journal of Rehabilitation.* 36:12–15, 1970.

17. Rosinek, M. *Skills Assessment Module.* Athens, GA.: Piney Mountain Press, Inc., 1985.

18. Spencer, K.C. Supported employment: The role of occupational therapy at the job site. In K. Jacobs (Ed.), *Occupational Therapy Practice.* Rockville, MD.: Aspen Publishers, Inc., 1990, pp. 74–82.

19. Trombly, C.A., and Scott, A.D. *Occupational Therapy for Physical Dysfunction.* Baltimore: Williams & Wilkins, 1977.

20. Valparspective, 2:1.

21. Watanabe, S. Activities Configuration. 1968 Regional Institute on the Evaluation Process, Final Report RSA-123-T-68. New York, American Occupational Therapy Association, 1968.

22. Wyrick, J. Demographic Survey. Work Programs Special Interest Section Annual Business Meeting. New Orleans: AOTA, April 29, 1990.

4

The Jacobs Prevocational Skills Assessment

This chapter presents an in-depth look at the Jacobs Prevocational Skills Assessment (JPSA), which was developed for a learning-disabled adolescent population at the Learning Prep School. The JPSA is composed of 15 tasks designed to assess performance in specific work-related areas. The rationale behind the JPSA will be explored in contrast to previously available evaluations. In addition, the assessment will be presented in its entirety, including graphics.

DEVELOPMENT OF THE JPSA

Despite the number of commercially available systems, there appeared to be no one evaluation universally applicable to the learning-disabled population because of their diverse visual, perceptual, motor, and language abilities and social, developmental, and academic profiles. For example, one learning-disabled student may be able to follow written directions, while another cannot read beyond a first-grade level but understands verbal instructions with visual demonstrations. Lynch et. al. [2] support this realization: "Despite the focus on assessment, vocational assessment for learning disabled students is an area in which little work has been done." For these reasons the JPSA was developed.

The JPSA was developed in 1979. Since that time it has seen many constructive changes as the result of clinical use. Many of the changes evolved from an effort to key words and tasks more toward "real" work. The revised instrument is presented in this book, along with some background on the instrument's evolution.

The JPSA is a *standard* instrument, with all the aforementioned limitations of this type of test. However, it has proved to be a useful screening tool for obtaining pertinent information for occupational therapy treatment planning and referrals. For example, from assessment results I have been able to suggest academic and vocational programming appropriate to the student's ability. The JPSA was not designed to be applicable to a wide variety of work-related programs with respect to age and disability; however, the general concept may serve as a model for designing a similar instrument, or the JPSA may be adapted to meet the particular needs of a therapist's clients.

Selection of Skill Areas

The basis for the development of any evaluation instrument is observation. A large part of occupational therapy training is directed toward honing this skill as an objective tool. Applying this skill to the preadolescent and adolescent learning-disabled population at the Learning Prep School revealed deficiencies in need of remediation in the following work-related areas:

I. Motor coordination
  A. Fine
  B. Gross
II. Eye-hand coordination
III. Conceptual skills
  A. Alphabet recognition and ordering
  B. Number
  C. Number quantity
  D. Money and money concepts
  E. Recognition of the student's own name
  F. Color
IV. Motor planning
V. Figure-ground discrimination
VI. Sorting ability
VII. Matching ability
VIII. Classification ability
IX. Sequencing ability
X. Problem solving
XI. Decision making
XII. Following directions with one, two, three, or more steps
  A. Oral directions
  B. Written directions
  C. Visual directions
XIII. Memory
  A. Auditory
  B. Visual
XIV. Task focus
XV. Work-related behavior

These original categories became the foundation for assessing work-related skills and behaviors. However, in the course of clinical implementation several basic categories were revised or deleted, and others were inserted. These changes facilitated a clearer distinction among areas needing remediation as reasonably independent variables. Certain distinctions were found too impractical for the therapist to make readily. For example, gross motor coordination was dropped as a separate category because its contribution to the overall validity of the assessment did not justify the sacrifice of brevity, another major criterion of the test. Furthermore, areas that represented developmentally sequential skills that would require many independent tasks to test were merged. For instance, the two categories of classification and sequencing became a single category. Additional variables including organizational skills and use of tools were added on the basis of clinical experience. Currently, the following categories are thought to represent the most useful information (definitions have been included for clarity):

1. Fine motor coordination: the ability to perform small movements (grasping, writing) in the most efficient manner
2. Eye-hand coordination: the ability to use eyes and hands together to perform a task
3. Motor planning: the ability to plan new or nonhabitual movements
4. Attention to detail: the ability to focus on the important aspects of one's visual field and "tune out" the unimportant background
5. Sorting: the ability to select by similar traits
6. Classification and sequencing: the ability to arrange items by class (e.g., all tools) and in an orderly succession
7. Decision making: the ability to consider evidence and reach some conclusion without undue delay
8. Problem solving: the ability to devise an appropriate solution for a new problem (It is my opinion that problem solving is a difficult skill to assess. Placing an individual in a situation that calls for this skill and observing how he or she responds is one method. Throughout the JPSA, such situations have been devised.)
9. Organizational skills: the ability to organize one's approach to and performance of an activity (e.g., the ability to use time and work space appropriately)
10. Use of tools: the ability to use common tools and equipment (e.g., a hammer and nails) appropriately
11. Ability to follow verbal, written, or visual directions
12. Practical daily living knowledge, including alphabet recognition and alphabetical ordering, number and number quantity, money and money quantity, reading, functional mathematics, telling time
13. Task focus: the ability to attend to an activity for a period of time
14. Behavioral observations, such as communication skills, perseverance, motivation, reliability, initiative, good posture, neat personal appearance, positive attitude toward the therapist and other students

Task Selection

The tasks chosen to assess the student's performance in these areas underwent a similar evolution. The following technical factors and theoretical considerations related to the school's population were the initial criteria for inclusion in the assessment:

Technical factors	Theoretical considerations
1. Compactness of task elements	1. Range of complexity level within and among individual tasks

2. Low cost of elements (optimally, those available in an occupational therapy department)
3. Ease of administration (minimal special training required)
4. Brevity

2. Adaptability to physical and cognitive limitations

3. High relation to work

4. High interest level for preadolescents and adolescents
5. Built-in rewards
6. Limited task duration (because of attentional difficulties)
7. Provision for comprehension of written, visual, and verbal instructions

The original tasks were nail inspection, alphabetical ordering, filing, using hammer and screwdriver, envelope stuffing, nut and bolt assembly, sorting and naming money, an activity involving matching and/or body awareness, four increasingly complex mazes, a kitchen activity involving sequencing, classification of food items, leather key ring assembly, and a cooking activity. In general these tasks proved to be reasonably useful. Several improvements have been made, however. These changes resulted from brainstorming with therapists and from using the assessment with a widening range of ages and disabilities.

A calculator was added to increase task complexity and because of the increasing use of calculators in the work environment. The tasks' names and vocabulary were modified to parallel those of the work setting. For example, *nail inspection* became *quality control, alphabetical ordering* became *filing, cooking activity* became *food preparation.*

The current tasks are (1) Quality control, (2) Filing, (3) Carpentry Assembly, (4) Classification, (5) Office Work, (6) Telephone Directory, (7) Factory Work, (8) Environmental Mobility, (9) Money Concepts, (10) Functional Banking, (11) Time Concepts, (12) Work Attitudes, (13) Body Scheme, (14) Leather Assembly, and (15) Food Preparation. Furthermore, these tasks can be categorized as Work Skills.

Recording Data

My criteria for the recording medium were that it be easy to use, that is, entry of data would require minimal disruption of the test procedure, and that the raw data be easily accessible for further analysis. The matrix tabular form (see profile sheet, Fig. 4-1) has proved ideal and has been retained through all the test content changes because of its conciseness.

TEST ELEMENTS

On the following pages the JPSA is described. First the profile sheet (scoring form) is discussed, and illustrations (suitable for photocopying) are presented (Fig. 4-1). The manual is then discussed. Its contents are presented in the Appendix at the end of this chapter. Descriptions of the 15 tasks are then given, along with examples of possible modifications. Next the materials necessary for the assessment are listed. Finally, a suggested format for summarizing the results of the assessment is given in the form of three case studies.

Profile Sheet

A single-page (8 1/2" × 14") checklist-style profile sheet was constructed with the respective categories—physical capacities, work behaviors, and work aptitudes—in columns across the top of the page and the individual tasks or work skills in rows along the side. If a specific physical capacity, work behavior, or aptitude is required in a task, the box where the skill and task intersect is checked. The placement of these checks was determined by numerous activity analyses of the tasks and was reviewed by numerous occupational therapists.

The therapist uses the profile sheet throughout the testing session to record results. When a specific physical capacity, work behavior, or aptitude is noted to be limited or absent during a specific task, the check in the corresponding box is circled. For example, if the student awkwardly manipulated tools (e.g., screwdriver, knife, pencil), then the fine motor coordination check would be circled in the appropriate tasks. If a student were easily "stumped" and unable to think of alternative approaches to a problem, the problem solving check would be circled in the corresponding tasks. On completion of the total assessment (after approximately 1–2 hours) a pattern of circled checks will be evident in the columns. Any physical capacity, work behavior, or aptitude with two or more circled checks will be an area for remediation in therapy. In the Behavioral Observation section, the therapist notes important test behaviors: motivation, perseverance, cooperative behavior, personal appearance, hand dominance. Treatment goals then can be established by integrating the limited or absent physical capacity, work behavior, or aptitude with the observations noted during the testing session. In addition, the therapist notes any modification of task instructions or adaptive equipment utilized.

The *time* required to complete each task is recorded on the profile sheet. A maximum average time for task completion is listed (see Fig. 4-28). These values were determined by testing a population sample of normal adolescents and then doubling their average time for each task. If the student reaches this maximum without completing the task, the therapist terminates the task.

Note: There are major limitations to the present time requirements. It is planned for Methods Time Measurement (MTM) industrial norming system to be developed on the JPSA. These figures will be made available through a journal article.

Manual

A manual (4" × 5") is used by the therapist throughout the testing procedure. The manual contains the general guidelines as well as the purpose, materials, and instructions for each of the 15 tasks. The manual in its entirety is printed as the Appendix to this chapter.

The Jacobs Prevocational Skills Assessment

WORK SKILLS	PHYSICAL CAPACITIES			
	Fine Motor Coordination	Eye-Hand Coordination	Motor Planning	Use of Tools
1. Quality Control	✔			
2. Filing A	✔			
B	✔			
C	✔			
3. Carpentry Assembly	✔	✔	✔	✔
4. Classification	✔			
5. Office Work A	✔	✔	✔	✔
B	✔	✔	✔	
C	✔	✔	✔	
6. Telephone Directory A	✔	✔		
B	✔	✔		
7. Factory Work	✔	✔	✔	
8. Environmental Mobility A	✔	✔	✔	
B				
9. Money Concepts A				
B				
C	✔			
D	✔			
10. Functional Banking A	✔	✔		
B	✔	✔		✔
11. Time Concept A				
B				
C				
12. Work Attitudes A				
B				
13. Assembly	✔			
14. Leather Assembly	✔	✔	✔	✔
15. Food Preparation	✔	✔	✔	✔

© 1979 Jacobs, K. (revised 1988)

Figure 4-1.   A blank JPSA form for the reader's use.

Task Focus	Visual	Written	Verbal	Organizational Skills	Decision Making	Sorting	Attention to Detail	Classification	Sequencing	Problem Solving	Practical Daily Living Knowledge	Behavioral Observations
✓			✓	✓	✓	✓	✓					
✓		✓		✓	✓	✓		✓	✓	✓		
✓		✓		✓	✓	✓	✓	✓	✓	✓		
✓		✓		✓	✓	✓		✓	✓	✓		
✓					✓		✓		✓			
✓			✓		✓			✓	✓			
✓			✓	✓				✓	✓			
✓	✓		✓	✓				✓	✓			
✓		✓		✓				✓	✓	✓		
✓			✓	✓			✓	✓			✓	
✓			✓								✓	
✓			✓		✓		✓		✓			
✓			✓	✓			✓		✓			
✓	✓		✓						✓			
✓			✓								✓	
✓			✓								✓	
✓			✓		✓		✓		✓		✓	
✓			✓	✓	✓		✓		✓		✓	
✓	✓		✓		✓		✓				✓	
✓			✓		✓		✓				✓	
✓			✓								✓	
✓			✓				✓				✓	
✓			✓						✓		✓	
✓			✓	✓	✓		✓	✓				
✓			✓		✓				✓			
✓	✓		✓	✓					✓			
✓	✓			✓			✓	✓				
✓	✓				✓			✓				

Figure 4-1.   (continued)

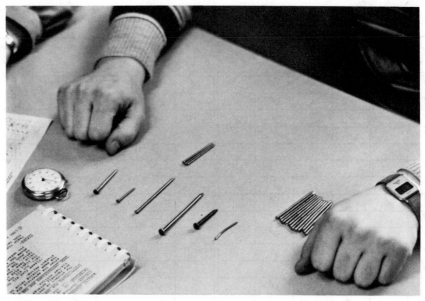

Figure 4-2.   Task 1, Quality Control. Student inspects nails.

Many of the tasks have been divided into parts of increasing difficulty. If a student is unable to do the first part of a task, the therapist should use his or her judgment as to whether to proceed with the next part or go on to the next task.

A brief description of each task, examples of task modifications, and graphics are presented below. A list of all materials needed for the assessment follows these descriptions.

Tasks
1. Quality Control

Twenty-six nails of various sizes are placed in a random pile on the table. The student is instructed to find all the nails that look the same as the one shown by the therapist (Fig. 4-2).

Modification: For students with poor or absent upper-extremity coordination, the therapist can pick up each nail individually and ask for a verbal or gestural yes or no response as to its sameness to the model nail.

2. Filing

In Part A, the therapist places a two-sided instruction card in front of the student to read silently (Fig. 4-3). The instructions have been typed on the card so as to have on the first side an incomplete sentence, which is completed on the second. The instruction card is removed, and the student is given a packet of 26 cards (Fig. 4-4), each bearing one word for each letter of the alphabet. The student is to alphabetize the cards and place them once again in a packet.

Modification: An alphabet can be provided as a guide for this part.

In Part B, the student is instructed to alphabetize 13 cards, each of which bears a last name and first initial in the left-hand corner, into a file box that contains *A* to *Z* separation cards (Fig. 4-5).

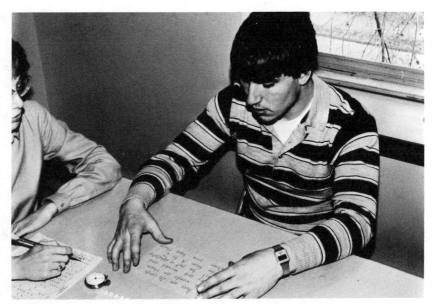

Figure 4-3.   Task 2, Filing, Part A. Student examines the instruction card before starting to alphabetize 26 cards.

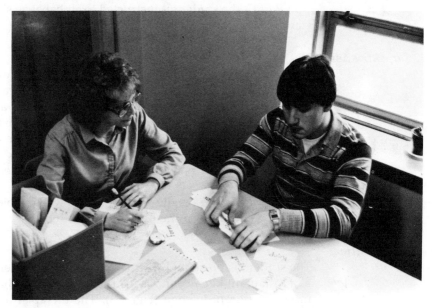

Figure 4-4.   Task 2, Filing, Part A. Alphabetizing 26 cards.

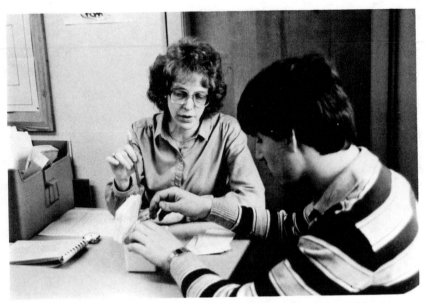

Figure 4-5.   Task 2, Filing, Part B. Student places 13 alphabetized cards in a file box.

In Part C, the student is instructed to alphabetize six cards with words starting with the same letter (e.g., money, match) (Fig. 4-6).

3. Carpentry Assembly

A wooden board with two nails and three screws (one blade-head and two Phillips screws) driven three-quarters of the way into the wood is placed in front of the subject. Two screwdrivers and a hammer are placed on either side of the board. The therapist instructs the student to name the tools and to use them to put the nails and screws all the way into the board. The second step of the task involves having a student position a nail independently and hammer it into the wood (Fig. 4-7).

Modifications: Clamp the wooden board to the table. Use an adaptive screwdriver. Build up the handles on the tools.

4. Classification

The student is presented with 17 pictures of items related or not related to a restaurant kitchen and is instructed to find all the items that belong in the restaurant kitchen (Fig. 4-8). The therapist then optionally asks questions about the pictures, for example, "Name the items shown." The therapist has an option to show a restaurant sketch.

5. Office Work

In Part A, the student is to staple business cards in a designated position on a sheet of paper (Fig. 4-9).

In Part B, the student is instructed to fold the sheets from Part A into thirds and place them in individual envelopes (Fig. 4-10).

Modification: Draw lines on the paper to indicate where to fold.

In Part C, the stuffed envelopes remain, and five piles of colored

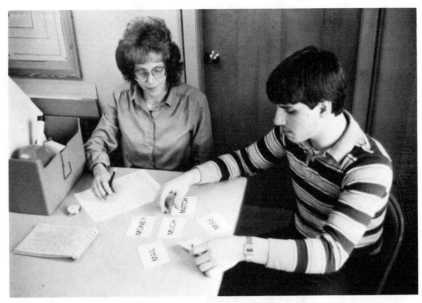

Figure 4-6.   Task 2, Filing, Part C. Student alphabetizes six words starting with the same letter.

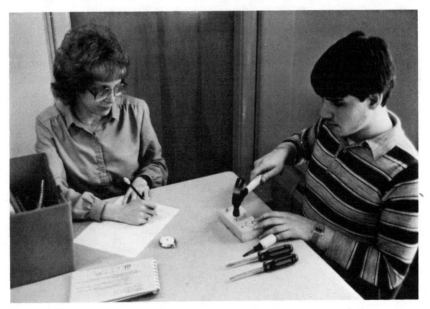

Figure 4-7.   Task 3, Carpentry Assembly. Student hammers nails into
wooden board.

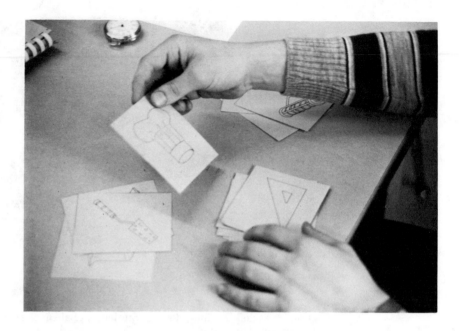

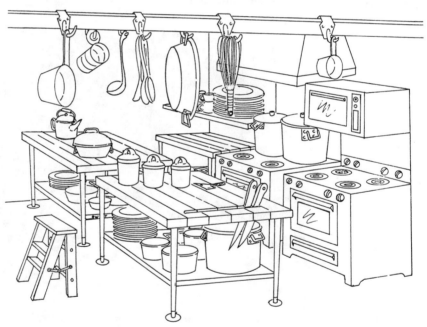

Figure 4-8.   Task 4, Classification. Student finds all the items that belong in a restaurant kitchen. The first drawing (for optional use) shows
a restaurant kitchen; the next three pages show 12 items that might be
found in a restaurant kitchen; the fourth and fifth drawings show five
non-kitchen items.

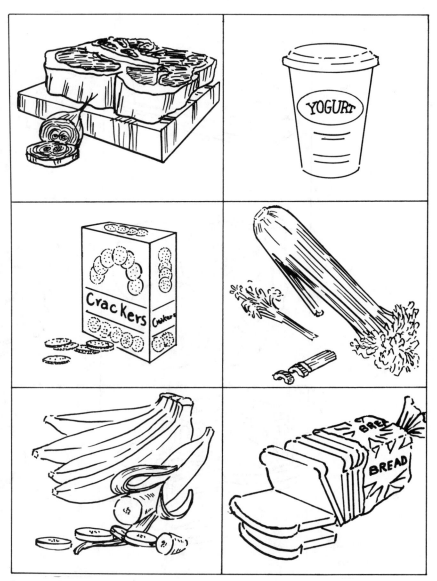

Figure 4-8.   (continued)

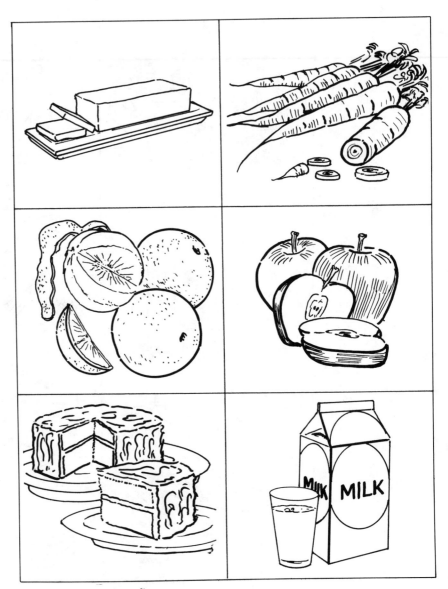

Figure 4-8.   (continued)

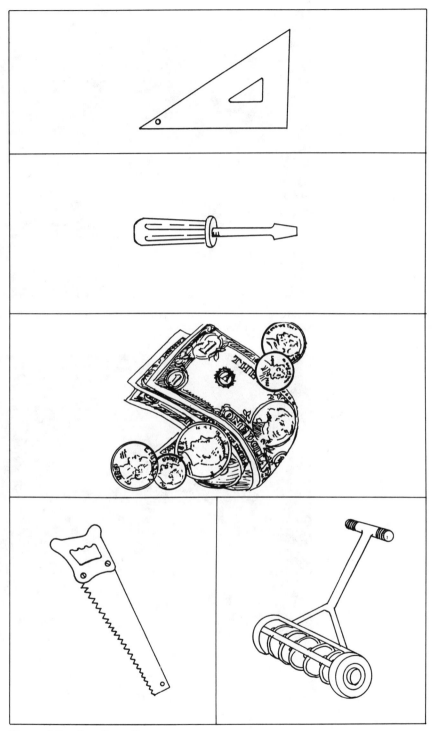

Figure 4-8.   (continued)

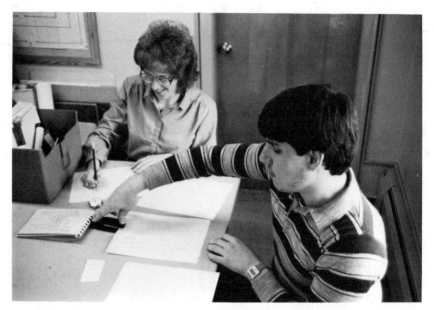

Figure 4-9.   Task 5, Office Work, Part A. Student staples business cards to sheets of paper.

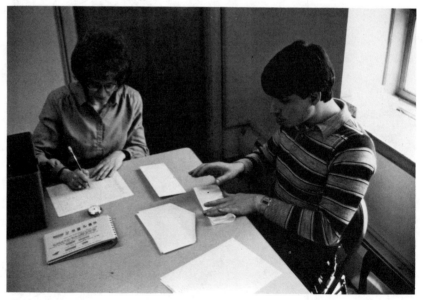

Figure 4-10.   Task 5, Office Work, Part B. Student folds stapled sheets and places them in envelopes.

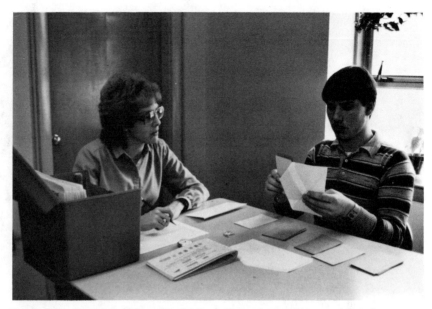

Figure 4-11.   Task 5, Office Work, Part C. Student follows written directions to collate colored paper and places the resulting piles in envelopes.

paper and paper clips are arranged on the table. Written directions are given to the student to read silently. The instructions tell the student to collate the colored paper, paper clip the resulting piles, and place them in the envelopes. Extra paper and paper clips have been deliberately added to test problem solving ability (Fig. 4-11).

Modification: Use larger paper clips. Use a color-coded instruction card, for example, with the word *green* written in green ink.

6. Telephone Directory

In Part A, the student is instructed to find the name of a company in a small telephone directory and write the name, address, and telephone number on a card (Fig. 4-12).

Modification: Write one address on a separate sheet for the student who is unable to use the directory.

In Part B, the directory is removed and the student is instructed to address a blank envelope from the information on the card from Part A. In addition, the student is asked to put his or her return address and a stamp on the envelope.

Modification: Present two envelopes addressed incorrectly and have the student indicate what is missing (e.g., zip code, return address).

7. Factory Work

The student is presented with a wooden board containing six flat-head bolts in various sizes, arranged in two rows. Two nuts are screwed onto the shank of each bolt until the end of the shank is flush with the nut. The two smallest bolts have been purposely given three nuts each to observe how the student responds to the task instruction of removing

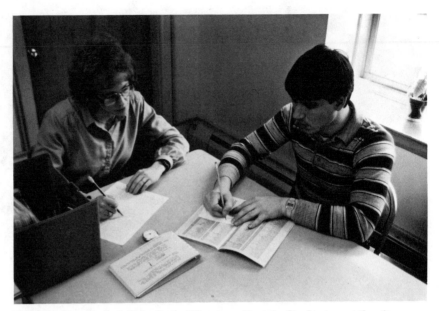

Figure 4-12.   Task 6, Telephone Directory, Part A. Student uses the directory to locate an address.

all the nuts from the bolts. The student is verbally instructed to remove all the nuts from the bolts and to place them in the cup provided. When this is completed, the student is instructed to put all the nuts back onto the bolt (Fig. 4-13).

Modifications: Clamp the board to the table. Use a modified version of the board containing a single row of the larger bolts, or instruct the student to remove the nuts only from the row of large bolts.

8. Environmental Mobility

In Part A, an opened street map of Washington, D.C., covered with a sheet of clear plastic of the same dimensions, is placed on the table. The therapist instructs the student to use a marking pen to mark the streets from the train station to the White House and from the White House to the Jefferson Memorial.

Modification: Simplify the instructions, for example, "Follow the streets from the White House to the Jefferson Memorial."

In Part B, after all the materials from Part A have been removed, the student is presented a card with directions and is instructed to follow them to perform a simple errand, for example, to retrieve an envelope from the therapist's mailbox (Fig. 4-14). Devise your own directions and have a colleague follow them before using them in the assessment. This should eliminate any confusion.

9. Money Concepts

In Part A, the student is asked to identify four coins and a dollar bill.

Modification: For nonverbal students, the therapist can point to each coin and ask, "Is this a penny?" and so on.

In Part B, the student is presented with four sets of coins of various denominations and is asked to state the value of each set (Fig. 4-15).

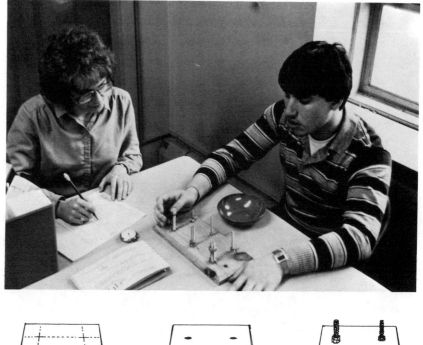

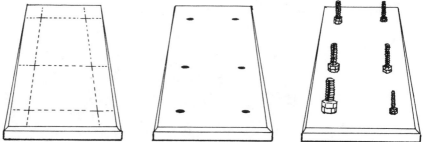

Figure 4-13.   Task 7, Factory Work. Student removes all nuts from bolts and then replaces them.

Modification: For the nonverbal student, write out answers, including the correct ones, on a card, and ask the student to point to the correct answer.

In Part C, a cash register receipt is placed on the table with a specified assortment of money. The therapist instructs the student to find the total on the receipt and read it aloud and then find the corresponding amount of money on the table (Fig. 4-16).

In Part D, there is a brief simulation. The money from Part C remains on the table. The therapist pretends to purchase an inexpensive magazine (priced under a dollar) from the student. The therapist hands the student a dollar bill and asks for the appropriate change. The solution should be calculated mentally (Fig. 4-17).

10. Functional Banking

In Part A, an enlarged bank check is presented, and the student must write out the answers to a set of questions pertaining to the check— the amount of the check, the date, the account number (Fig. 4-18).

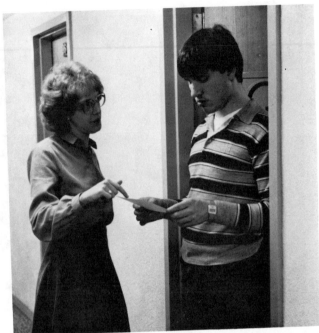

Figure 4-14.   Task 8, Environmental Mobility, Part B. Therapist instructs student to follow written directions to perform a simple errand.

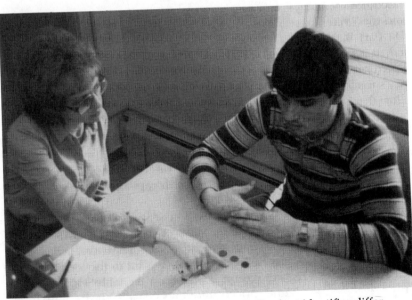

Figure 4-15.   Task 9, Money Concepts, Part B. Student identifies different coins.

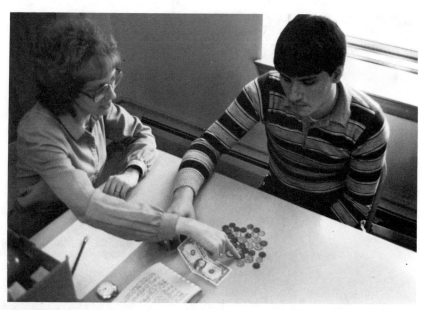

Figure 4-16.   Task 9, Money Concepts, Part C. Student finds the amount of money on the table that corresponds to that from the cash register receipt.

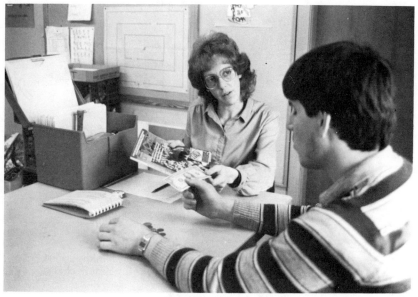

Figure 4-17.   Task 9, Money Concepts, Part D. Student presents therapist with the correct amount of change after purchase of a magazine.

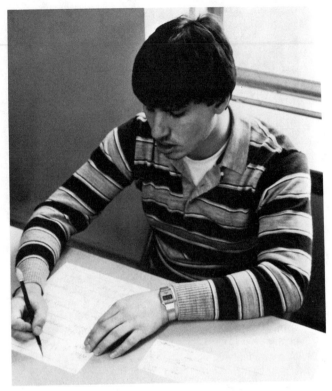

A

| NO. 175 | $ 3.99 | | KAREN JACOB-GOLD | NUMBER |
| Jan. 2 19 83 | | | ANY STREET | 175 |

B

Figure 4-18.   Task 10, Functional Banking, Part A. A: Student answers questions about a bank check. B: Sample check.

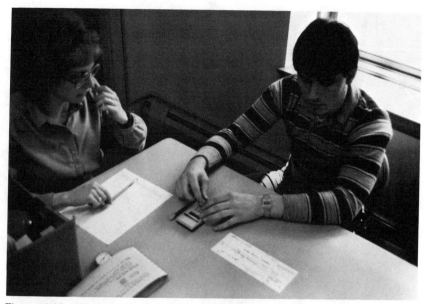

Figure 4-19. Task 10, Functional Banking, Part B. Using a calculator, student finds the balance in a checking account.

In Part B, the student is instructed to use a calculator to find the balance in the checking account after the check is paid (Fig. 4-19).

Modification: For students with fine motor difficulties, Sharp* makes an excellent solar-cell calculator, model QS-2125, with large keys and an angled base. This calculator can be useful in the clinic as well.

11. Time Concepts

In Part A, the student is presented three pictures of a clock face, each showing a different time. The therapist instructs the student to read each time (Fig. 4-20).

In Part B, two pictures of clocks are presented together, and the student is asked to decide which clock has the later time.

In Part C, a picture of a digital clock reading 12:40 is placed on the table, and the student is asked what time it will be in 30 minutes.

12. Work Attitudes

This task is concerned with the student's work attitude and decision-making ability.

In Part A, the therapist randomly places before the student five cards, each depicting a step in a sequence of purchasing a meal at a fast-food shop. The student is asked to place the cards in correct order (Fig. 4-21).

Modification: Present a three-card sequence.

In Part B, the task is a totally verbal one, which requires the student to devise solutions to three small vignettes relating to work. For example, "You are working at the grill at McDonald's when a fire starts. What do you do?"

*Sharp Electronics Corporation, 10 Sharp Plaza, Paramus, New Jersey 07652.

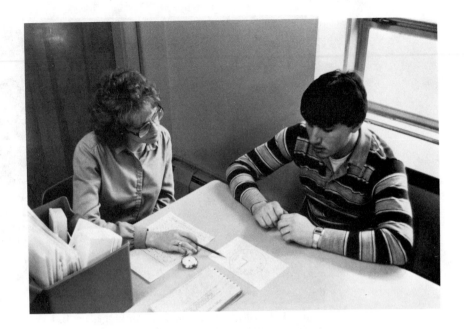

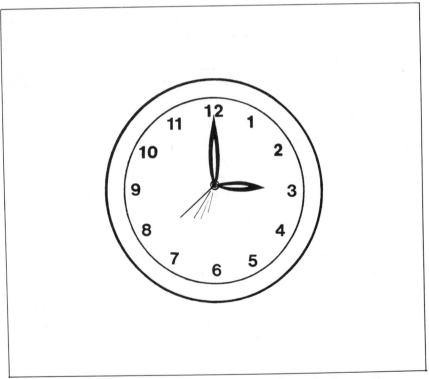

Figure 4-20.   Task 11, Time Concepts, Part A. Student tells time on the clock.

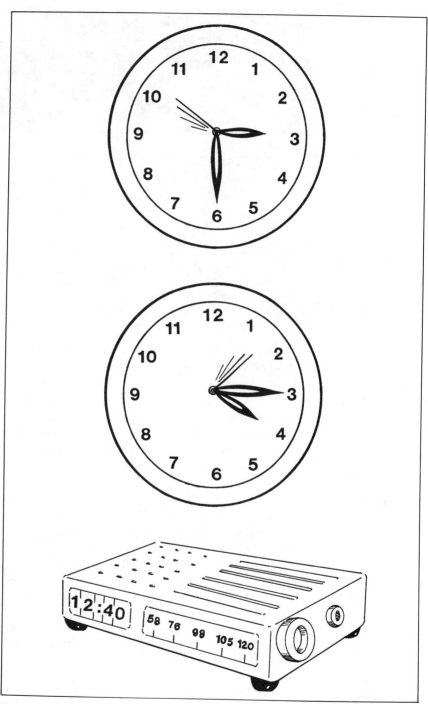

Figure 4-20.   (continued)

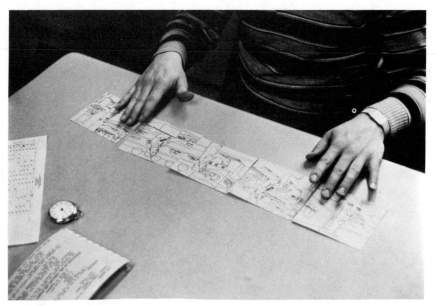

Figure 4-21.   Task 12, Work Attitudes, Part A. Student arranges in sequence five cards illustrating purchase of a meal at a fast-food shop.

Modification: To adapt for a nonverbal student, print up a card with several solutions to each vignette for the student to choose from.

13. Body Scheme

The student is shown a drawing of a teenaged boy for 15 seconds. Upon its removal, five identical drawings that have been cut up (i.e., five heads, ten arms, etc.) are presented. The student reassembles the parts (Fig. 4-22).

14. Leather Assembly

The therapist demonstrates the construction of a simple leather key ring and instructs the student to make a similar one (Fig. 4-23). A reward feature has been integrated into this task: The student is allowed to keep the key ring. (Through the years of test use, I have found this task provides the foundation for spin-off activities in treatment, such as the purpose of keys. This is the first experience some students have with keys!) Since the main purpose of this task is to reward the student, the therapist should assist the student if he or she is having difficulty.

Modifications: Increase the size of the rivets. Eliminate the extra sets of rivets.

15. Food Preparation

The student is requested to follow five visual instructions to make honey butter (Fig. 4-24). This is an enjoyable final activity for the testing session and gives the therapist the chance to speak informally with the student. The option of eating the honey butter on crackers is another form of positive reward.

Modification: Use adaptive equipment, for example, stabilize bowl.

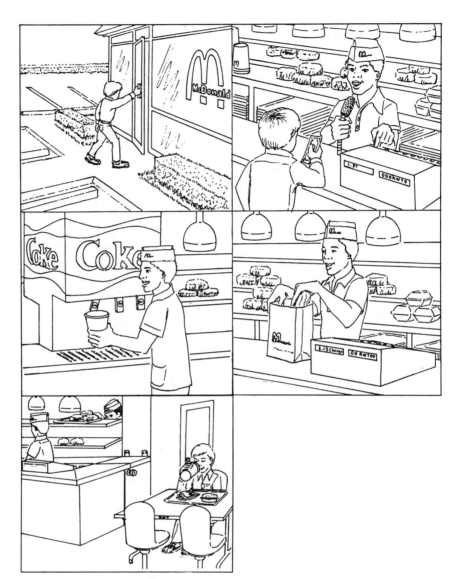

Figure 4-21.   (continued)

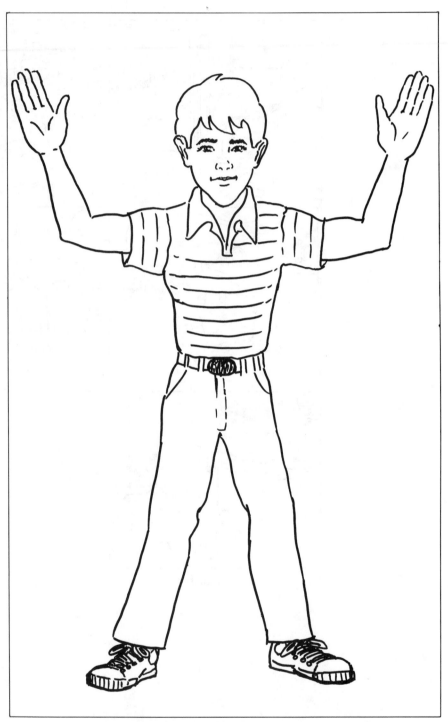

Figure 4-22.   Task 13, Body Scheme. Student is shown an intact drawing
of a boy. The drawing is then removed, and the student is given a cut-up
version of the same drawing to put together correctly. The drawing used
in this task is to be photocopied—one copy to remain intact, the five other
copies to be cut up into parts for reassembly.

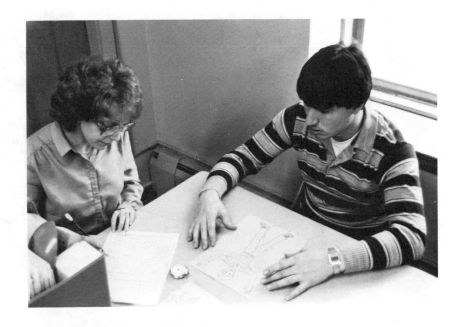

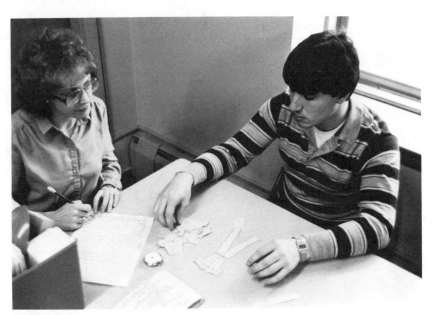

Figure 4-22.   (continued)

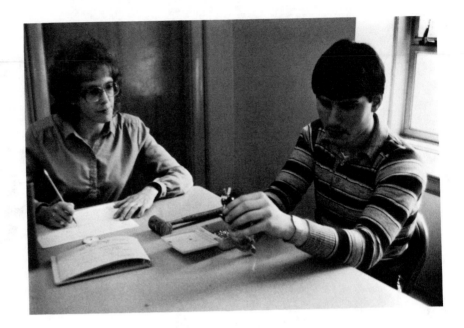

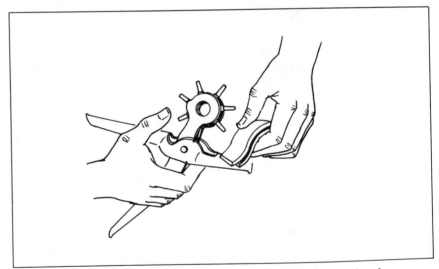

Figure 4-23.   Task 14, Leather Assembly. Following the instructional drawings shown here, the therapist demonstrates to the student how to make a simple leather key ring. Immediately following this demonstration, the student makes a leather key ring

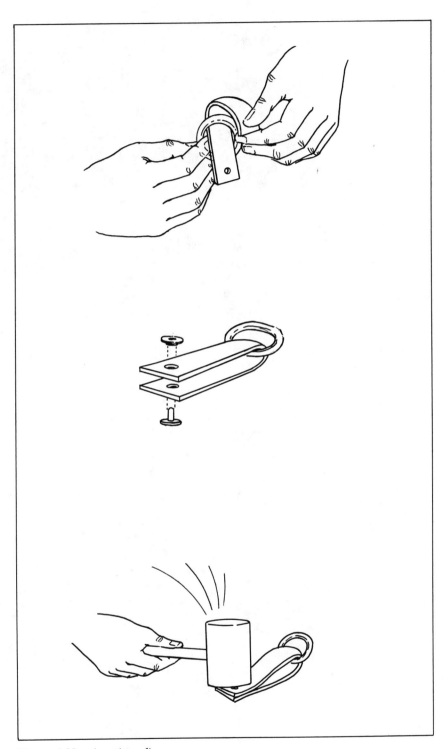

Figure 4-23.   (continued)

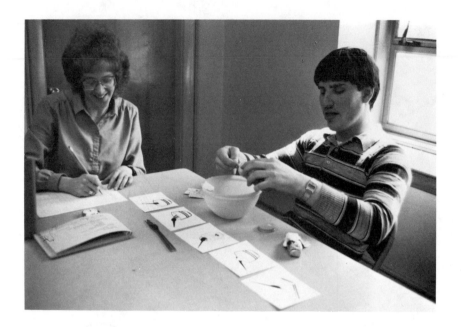

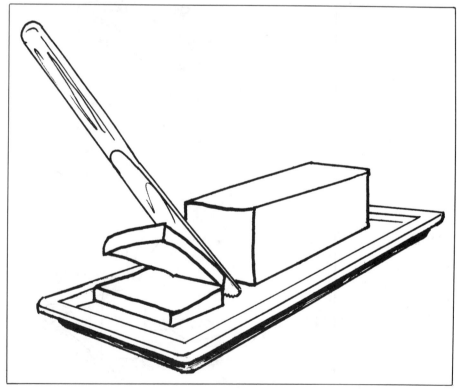

Figure 4-24. Task 15, Food Preparation. Following the directions on five cards, student prepares honey butter.

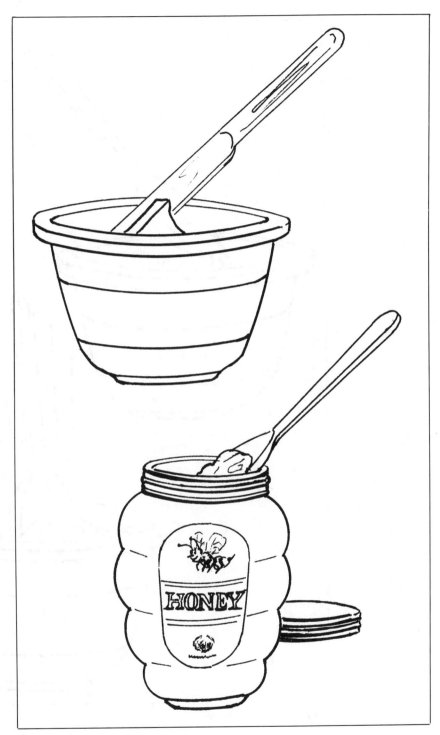

Figure 4-24.   (continued)

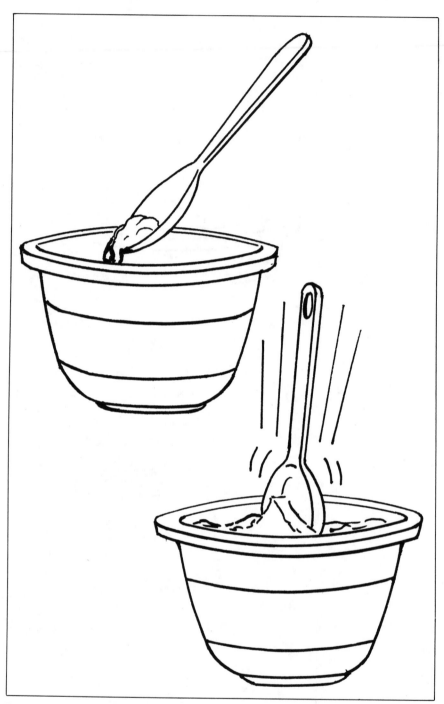

Figure 4-24. (continued)

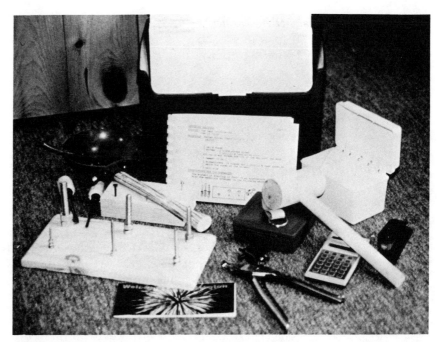

Figure 4-25.   All the items necessary for the JPSA, shown with the plastic carrying case.

Materials Required

All the materials for the assessment are readily available from an occupational therapy department, hardware store, and stationery shop (Fig. 4-25). The total cost of the materials if you were to purchase each item is approximately $50. All illustrations and the profile sheet have been provided in this book, and you may copy them for your use. Please note that illustrations have specific sizes and may need to be enlarged.

A "shopping list" by task for all the materials needed to construct a JPSA follows. All the materials can be carried in a plastic carrying case, with each task neatly housed in a labelled vertical file folder. When assembled, the JPSA is easily transportable, weighing only 12 pounds. Some task materials (e.g., hammers, wooden board) that are too large for the file folders can be positioned inside the carrying case.

General Items

1   plastic carrying case (10 1/2" × 9" × 12")

17   vertical file folders (9 1/2" × 11 3/4" × 1 1/2" expansion) (one for each of the 15 tasks and one each for the manual and profile sheets)

17   3 1/2" × 1/2" self-sticking file folder labels

20   profile sheets (see Fig. 4-1).

1   manual (see Appendix) (Suggestion: I keep an extra copy of the instructions for each task in the file folder for the task for easy reference.)

1   stopwatch or clock with a second hand.

Items Needed to Construct Assessment
> 1   pair of scissors
> 1   hand or power drill

Optional Procedures
> Instruction cards and graphics can be laminated very inexpensively at a copy shop to increase their longevity. The manual can be spiral bound inexpensively, again at a copy shop.

Task 1. Quality Control
> 16   2½″ nails
> 10   odd-size and bent nails

Task 2. Filing
> 26   white cards (3″ × 5″), each bearing one of the following words: age, book, chef, date, employee, form, greater, help, in, janitor, keep, left, mechanic, nurse, off, pencil, quick, read, store, typist, use, visit, work, Xerox, year, zip
> 1   two-sided instruction card (4¼″ × 5½″) with the following:

[side 1] HERE ARE 26 CARDS WITH WORDS ON THEM. THEY ARE MIXED AND MUST BE PUT IN ALPHABETICAL ORDER FROM A TO Z. WHEN YOU HAVE THEM

[side 2] ARRANGED, PUT THEM IN A PACK AS THEY ARE RIGHT NOW. ANY QUESTIONS? IF NOT, BEGIN.

> 1   plastic file box (5¼″ × 3½″ × 3″)
> 1   set of *A* to *Z* guides for 3″ × 5″ index cards
> 1   instruction card (4¼″ × 5½″) with the following on one side:

HERE ARE 13 CARDS WITH LAST NAMES. PUT THESE CARDS IN ALPHABETICAL ORDER IN THE FILE BOX.

> 13   white lined (3″ × 5″) index cards each bearing one of the following names in the left-hand corner:

ADAMS, C.; BANKS, C; DINAN, K.; EVANS, W.; GREEN, G.; GRAY, A.; HALL, J.; JONES, L.; JOHNSON, J; MANN, D.; PETERS, C.; STEVENS, P.; WILLIAMS, E.

> 6   white (3″ × 5″) cards, each with one of the following words written in capital letters:

MONEY, MATCH, MAIL, MAIN, MISS, MUCH

> 1   instruction card with the following information printed on one side:

HERE ARE 6 CARDS WITH WORDS, PUT THESE CARDS IN ALPHABETICAL ORDER IN THE FILE BOX.

Task 3. Carpentry Assembly
> 1   pine board (6″ × 4″ × 4″)
> 1   hammer (4 oz)
> 1   blade-head screwdriver
> 1   Phillips-head screwdriver

1   6″ × 2″ Phillips screw
1   6″ × 2″ flat-head blade screw
1   6″ × 1½″ Phillips screw
1   1″ 4d nail
1   1½″ 4d nail
1   2″ 4d nail

The wooden board, nails, and screws are typically consumable items; however, it may be possible to recycle the screws and the board.

Task 4. Classification

1   9″ × 12″ illustration of a restaurant kitchen (see Fig. 4-8)
17 4½″ × 5″ cards: 12 drawings relating to a restaurant kitchen; 5 unrelated drawings

Task 5. Office Work

1   standard-size stapler
6   standard-size business cards
5   sheets (8½″ × 11″) white paper
5   business size white envelopes
17 sheets (3½″ × 6″) red construction paper
5   sheets (3½″ × 6″) pink construction paper
5   sheets (3½″ × 6″) green construction paper
11 sheets (3½″ × 6″) orange construction paper
5   sheets (3½″ × 6″) yellow construction paper
6   standard-size paper clips
1   two-sided instruction card (4½″ × 5½″) with the following information printed in bold type

[side 1] YOU ARE TO TAKE 3 RED CARDS, 2 ORANGE CARDS, 1 GREEN CARD, 1 PINK CARD, AND 1 YELLOW CARD AND PLACE THEM IN A PILE. TAKE ONE

[side 2] PAPER CLIP AND CLIP THE PILE TOGETHER. MAKE 4 MORE PILES FOLLOWING THE SAME PROCEDURE. PUT EACH PILE INTO AN ENVELOPE.

The business cards and white paper are consumable. When you are assembling your materials, you may want to gather a stock of these items. To eliminate the cost of purchasing business cards and white paper, I have approached local printers and copy shops asking for donations of these supplies. Many companies are happy to give away these surplus items.

Task 6. Telephone Directory

1   9″ × 11″ telephone directory
1   1 pencil
1   3″ × 5″ index card with the following information:

NAME ⎯⎯⎯⎯⎯⎯⎯⎯⎯⎯⎯⎯⎯⎯⎯⎯⎯⎯⎯⎯⎯⎯⎯⎯⎯⎯⎯
ADDRESS ⎯⎯⎯⎯⎯⎯⎯⎯⎯⎯⎯⎯⎯⎯⎯⎯⎯⎯⎯⎯⎯⎯⎯⎯
⎯⎯⎯⎯⎯⎯⎯⎯⎯⎯⎯⎯⎯⎯⎯⎯⎯⎯⎯⎯⎯⎯⎯⎯⎯⎯⎯⎯⎯⎯
TELEPHONE NUMBER ⎯⎯⎯⎯⎯⎯⎯⎯⎯⎯⎯⎯⎯⎯⎯⎯⎯⎯

1   white business-size envelope
1   pen
1   stamp

The index card, envelope, and stamp are consumable. Again, to cut down on expenses, approach paper suppliers or stationery shops for donations of envelopes and index cards. Stickers found in ads from record companies or from the Easter Seal Society can be substituted for stamps.

Task 7. Factory Work

1   $5\frac{1}{2}''$ × $11''$ × $1''$ wooden board (see Fig. 4-13)
1   $\frac{5}{16}''$ × $3''$ carriage bolt and 2 matching nuts
1   $\frac{3}{8}''$ × $3''$ carriage bolt and 2 matching nuts
1   $\frac{1}{2}''$ × $3''$ carriage bolt and 2 matching nuts
1   $\frac{1}{4}''$ × $3''$ machine screw and 2 matching nuts
1   $\frac{8}{32}''$ × $3''$ machine screw and 3 matching nuts
1   $\frac{6}{32}''$ × $3''$ machine screw and 3 matching nuts
1   small plastic bowl (You may substitute a small plastic margarine container.)

Task 8. Environmental Mobility

1   map of Washington, D.C., ($14''$ × $23''$)*
1   broad-tip black marking pen or black crayon
1   piece of clear plastic ($14''$ × $23''$)
1   business-size white envelope
1   instruction card ($5''$ × $7''$). Develop your own for your own setting. The card might read as follows:

GO OUT THE DOOR.
TURN RIGHT.
WALK THROUGH THE DOOR.
GO DOWN TWO FLIGHTS OF STAIRS.
YOU WILL BE ON THE FIRST FLOOR.
TURN RIGHT.
GO THROUGH THE DOOR.
WALK DOWN THE HALL.
JUST BEFORE THE DOOR IN THE HALL, TAKE A LEFT AND AN IMMEDIATE RIGHT.
WALK DOWN THE HALL UNTIL YOU SEE THE MAILBOXES ON THE LEFT.
LOOK IN THE MAILBOX MARKED
[therapist's last name].
BRING BACK THE WHITE ENVELOPE THAT IS IN THE MAILBOX.

Task 9. Money Concepts

4   pennies
3   nickels
6   dimes
5   quarters
1   dollar bill

*Available free from National Parks Service, Washington, D.C. Ask for the "Welcome to Washington, D.C." map.

1   cash register receipt with a total reading between $2.11 and 2.24
1   inexpensive magazine (priced under a dollar)

Task 10. Functional Banking

1   3½" × 10" bank check (see Fig. 4-18B)
1   #2 pencil
1   inexpensive calculator
1   8½" × 11" sheet of white paper with the following information in bold print:

NAME _____

1. What is the date on the check? _____
2. What is the amount of the check? _____
3. To whom is the money being paid? _____
4. What is the account number? _____
5. Whose account will the money come from? _____

Task 11. Time Concepts

1   3" × 5" card with a picture of a clock reading 3:00
1   3" × 5" card with a picture of a clock reading 3:30
1   3" × 5" card with a picture of a clock reading 4:15
1   3" × 5" card with a picture of a digital clock reading 12:40 (see Fig. 4-20).

Task 12. Work Attitudes

5   3½" × 4½" cards, each depicting a step in the sequence of a student walking into a fast-food shop and purchasing a meal (see Fig. 4-21)

Task 13. Body Scheme

1   8½" × 11" sheet of paper with a drawing of a teenaged boy (see Fig. 4-22)
5   identical drawings cut into the following parts: 5 heads, 5 torsos, 10 arms, 5 pairs of legs, 10 feet

Task 14. Leather Assembly

1   standard-size rotary leather hole punch
1   wooden leather mallet (1 1/2" × 4")
2   key rings
6   sets of small rivets
2   1" × 3" 7-oz leather strips
1   plastic box (4" × 4" × ½") to hold rivets, leather, and key rings

The leather, key rings, and rivets are consumable items. The leather strips, however, can be cut from scrap leather. Make sure that you are using a sharp hole punch to facilitate use.

Task 15. Food Preparation

1   stick of margarine (Take it out at the beginning of the testing session to soften.)
1   small jar of honey

1   small mixing spoon
1   teaspoon
1   butter knife
1   small plastic bowl
1   box of crackers (Keep these on hand, but leave only a small package in the assessment box.)
5   4¼" × 5 1/2" instruction cards (see Fig. 4-24)

Writing The Evaluation Report

When the test is completed, the therapist has sufficient information to devise a treatment plan. To expedite the write-up procedure and to facilitate clarity in communicating results, I have devised a format that is concrete yet descriptive enough for both educators and laypersons to comprehend. This format is illustrated in the sample evaluation reports that follow this section.

After the therapist has reviewed the profile sheet and calculated the number of circled checks in each column, he or she is able readily to complete the report. This typically takes 15 to 30 minutes, depending on the complexity of results.

The completed version of the evaluation report, including the profile sheet, is placed in the student's chart, with copies sent to pertinent individuals: parents, teachers, academic supervisor, other therapists. In addition, when appropriate, the therapist may verbally convey results to these persons.

The following are examples of completed evaluation reports, which may help to clarify the JPSA. The first example describes a student I will call Stacey, who will be further discussed in Chapter 5. I hope these discussions will assist you in conceptualizing the dynamics of the occupational therapist's role in an educational setting directed at work-related programming.

Sample Evaluation Report 1*
Name: Stacey
Chronological age: 15 years
Stacey was given the Jacobs Prevocational Skills Assessment on February 15 and 17 and March 1, 1984.

Evaluation Battery
The assessment consists of 15 informal tasks involving functional ability in the following skill areas: fine motor coordination, eye–hand coordination, motor planning, attention to detail, sorting, classification and sequencing, decision making, problem solving, organizational skills, use of tools, ability to follow directions, conceptual skills, task focus, and behavioral observations (Fig. 4-26)

Impressions and Observations
Stacey was cooperative and had pleasant interaction skills. She appeared motivated to perform well and maintained good task focus throughout the test session. At times when the task was difficult, she appeared anxious and seemed to lack confidence in her abilities. Before the evaluation Stacey was able to take an active, responsible role in scheduling the test sessions.

Stacey was unsystematic in her approach to most tasks, showing difficulty in

*Sample Evaluation Reports 1 and 2 were provided by Nancy Mazonson, M.S., OTR.

The Jacobs Prevocational Skills Assessment

WORK SKILLS	PHYSICAL CAPACITIES			
	Fine Motor Coordination	Eye-Hand Coordination	Motor Planning	Use of Tools
1. Quality Control	✔			
2. Filing A	✔			
B	✔			
C	✔			
3. Carpentry Assembly	✔	⊘	⊘	✔
4. Classification	✔			
5. Office Work A	✔	✔	✔	✔
B	✔	✔	✔	
C	⊘	✔	✔	
6. Telephone Directory A	✔	✔		
B	✔	✔		
7. Factory Work	⊘	✔	✔	
8. Environmental Mobility A	✔	✔	✔	
B				
9. Money Concepts A				
B				
C	✔			
D	✔			
10. Functional Banking A	✔	✔		
B	✔	✔		✔
11. Time Concept A				
B				
C				
12. Work Attitudes A				
B				
13. Assembly	✔			
14. Leather Assembly	⊘	✔	✔	✔
15. Food Preparation	✔	✔	✔	⊘

© 1979 Jacobs, K. (revised 1988)

✔ sitting posture cooperative, pleasant

Figure 4-26.   The JPSA form completed for Stacey's evaluation.

	WORK BEHAVIORS					WORK APTITUDES					Behavioral Observations
		Ability to Follow Directions									
Task Focus	Visual	Written	Verbal	Organizational Skills	Decision Making	Sorting	Attention to Detail	Classification Sequencing	Problem Solving	Practical Daily Living Knowledge	
(✓)			(✓)	(✓)	✓	✓	(✓)				↓ use of model
✓		(✓)		(✓)	✓	✓		(✓)	(✓)	(✓)	↓ scanning
✓		(✓)	✓		✓	✓	✓	✓	✓	(✓)	
✓		(✓)	✓		(✓)	✓		✓	✓	(✓)	
✓					✓		✓		✓		awkward tool use
✓			✓		✓			✓	✓		
✓				✓	(✓)			✓	✓		
✓	✓		✓	✓				✓	✓		
✓		✓		(✓)				✓	✓	(✓)	became disorganized
✓			✓	✓			✓	✓		✓	
✓			✓	✓						✓	poor handwriting
✓			✓		✓		✓		✓		needed cue to replace bolts
✓			✓	✓			✓		✓		
✓		(✓)		(✓)					✓		
✓			✓							(✓)	has very basic understanding
✓										(✓)	
✓			✓		✓		✓		✓	(✓)	needed cues
✓			✓	✓	✓		✓		✓	(✓)	↓ concept making change
✓		✓	✓		(✓)		✓			✓	change
✓		(✓)			✓		✓			✓	appears familiar with use of calculator
✓			✓							✓	
✓			✓				✓			✓	
✓			✓						✓	✓	slow, but answered correctly
✓			✓	✓	✓		✓	✓			disorganized use of table space
✓			✓		✓				✓		
✓	✓		✓	✓					✓		
✓	✓						✓	✓			
✓	✓				(✓)			(✓)			awkward use of tools

↓ self confidence disorganized

Figure 4-26.   (continued)

sequencing and organization. She had difficulty in following two- or three-step written or oral directions, which may be related to problems in reading comprehension and in memory. Stacey seemed to be able to follow best a combination of oral and visual directions. She used visual cues in problem solving to compensate for memory problems. Stacey's manipulation of small objects appeared awkward, and she seemed to have problems with visual scanning.

Strengths

1. Cooperative, motivated
2. Adequate work attitudes
3. Adequate task focus
4. Ability to use visual cues for beginning problem solving
5. Beginning-level concepts of money

Weaknesses

1. Poor organizational skills
2. Inconsistent in following multistep directions
3. Poor memory
4. Poor visual scanning
5. Weak in acknowledging difficulties
6. Weak in problem solving and decision making
7. Poor in matching
8. Poor in alphabetizing
9. Poor fine motor coordination
10. Weak in classification and sequencing

Recommendations

It is recommended that Stacey be placed in a highly supervised work setting to improve the following procedures: organization, problem solving, sequencing, and decision making. It is recommended that Stacey be seen in a small group twice per week in occupational therapy to work on functional money skills, direction following, and the ability to assess strengths and weaknesses.

Sample Evaluation Report 2*

Name: Keith
Chronological age: 17 years
Keith was given the Jacobs Prevocational Skills Assessment on February 24, 1984.

Evaluation Battery

The assessment consists of 15 informal tasks involving functional ability in the following skill areas: fine motor coordination, eye-hand coordination, motor planning, attention to detail, sorting, classification and sequencing, decision making, problem solving, organizational skills, use of tools, ability to follow directions, conceptual skills, task focus, and behavioral observations (Fig. 4-27).

Impressions and Observations

Keith was cooperative and pleasant throughout the testing session. He presented himself as a charming, mature young gentleman and engaged easily in social conversation.

During the test Keith said that he understood instructions; however, his performance showed otherwise. He did not ask for assistance with tasks or clarification of instructions when it was clear that he was unsure how to continue with the test items. Keith worked close to the table at a very slow, steady pace. His task focus was good.

Keith had difficulty following two- and three-step oral, written, and visual directions. Performance of tasks involving visual and oral directions broke down when an auditory or visual memory component was introduced.

The Jacobs Prevocational Skills Assessment

WORK SKILLS	PHYSICAL CAPACITIES			
	Fine Motor Coordination	Eye-Hand Coordination	Motor Planning	Use of Tools
1. Quality Control	✓			
2. Filing A	✓			
B	(✓)			
C	✓			
3. Carpentry Assembly	(✓)	(✓)	✓	✓
4. Classification	✓			
5. Office Work A	(✓)	✓	✓	✓
B	(✓)	✓	(✓)	
C	(✓)	✓	✓	
6. Telephone Directory A	✓	✓		
B	✓	✓		
7. Factory Work	(✓)	✓	(✓)	
8. Environmental Mobility A	✓	✓	✓	
B				
9. Money Concepts A				
B				
C	✓			
D	✓			
10. Functional Banking A	✓	✓		
B	✓	✓		✓
11. Time Concept A				
B				
C				
12. Work Attitudes A				
B				
13. Assembly	(✓)			
14. Leather Assembly	(✓)	✓	(✓)	✓
15. Food Preparation	✓	✓	✓	✓

© 1979 Jacobs, K. (revised 1988)

conversant, pleasant, nicely groomed

Figure 4-27.   The JPSA form completed for Keith's evaluation.

Task Focus	Visual	Written	Verbal	Organizational Skills	Decision Making		Sorting	Attention to Detail	Classification Sequencing	Problem Solving	Practical Daily Living Knowledge	Behavioral Observations
✓			(✓)	(✓)	✓		✓	(✓)				became disorganized
✓		✓		✓	(✓)		✓		✓	✓	(✓)	poor use of model
✓		✓		✓	✓		✓	✓	✓	✓	✓	slow, labored
✓		✓		✓	✓		✓		✓	✓	(✓)	
✓					✓			✓	(✓)			
✓		✓			(✓)				(✓)			awkward with tools
✓				✓	✓				✓	✓		
✓	✓		✓	✓					✓	(✓)		poor folding
✓		✓		(✓)					✓	✓	✓	disorganized easily
✓			✓	✓				✓	✓		(✓)	
✓			✓	✓							✓	writing slowly, but neat.
✓			✓		✓		✓		✓			extremely slow motions
✓		(✓)	✓				✓			(✓)		required cues (memory)
✓	✓		✓							(✓)		required assistance
✓			✓								✓	
✓			✓								(✓)	
✓		(✓)			(✓)		✓		✓		(✓)	
✓		(✓)	✓		✓		✓		✓		(✓)	lacks understanding
✓		✓	✓		✓		✓				(✓)	of basic change
✓			✓		✓		✓				(✓)	making
✓			✓								✓	
✓			✓				✓				✓	
✓			(✓)						✓		(✓)	difficulty with digital
✓			✓	✓	✓		✓	✓				O.k.
✓			✓		✓				✓			approp. resposes
✓	(✓)		✓						(✓)			unsystematic trial + error
✓	(✓)			✓			✓	✓				awkward, appeared confused
✓	✓				(✓)		✓					unsure-needed cues

Figure 4-27.   (continued)

Fine motor coordination is a problem area for Keith. While he was able to complete all tasks, fine motor movements were slow and labored and appeared to require concentration.

Keith's conceptual skills of alphabetizing and money use were limited. Difficulty arose when he was asked to alphabetize words beginning with the same letter. He was also unable to perform simple calculations involving coin values under $1.00. He had difficulty with matching skills but was able to complete concrete tasks involving classifying and sequencing.

Keith's performance broke down when multiple visual stimuli were presented, perhaps because of difficulty with attention to detail and visual perception.

Strengths
1. Cooperative and friendly
2. Socially pleasant
3. Good task focus
4. Good classification and sequencing skills
5. Adequate sorting of concrete items
6. Functional eye–hand coordination

Weaknesses
1. Poor fine motor coordination
2. Weak in problem solving and decision making
3. Inability to recognize or verbalize his needs
4. Difficulty following oral, written, and visual directions
5. Poor memory
6. Weak in alphabetizing
7. Poor in money use
8. Weak in using written directions
9. Difficulty with attention to detail
10. Poor motor planning

Recommendations
It is recommended that Keith continue with his present occupational therapy schedule of two small group sessions per week and his volunteer job in the school resource room (filing, photocopying, acting as a receptionist) once per week with consultation provided by the occupational therapist. It is also recommended that in all classrooms and workshops material be presented using a combined format of simplified oral, visual, and written directions.

Suggested Goals and Treatment
1. To improve fine motor coordination; proper use of oral, written, and visual directions; problem solving; and decision making through fabrication of a date book and other age-appropriate craft and leisure activities.
2. To improve fine motor coordination and motor planning skills (incorporating memory) through babysitter's training course and other work-related training, such as cooking and sewing.
3. To increase attention to detail, alphabetizing, communication, problem-solving, and decision-making skills, Keith will participate in school yearbook activities and continue part-time work in the resource room, where occupational therapy consultation will be provided.
4. To improve Keith's ability to verbalize his needs through proper feedback and reinforcement during the above activities.

Since the JPSA is useful as a screening tool, information obtained can be most beneficial when used in combination with other evaluations.

Sample Evaluation, Report 3 illustrates the use of some of the tasks from the JPSA in combination with results from the Skills Assessment Module (SAM) (see Chapter 3). Note that Figure 4-28 reflects a maximum average time for task completion, which may be useful in comparing clients' test results.

Sample Evaluation, Report 3
Name: Jesse
Age: 17 years
Jesse was given the following evaluations: the Skills Assessment Module; seven of the 15 work samples from the Jacobs Prevocational Skills Assessment; an Activity Configuration; and an Activity of Daily Living (ADL).

Descriptions of Evaluations
The Skills Assessment Module (SAM) is designed to assess a student's affective, cognitive, and psychomotor abilities in relation to skills required in vocational training programs. SAM consists of three paper pencil tests: Learning Styles Inventory, Revised Beta Examination, and Auditory Directions Screen; and 12 hands-on modules or work samples.

Learning Styles Inventory is an evaluation instrument formulated to help determine the learning styles of students. It is divided into three main areas: (1) information gathering, (2) work conditions, and (3) expressive preference. The test is in the form of a self-report in which the student ranks statements that best reflect his or her feelings.

Revised Beta Examination Second Edition (Beta-II) is a nonverbal measure of intellectual ability for the general population.

Auditory Directions Screen (ADS) is an oral directions test which assesses an individual's ability to follow oral directions.

The 12 hands-on modules or work samples provide information for identifying the student's general areas of vocational strengths and weaknesses. These modules are Mail Sort, Alphabetizing Cards, Etch-A-Sketch Maze, Payroll Computation, Patient Information Memo, Small Parts Assembly A and B, Ruler Reading, Pipe Assembly, O-Rings, Block Design, Color Sort, and Circuit Board.

The Jacobs Prevocational Skills Assessment (JPSA) assesses various work behaviors, skills and aptitudes, and physical capacities of learning-disabled adolescents. It consists of 15 work samples, such as Functional Banking and Carpentry Assembly. The tasks within the work samples involve functional abilities in the following areas: fine motor coordination, eye-hand coordination, motor planning, use of tools, task focus, ability to follow directions (verbal, written, and visual), organizational skills, decision making, sorting, attention to detail, classification, sequencing, problem solving, practical daily living knowledge, and work behaviors.

Jesse was given the following JPSA work samples: #6—Telephone Directory, #9—Money Concepts, #10—Functional Banking, #11—Time Concepts, #12—Work Attitudes, #13—Body Scheme, and #14—Leather Assembly. The Activity Configuration consisted of Jesse listing hourly activities for a typical week, with personal assessments of the nature of the activity (recreation, school, etc.). For the ADL, Jesse was observed eating lunch in a restaurant.

Impressions and Observations
Jesse was cooperative and had pleasant interaction skills. He appeared motivated to perform the various evaluation tasks and maintained a good-to-excellent task focus throughout the five hours of testing. It was only during activities which required fine dexterity or visual spatial processing that Jesse appeared fatigued and frustrated.

Task	Time in Minutes
1. Quality Control	2
2. Filing A	10
B	5
C	3
3. Carpentry Assembly	5
4. Classification	2
5. Office Work A	8
B	6
C	8
6. Telephone Directory A	6
B	10
7. Factory Work	12
8. Environmental Mobility A	5
B	(variable) 10
9. Money Concepts A	2
B	5
C	5
D	5
10. Functional Banking A	10
B	4
11. Time Concept A	1
B	2
C	2
12. Work Attitudes A	5
B	5
13. Assembly	10
14. Leather Assembly	12
15. Food Preparation	8

Figure 4-28.   The JPSA profile sheet, here shown filled out in the column at the far right with the maximum time limit in minutes for each task.

Evaluation Results: Skills Assessment Modules (SAM)

Learning Styles Instrument
This instrument delineates nine learning styles. A score of 32–40 indicates that the style is a major learning style for the student. A student does not necessarily have only one learning style. The results of Jesse's Learning Styles Inventory indicated that he feels comfortable with the following learning styles:

1. Visual Language—This is a student who learns well from seeing words in books, on the chalkboard, in charts, or in workbooks. He may even write words down that are given to him orally, because he remembers and uses information better if he has read it.
2. Visual Numerical—This student has to *see* numbers to work with them. He is more likely to remember and understand math facts if he has seen them.
3. Auditory-Visual-Kinesthetic Combination (A-V-K)—The A-V-K student learns best by experience. He definitely needs a combination of stimuli. The manipulation of material along with the accompanying sights and sounds (words and numbers seen and spoken) will make a big difference to him. He may not be able to understand or be able to keep his mind on his work unless he is totally involved. He seeks to handle, touch, and work with what he is learning.

Beta-II
This portion of the SAM contains six tests intended to measure different aspects of nonverbal ability.

Test 1—Mazes
Test 2—Coding
Test 3—Paper Form Boards
Test 4—Picture Completion
Test 5—Clerical Checking
Test 6—Picture Absurdities

Jesse obtained a Beta-II IQ score of 60. A plausible explanation for this depressed score may be found in some of the individual test scores. Although it is stressed in the Beta-II manual that one should not look at individual test scores, doing so provides some explanation for Jesse's score. For example, he had difficulty with both Test 1 (Mazes) and Test 3 (Paper Form Boards). His raw score of 0 on each test may be contributed to the fact that both tests had a visual-perceptual requirement, which is an area of difficulty for Jesse.

Auditory Directions Screening
The ADS provides a quick method of screening a student's need for activities involving the use of auditory skills. Although the ADS is psychometrically normed, it is not intended to be used as a scientific indicator of the future success or failure of a student. Jesse's total number of errors was six. This score would indicate that he needs improvement with auditory skills.

Hands-on Modules or Work Samples
1. *Mail Sort*—Jesse sorted preaddressed postcards by zip code. This work sample assesses digital discrimination. He worked consistently with bilateral hand use. Although he initially had difficulty visually locating the zip code numbers over the mail slots, he completed the task with 80% accuracy.
2. *Alphabetizing Cards*—Jesse filed preaddressed postcards alphabetically. This work sample assesses clerical/verbal perception. He worked quickly, with an excellent task focus. Six errors were observed.
3. *Etch-A-Sketch Maze*—Jesse was instructed to follow a pattern by simultaneously turning two dials quickly and accurately. This work sample assesses motor coordination. Jesse was able to use the dials bilaterally but was unable to stay within the lines of the maze.

4. *Payroll Computation*—Jesse was instructed to compute employees' earnings with the aid of a calculator. This work sample assesses clerical/numerical perception. Jesse used the adding machine appropriately to complete the calculations with 100% accuracy.

5. *Patient Information Memo*—Jesse was instructed to read, analyze, and transcribe written material. This work sample assesses the ability to follow written instructions. Jesse appeared to enjoy this task, saying, "This is neat." Jesse's handwriting was legible and he had only 10 errors. His task focus was excellent.

6. *Small Parts*—Jesse was instructed to manipulate small objects on a board using small tools. He had great difficulty with these tasks and was unable to appropriately use the screwdriver and tweezers. The work sample assesses aiming and finger dexterity.

7. *Ruler Reading*—Jesse was instructed to read a ruler and measure to the nearest sixteenth of an inch. This task assesses measurement ability. Although he diligently worked on this task, he did not mark off the correct measurement on the line, but rather rewrote the measurement on the line.

8. *Pipe Assembly*—Jesse was instructed to assemble a pipe and faucet assembly with appropriate tools according to a printed diagram. This task assesses manual dexterity. He was unable to follow the diagram (two-dimensional) to assemble the pipe and faucet. In particular, he had difficulty positioning the pipes in their appropriate order and then screwing them together.

9. *O-Rings*—Jesse was instructed to sort objects of similar material according to size. This work sample assesses form perception. He performed this task very quickly; however, 75 percent of the rings were mismatched.

10. *Block Design*—Using a set of colored blocks, Jesse was asked to construct designs based on a printed diagram. This task assesses spatial perception. He initially assembled the blocks in one line, but after cueing he constructed the blocks one on top of the other. He was unable to replicate the three-dimensional design from the two-dimensional printed diagram.

11. *Color Sort*—Jesse was instructed to sort seven different colors by identifying the central color in a pattern. This work sample asssess color discrimination. Initially, he was confused on what colors to match. After a demonstration, he proceeded to complete the task with only one error.

12. *Circuit Board*—Jesse was instructed to wire a circuit by following a color-coded pattern. This task assesses ability to follow diagrammed instructions. Jesse was unable to replicate the two-dimensional design from the diagram onto the circuit board.

Seven work samples from the Jacobs Prevocational Skills Assessment (JPSA) were administered:

#6 Telephone Directory—This task involves the use of a telephone directory to obtain information to address an envelope. Jesse initially had difficulty using the directory; however, with instruction from the therapist in its use, he was able to complete this activity without difficulty.

#9 Money Concepts—This task involves coin identification, adding coins, and making change. Jesse was able to correctly identify a penny, nickel, dime, quarter, and dollar. He was able to read the total from a cash register receipt, but was unable to find that amount from the coins presented or calculate how much money was presented. Jesse was unable to mentally calculate $1.00 − $.69 = $.31.

#10 Functional Banking—This task involves identification of information on a bank check and simple account balancing using a calculator. Jesse was able to comprehend the five questions regarding a bank check, including "What is the amount of the check?" He answered these questions correctly using legible printed handwriting. He was able to use the calculator without difficulty, al-

though he problem-solved aloud whether the solution to the problem was addition or subtraction.

#11 Time Concepts—This task involves identifying time on a clock, time comparisons, and simple problem solving. Jesse initially stated that he could not read a face clock. After prompting, he was able to identify times on two face clocks and one digital clock. He was unable to mentally calculate a time comparison activity.

#12 Work Attitudes—This task involves sequencing five cards depicting a student making a purchase at a fast-food restaurant. Jesse was able to sequence correctly three of the five cards. The second part of this task consists of three auditory vignettes designed to ascertain work attitude. One example is: "You have 15 minutes left to work. Your friend comes into McDonald's and says, 'No one is looking. Why don't you leave work now?' What do you do?" Jesse provided appropriate responses to all questions.

#13 Body Scheme—This task involves assembling five models of a person from visual memory. Jesse was able to assemble only one model correctly. Errors involved reversed direction placement of arms and shoes.

#14 Leather Assembly—This task involves the assembling of a simple leather key ring from visual demonstration. Jesse approached this task enthusiastically, although he was unable to use the leather hole punch and had difficulty manipulating and setting the rivets.

Activity Configuration
Jesse described his typical week day as follows:

6:00 AM	Wake up, dress, eat breakfast, retrieve lunch from refrigerator and put into a bag
7:20 AM	Take bus from home
8:30 AM–3:00 PM	Attend school
3:30 PM	Arrive home
3:30–6:30 PM	Complete homework Work on computer, playing games
6:30 PM	Dinner Watch TV Spend time with parents
9:30 or 10:00 PM	Bed

Activities of Daily Living
Jesse was able to read from a menu and appropriately order his meal. His posture at the table and utensil use were awkward. In addition, Jesse had difficulty independently organizing his table space. He was very conversive during the meal.

Strengths
1. Cooperative and friendly
2. Highly motivated
3. Good task focus
4. Able to verbalize
5. Able to use both a calculator and adding machine to accurately solve functional multiplication and subtraction problems
6. Able to read and comprehend written testing directions and instructions
7. Able to print legibly
8. Beginning-level concepts of money
9. Good work attitudes
10. Interested in and able to use both the Apple IIe and IBM (PS2) computers

Weaknesses
1. Awkward use of tools (e.g., hammer, screw driver, wrench, and utensils)
2. Decreased strength in left hand
3. Difficulty with fine motor coordination

4. Difficulty with spatial orientation (visual–spatial awareness)
5. Difficulty with motor planning
6. Limited avocational activities

Recommendations

The following recommendations have been based on information gathered from the evaluation, review of medical and school records, and the mother's informal report.

By age 17, all of Jesse's programming should be focusing on *functionality*, to assist him in making the transition over the next few years from student to independent adult—ideally a competitively employed worker. To this end, it is highly recommended that Jesse enter into a school-based work study program. The evaluation results indicate that Jesse could be successful in a work study placement that is highly *structured* and designed to meet his individual needs. For example, work study programming could initially be incorporated into occupational therapy services.

It is suggested that Jesse's present occupational therapy programming could be more effective if provided at the work study job site, with the occupational therapist in the role of a job coach. Ideally, the occupational therapist would work with Jesse two times a week for one-hour sessions at the job site. If arrangements for occupational therapy services cannot be made for the job site, a job coach should be provided during the initial placement period. Once Jesse has developed confidence in his ability to perform the duties of his job, the amount of time and days on the job should be increased, while the presence of the job coach is decreased.

Although it is believed that Jesse could be successful working in settings performing food service and/or janitorial duties, he is not very motivated or interested in these types of positions. He is, however, interested in activities that involve computers. It was revealed during testing that Jesse can successfully perform activities that involve reading written material and transcribing information from this material onto a form entry format. Such activities lend themselves nicely to a computer. Jobs requiring these activities include receptionist and inventory data entry processor, jobs that might be found in an auto supply store or insurance company. Jesse's interest in computers is a strength which needs to be reinforced in both the school and home environments and eventually should be incorporated into his work environment.

It is highly recommended that Jesse receive occupational therapy programming two times per week for 45–60 minutes in a group environment. Working in a group will provide Jesse the opportunity to hone appropriate work behaviors, such as socialization skills.

Suggestions for the School Environment

1. To provide, initially on a limited basis (e.g., two times a week for 1–2 hours/day), a highly structured work study placement.
2. To provide a job coach, ideally the occupational therapist, during the initial placement on the job.
3. To provide functional academic and vocational programming.
4. To provide therapeutic intervention focusing on functionality and the development of compensatory strategies.
5. To provide a curriculum in computers.
6. To provide occupational therapy in a group session, two times a week for 45–60 minutes each (if occupational therapy is not incorporated into the work study placement).

Suggestions for the Home Environment

1. To develop, with Jesse's assistance, a list of chores that he will perform routinely. Ideally, the list should be made into a grid chart, which can be checked once a chore is completed. Suggested chores: setting the table, loading and unloading the dishwasher, folding laundry and putting it away, vacuuming, and assisting in meal preparation. Chores are an

ideal way of developing appropriate work behaviors and can be viewed as a job within the home environment.

2. To encourage Jesse's use of the computer, in particular, reinforcing the use of reading material and transcribing information into the computer in a form entry format.
3. To foster avocational activities and involvement with peers.
4. To explore the feasibility of Jesse obtaining a volunteer job, for instance, with a senior citizen center.

Thank you for this consultation.

Karen Jacobs, M.S., OTR/L, FAOTA
Occupational therapist

Appendix 4-1: Jacobs Prevocational Skills Assessment Manual

In this section, the manual for the Jacobs Prevocational Skills Assessment is presented. You may photocopy these pages; spiral binding will facilitate use.

Introduction of Assessment to Student
The therapist should read the following to the student before beginning the assessment:

"I am going to be giving you an OT assessment, which consists of 15 different tasks relating to work. Each task is timed, and I will let you know during each task when your time is up. Please try each task and do the best you can. Throughout the assessment I will be writing some notes to help me remember what you have done. After you have completed the whole assessment, we will set up another time to meet. At that meeting I will be able to explain the results to you. Do you have any questions before we begin? [Wait for a response.] Then let's begin."

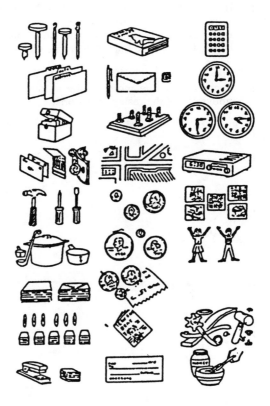

1

Quality Control
Purpose
  Sorting

Materials
  16 2½" nails
  10 odd-size and bent nails

Instructions
  The student is seated to the left of the therapist. The 26 nails are randomly arranged on the table in front of the student, at his or her midline.
  After the materials are arranged, the therapist picks up one of the 2½-inch nails in his or her right hand and shows it to the student, saying:

  Please find all the nails that look the same as this nail. Put all the same nails here. [Point to the right side of the table.] Put all the different nails here. [Point to the left side of the table.] The different nails are ones that are bent or much thinner or thicker than this nail. [Show the student one of the 2½-inch nails in the pile.] Do you understand? [Wait for a response.] Please begin. [Place model nail below pile of nails.]

Timing
  Begin timing the moment the student has acknowledged that he or she understands the task instructions.

2

Task 2

Filing
Purpose
   Sequencing
   Conceptual skills

Part A

Materials
   26 white cards (3″ × 5″), each bearing one word beginning with each letter of the alphabet. Most of the words are related to work.
   Instruction card (4¼″ × 5½″)

Instructions
   If the student is unable to read, the therapist should read instructions aloud. For students who have difficulty comprehending verbal instructions, the therapist may demonstrate both parts.

   A written instruction card is placed on the table directly in front of the student, 6 inches from the front of the table. The therapist instructs the student to read the card silently. After the student has read it, the card is removed. The therapist places on the table directly in front of the student, 6 inches from the edge of the table, a well-shuffled stack of cards. The therapist asks, "Do you have any questions? [Wait for a response.] Please begin."

Part B
   Parts B and C are presented to the student only if he or she was able to attempt the preceding part.

Materials
   1 (5¼″ × 3½″ × 3″) plastic card file
   1 set of A to Z guides for 3″ × 5″ index cards
   13 white lined (3″ × 5″) index cards each bearing a different name with a
      first initial
   1 instruction card (4¼″ × 5½″)

Instructions
   Written instructions are placed in front of the student as in Part A. After the student has read the instructions silently, the card is removed. The therapist arranges the materials as shown below and asks, "Do you understand? [Wait for a response.] Please begin."

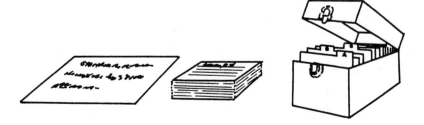

3

Part C

Materials

6 white cards (4" × 3") each bearing one of the following words written in bold capital letters: MONEY, MATCH, MAIL, MAIN, MISS, MUCH
1 instruction card (4¼" × 5½")
1 plastic card file and *A* to *Z* guides from Part B

Instructions

Written instructions are placed in front of the student as in Parts A and B. After the student has read the instructions silently, the card is removed. The therapist arranges the materials as in Part B and asks, "Do you understand? [Wait for a response.] Please begin."

Timing

Begin timing the moment after you say *begin* in each part.

4

Task 3

Carpentry Assembly
Purpose
   Eye-hand coordination
   Use of tools

Materials
   1 pine board (6″ × 4″ × 4″) with nails and screws as shown below (two nails
      and three screws are ¾ of the way into the wood):
   1 hammer (4-oz.)
   1 blade-head screwdriver
   1 Phillips-head screwdriver
   1 6″ × 2″ Phillips screw
   1 6″ × 2″ flat-head blade screw
   1 6″ × 1½″ Phillips screw
   1 1″ 4d nail
   1 1½″ 4d nail
   1 2″ 4d nail (single nail placed in board by student)

Instructions
   The student stands in front of a table of appropriate height, with materials
   arranged as shown below:

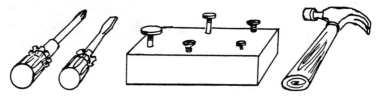

   The therapist asks the student the following questions:

   "What is this?" [Point to the blade-head screwdriver.]
   "What is this?" [Point to the Phillips-head screwdriver.]
   "What is this?" [Point to the hammer.]

   If the student is unable to name the tools, the therapist should say:

   Show me the screwdriver.
   Show me the hammer.

   The therapist then says

   "Use the hammer and screwdrivers to make all the nails and screws flat into
   the wood. Do you understand? [Wait for a response.] Please begin."

   After the student has completed this part, the therapist says

   "Hammer this nail [places a single nail on the table] into the wood. Do you
   understand? [Wait for a response.] Please begin."

Timing
   Begin timing the moment after you say *begin*.

5

Task 4

Classification

Purpose
   Classification

Materials
   1 illustration (9″ × 12″) of a restaurant kitchen (optional use)
   12 cards (4½″ × 5″), each bearing a drawing of an item related to a restaurant kitchen
   5 cards (4½″ × 5″), each bearing a drawing of an item unrelated to a kitchen

Instructions
   The therapist arranges the materials as shown:

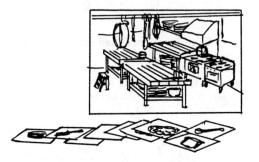

   The therapist says:

   "Find all the cards with items that belong in a restaurant kitchen. Place these cards here. [Point to an area to the right of the materials.] Do you understand? [Wait for a response.] Please begin."

Timing
   Begin timing the moment after you say *begin*.

Task 5

Office Work

Purpose
Organizational skills
Use of tools (Part A)
Ability to follow written directions (Part C)

Part A

Materials
1 standard-size stapler
6 standard-size business cards
5 sheets white paper (8½″ × 11″)

Instructions
Each part is first demonstrated by the therapist. The therapist demonstrates this part while saying the following:

"This is a job that you might do if you worked in an office. Take one business card and staple it at the top of a piece of paper, like this. [The card is also centered at the top of the sheet.] Now you do the same with the other sheets."

Arrange the materials for Part A as shown below:

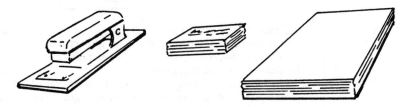

Part B

Materials
5 white sheets with stapled cards from Part A
5 business-size white envelopes

Instructions
Arrange materials as shown below:

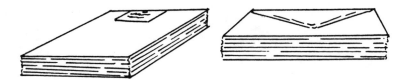

7

The therapist demonstrates this part while saying the following:

"Take one sheet at a time and fold it into thirds. Put this folded sheet into one of the unsealed envelopes. Then put the envelope here. [Point to the right side of the table, 12 inches from the front.] Now you do the same with the other sheets and envelopes."

Part C

Materials
17 sheets of red construction paper (3½" × 6")
 5 sheets of pink construction paper (3½" × 6")
 5 sheets of green construction paper (3½" × 6")
11 sheets of orange construction paper (3½" × 6")
 5 sheets of yellow construction paper (3½" × 6")
 1 two-sided instruction card (4¼" × 5")
 6 standard-size paper clips
Part B materials (envelopes filled with folded sheets)

Instructions
Arrange the materials as shown below:

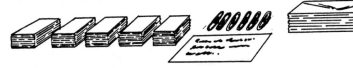

The therapist points to the stacks of paper one at a time from left to right, asking the student to name the color of each stack.

Then the therapist places the instruction card on the table and instructs the student to read it silently.

After the student has read the card, the therapist asks, "Do you have any questions? [Wait for a response.] Please begin." The instruction card remains on the table throughout this part.

Timing
Begin timing the moment after you complete giving the task instructions.

8

Telephone Directory
Purpose
  Figure-ground discrimination
  Organizational skills
  Conceptual skills
  Fine motor coordination

Part A

Materials
  1 telephone directory (9″ × 11″)
  1 #2 pencil
  1 index card (3″ × 5″) with the following information in bold print:
  NAME _____
  ADDRESS _____
  _____
  TELEPHONE NUMBER _____

Instructions
  Arrange the materials as shown

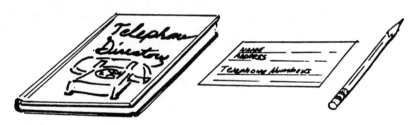

Before performing the assessment, the therapist should look through the telephone directory and select a company name that is written in bold print. This name will be used in both parts of this task.

After the materials are arranged the therapist says:

"Here is a telephone directory. Use the telephone directory to look up the address and telephone number of [selected name]. When you have found the address and telephone number, write them on this index card. [Point to the card.] Do you understand? [Wait for a response.] Please begin."

Part B

Materials
  1 white business-size envelope
  1 pen
  1 postage stamp
  1 index card with information from Part A

Instructions
  Arrange the materials as shown below:

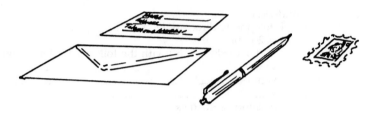

  The therapist says the following:

  "Now we want to send this envelope to [selected name]. Please write the name and address of [name] on the envelope. Write your return address and put this stamp on the envelope, too. Do you understand? [Wait for a response.] Please begin."

Timing
  Begin timing the moment after you say *begin*.

10

Task 7

Factory Work
Purpose
   Fine motor coordination
   Matching
   Problem solving

Materials
   1 5½" × 11" × 1" wooden board
   1 ⁵⁄₁₆" × 3" bolt with 2 matching nuts
   1 ⅜" × 3" with 2 matching nuts
   1 ½" × 3" bolt with 2 matching nuts
   1 ¼" × 3" bolt with 2 matching nuts
   1 ⁸⁄₃₂" × 3" screw with 3 matching nuts
   1 ⁶⁄₃₂" × 3" screw with 3 matching nuts
   1 small plastic bowl

Instructions
   The student is seated, and the therapist arranges the materials as shown:

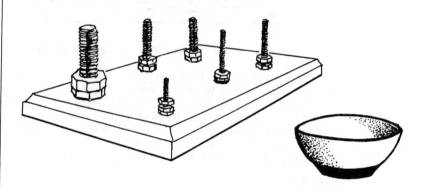

The therapist reads aloud the following directions for the student:

"There are six bolts with nuts on them. [Point to the wooden board.] Take *all* the nuts off the bolts and put them into this bowl. [Point to the bowl.] After *all* the nuts are in the bowl, put them all back on the bolts. Do you understand? [Wait for a response.] Please begin."

Timing
   Begin timing the moment after you say *begin*.

Task 8

Environmental Mobility
Purpose
   Motor planning
   Problem solving
   Ability to follow written directions

Part A

Materials
   1 map of Washington, D.C. (14″ × 23″)
   1 broad-tip black marking pen
   1 piece of clear plastic cut to the dimensions of the map (14″ × 23″)

Instructions
   The materials are arranged as shown below:

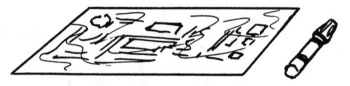

   The therapist reads the following instructions aloud:

"Please use this marking pen [point to the marking pen] to show the route
you would follow when you arrive in Washington, D.C., at the train station
[point to the train station on the map] and then want to see the sights first
at the White House [point to the White House on the map] and then at the
Jefferson Memorial [point to the Jefferson Memorial on the map]. Please
remember to follow the streets and not to cross over the lines. Do you have
any questions? [Wait for a response.] Please begin."

Part B

Materials
   1 instruction card (5″ × 7″)
   1 envelope

Instructions
   Before beginning this part, the therapist should have devised an instruction
card with a simple step-by-step errand. If the errand is to retrieve an item
(the envelope), be sure to place the item in its appropriate place before the
task.
   The therapist hands the student the instruction card and says:

"Please follow the written directions on the card to do an errand for me. Do
you understand? [Wait for a response.] Please begin."

   If the student is unable to read or comprehend instructions, the therapist
should accompany the student on this task while reading instructions aloud
for the student to follow.

Timing
   Begin timing the moment after you say *begin*.

12

Task 9

Money Concepts

Purpose

Conceptual skills: number and number quantity, money and money quantity

Part A

Materials
  1 penny
  1 nickel
  1 dime
  1 quarter
  1 dollar bill

Instructions

First, the therapist should shake the container holding the materials and ask the student, "What does this sound like?"

The therapist removes one penny and places it on the table in front of the student 6 inches from the front of the table and asks, "What is this?"

The therapist removes one nickel from the file and places it on the table to the right of the penny and asks, "What is this?"

The therapist carries out the same procedure with the dime, quarter, and dollar.

Part B

Materials
  4 pennies
  2 nickels
  3 dimes
  2 quarters

Instructions

All coins from Part A are removed. The therapist places four pennies on the table 6 inches from the front of the table and centered at the student's midline, and asks, "How much is this?"

The therapist removes three of the pennies and positions two nickels to the right of the penny. The therapist asks, "How much is this?"

The therapist removes all the coins and places one dime and one quarter in a row on the table 6 inches from the front of the table at the student's midline. The therapist asks, "How much is this?"

The therapist leaves these coins on the table and places one quarter, two dimes, two nickels, and four pennies in a row next to them. The therapist asks, "How much is this?"

Part C

Materials
  1 cash register receipt with a total between $2.11 and $2.24
  1 dollar bill
  5 quarters
  6 dimes
  3 nickels
  4 pennies

Instructions
  All material from Part B are removed. The therapist arranges the materials as shown:

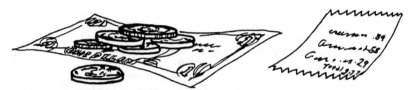

  The therapist says, "Please find the total on the cash register receipt and read it out loud."

  The therapist continues, "Please find the exact amount of money that you just read on the receipt [Point to the pile of money]."

Part D

Materials
  1 inexpensive magazine (priced under a dollar)
  All the money from Part C

Instructions
  The cash register receipt is removed from the table; all the money remains. The therapist holds the magazine in his or her left hand and says:

  "You are a sales clerk in a store, and I am a customer who would like to buy this magazine. Here is a dollar. [Hand the student the dollar bill from the pile of money on the table.] Please give me the correct change. [Hold out your hand with palm up.]"

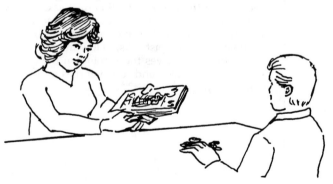

Timing
  Begin timing after you have completed each question that calls for a response from the student.

14

Task 10

Functional Banking
Purpose
   Conceptual skills
   Ability to follow written directions
   Use of tools

Part A

Materials
   1 bank check (3½″ × 10″)
   1 #2 pencil
   1 8½″ × 11″ sheet of white paper with the following information in bold
   print:
   NAME _____
   1.   What is the date on the check? _____
   2.   What is the amount of the check? _____
   3.   To whom is the money being paid? _____
   4.   What is the account number? _____
   5.   Whose account will the money come from? _____

Instructions
   The therapist arranges the materials as shown below:

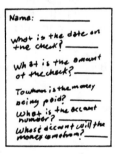 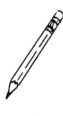

The therapist then says:

"Here is a bank check. [Point to the check.] The questions on this paper
[point to the paper] are about the bank check. Write the correct answers for
each question. Do you have any questions? [Wait for a response.] Please
begin."

15

Part B

Materials
   1 calculator
   1 bank check from Part A
   1 #2 pencil

Instructions
   The therapist removes the question sheet from Part A and arranges the materials as shown:

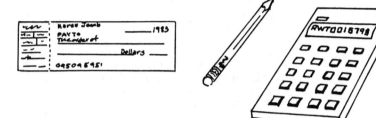

   The therapist instructs the student:

   "Please use this calculator [point to calculator] to find the balance in this account after the check is paid. Please tell me the amount out loud. Do you have any questions? [Wait for a response.] Please begin."

Timing
   Begin timing the moment after you say *begin*.

16

Task 11

Time Concepts
Purpose
   Conceptual skills

Part A

Materials
   1 3″ × 5″ card with a drawing of a clock reading 3:00 (clock #1)
   1 3″ × 5″ card with a drawing of a clock reading 3:30 (clock #2)
   1 3″ × 5″ card with a drawing of a clock reading 4:15 (clock #3)

Instructions
   The therapist places clock 1 on the table 6 inches from its edge and centered
   in front of the student. The therapist asks, "What time is it?" [Point to the
   clock.]
   The therapist follows a similar procedure with clocks 2 and 3.

Part B

Materials
   Clocks 2 and 3

Instructions
   Clocks 2 and 3 are placed next to each other on the table 6 inches from its
   edge and centered in front of the student. The therapist says, "It is in the
   afternoon. Which clock has the later time?"

Part C

Materials
   1 3″ × 5″ card with a drawing of a digital clock reading 12:40

Instructions
   All items from Part B are removed, and the digital clock card is placed on
   the table 6 inches from the edge and centered in front of the student. The
   therapist says:

   "Please look at this clock. If you are taking a break at this time [point to
   clock], what time would it be after 30 minutes?"

Timing
   Begin timing the moment after you have completed each question.

17

Task 12

Work Attitudes
Purpose
  Sequencing
  Work attitude
  Decision making

Part A

Materials
  5 cards (3½″ × 4¼″) each depicting a step in a sequence of a student purchasing food at a fast-food restaurant

Instructions
  The therapist places the five cards randomly on the table within the student's
  reach and says:

  "These picture cards tell a story, but the pictures are all mixed up. Please put
  them in order from start [point to the left side of the table] to finish [points
  to the right side of the table]. Do you have any questions? [Wait for a
  response.] Please begin."

Part B

Materials
  None

Instructions
  The therapist removes the cards from the table and says:

  "You are working at McDonald's. Your job is to keep the shop clean. You
  are going on your lunch break when a customer drops a cup of coffee on the
  floor. What should you do?" [Wait for response and then go on to next
  question.]

  "You have 15 minutes left to work. Your friend comes into McDonald's and
  says, ' "No one is looking. Why don't you leave work now?' What do you
  do?" [Wait for a response and then go on to next question.]

  "You are working at the grill at McDonald's when a fire starts. What do you
  do?"

Timing
  Begin timing after you have completed giving each question.

18

Task 13

Body Scheme
Purpose
    Organizational skills
    Visual memory
    Position in space

Materials
    1 8½" × 11" drawing of a teenage boy
    5 drawings of the boy cut into the following parts: 5 heads, 5 torsos, 10 arms, 5 pairs of legs, 10 feet

Instructions
    The drawing of the boy is placed on the table 6 inches from the edge and centered in front of the student. The therapist says:

    "Here is a picture of a boy. Look at this picture carefully." [Leave the picture on the table for 15 seconds and then remove it from the student's view.]

    Arrange the five cut drawings of the boy on the table randomly and say:

    "Put these pieces together to make copies of the boy that was on the paper that was shown before. Do you have any questions? [Wait for a response.] Please begin."

Timing
    Begin timing the moment after you say *begin*.

19

Task 14

Leather Assembly
Purpose
  Organizational skills
  Fine motor coordination
  Use of tools
  Reward (student keeps finished product)

Materials
  1 standard-size rotary leather hole punch
  1 wooden leather mallet (1½″ × 4″)
  2 key rings
  6 sets of small rivets
  2 1″ × 3″ 7-oz leather strips
  1 plastic box (4″ × 4″ × ½″) to hold rivets, leather, and rings

Instructions
  Before giving this task, the therapist should be familiar with the construction of the key ring (see Fig. 4-23).
  All materials are placed randomly on the table. Before beginning the assembly, the therapist says, "Watch what I do so you can do the same after I finish."
  The therapist then demonstrates the construction of the key ring without speaking. When it is completed, the therapist says, "Now you make the same key ring." [Point to the model key ring and then remove it.]

Timing
  Begin timing after you have completed the instructions.
  Please note that since one of the purposes of this task is to reward the student, you should assist the student in completing the task if he or she is having difficulty.

Task 15

Food Preparation

Purpose
  Ability to follow visual directions
  Use of tools
  Reward

Materials
  1 stick of softened margarine
  1 small jar of honey
  1 small mixing spoon
  1 teaspoon
  1 butter knife
  1 small plastic bowl
  1 box of crackers
  5 4¼" × 5½" cards showing how to make honey butter

Instructions
  The illustration cards are placed on the table in a row from card 1 to card 5. All other materials are arranged randomly on the table. The therapist instructs the student:

  "Please follow the cards to make honey butter. When you have finished making the butter, spread some on *two* crackers. You may eat the crackers with the butter when you are finished. Do you understand? Please begin."

Timing
  Begin timing the moment after you say *begin*.

21

REFERENCES

1. Gerber, P. J. "Learning Disabilities and Vocational Education—Realities and Challenges," in K. P. Lynch, W. E. Kiernan, and J. A. Starks (Eds.). *Prevocational and Vocational Education for Special Needs Youth: A Blueprint for the 1980s.* Baltimore: Paul H. Brookes, 1982. Pp. 185–197.
2. Lynch, K. P., Kiernan, W. E., and Stark, J. A. (Eds.). *Prevocational and Vocational Education for Special Needs Youth: A Blueprint for the 1980s.* Baltimore: Paul H. Brookes, 1982.

Work-Related Programs for Children and Adolescents

My Other Brother Daryl

Let me introduce you to Daryl.
He is 18 years old, TMH (30–40 IQ).
Been in school for 12 years.
Never been served in any setting other than elementary school.
He has had a number of years of "individual instruction."
He has learned to do a lot of things.
Daryl can now do lots of things he couldn't do before!
He can put 100 pegs in a board in less than 10 minutes while in his seat with 95 percent accuracy.
   But, he can't put quarters in vending machines.
Upon command he can "touch" nose, shoulder, leg, foot, hair, ear. He's still working on wrist, ankle, hips.
   But, he can't blow his nose when needed.
He can now do a 12 piece Big Bird puzzle with 100 percent accuracy and color an Easter Bunny and stay in the lines!
   But, he prefers music, but was never taught how to use a radio or record player.
He can now fold primary paper in halves and even quarters.
   But, he can't fold his clothes.
He can sort blocks by color; up to 10 different colors!
   But, he can't sort clothes; white from colors for washing.
He can roll Play Dough and make wonderful clay snakes!
   But, he can't roll bread dough and cut out biscuits.
He can string beads in alternating colors and match it to a pattern on a DLM card!
   But, he can't lace his shoes.
He can sing his ABC's and tell me names of all the letters of the alphabet when presented on a card in upper case with 80 percent accuracy.
   But, he can't tell the men's room from the ladies' room when we go to McDonald's.
He can be told it's cloudy/rainy and take a black felt cloud and put it on the day of the week on an enlarged calendar (with assistance).
   But, he still goes out in the rain without a raincoat or hat.
He can identify with 100 percent accuracy 100 different Peabody Picture Cards by pointing!

But, he can't order a hamburger by pointing to a picture or gesturing.
He can walk a balance beam frontwards, side-ways or backwards!
But, he can't walk up the steps of bleachers unassisted in the gym to go to a basketball game.
He can count to 100 by rote memory!
But, he doesn't know how many dollars to pay the waitress for a $2.50 McDonald's coupon special.
He can put the cube in the box, under the box, beside the box and behind the box.
But, he can't find the trash bin in McDonald's and empty his trash into it.
He can sit in a circle with appropriate behavior and sing songs and play "Duck, Duck, Goose."
But, nobody else in his neighborhood his age seems to want to do that.
I guess he's just not ready yet!

—*Peter Lewis*[11]

This prose poem epitomizes the need for initiating work programming that is functional at a young age rather than teaching splinter skills.

OCCUPATIONAL CHOICE PROCESS

In the transition from childhood to adulthood, a person undergoes an important process of occupational choice: exploration, tentative choice, and realistic definite choice. Maurer has suggested that we learn how to work through a sequential process that begins in childhood [9, 10] (Table 5-1). She notes that the rate of learning and the age of achievement of various stages may vary among individuals.

Because occupational choice is a dynamic process, programming must

Table 5-1.   Developmental Tasks in Prevocational Development

Age (years)	Task	Sample Activities
5–10	Identification with a worker	Role modeling in play and fantasy Imitation of workers
?–adolescence	Learning about work	Observing the environment
?–adolescence	Getting along with peers	Interaction with others in play and work
10–15	Formation of basic habits	Organization of time and behavior Part-time jobs School work Chores
?–18	Self-concept elaboration, including:	Reactions of significant others
11–12	Interests	Identifying likes and dislikes
13–14	Capacities	Awareness of what person does well
15–16	Values	Selecting what is important in life
?–adolescence	Relation to authority	Obeying parents Obeying other adults, teachers Adjusting to supervision

From P. A. Maurer, in K. Reed and G. Sanderson, *Concepts of Occupational Therapy* (2nd ed.). Baltimore: Williams & Wilkins, 1983.

begin at an early age, with the introduction of activities to foster career awareness and the exploration of vocational capabilities and interests. Although such awareness and exploration must be reinforced with "normal" children, it is particularly critical for programming to be presented developmentally and initiated at an early age for children with special needs. This is because in many cases these children receive limited exposure to the world of work, have limited career expectations on the part of parents and society, and take longer to incorporate a new skill into their behavioral repertoire.

HOME ENVIRONMENT

Exposure to the world of work should begin at home by being integrated into the preschool child's play activities. The child should be provided with toys, games, and books that have work themes and promote positive work concepts. (Appendix 5-1). Role-playing a worker can be encouraged by having available dress-up clothing and materials that resemble those of various jobs. Lynch and associates have proposed a constellation of activities that can be considered in a developmental sequence of work-related programming [7] (Table 5-2).

Repetition and practice are vitally important to children with special needs. They should be provided the opportunity to regularly participate in home chores, such as vacuuming, caring for a pet, throwing out the garbage, making beds. Chores should be graded and once mastered, be increased in quantity, duration, and level of difficulty (for example, progressing from assisting with emptying the dishwasher, to removing one's own dishes from the table after a meal, to independently setting the table, to preparing one's own lunch) [6].

Family involvement is important to developing positive work concepts. However, too often, well-meaning people tend to do for a child tasks that the child could accomplish if expectations were not based on time, tolerance, or temperament. Most of the time, the child can accomplish a chore independently if given enough time or if tasks are graded into less complex steps.

Typical first jobs, such as delivering newspapers or selling lemonade on the street corner, should be encouraged. Visits to the parents' work places, with explanations of the job and its tools, can provide exposure to work roles and a positive work concept. Visits to other types of jobs will provide the child with even greater exposure and exploration to the world of work (Fig. 5-1).

SCHOOL ENVIRONMENT

Beginning in kindergarten, the school environment should also foster the development of appropriate work behaviors, work skills, aptitudes, and physical capacities. This process involves the development of functional curricula based on business enterprises and simulated in the school or at actual job sites. While on-site job training is preferred, it is not always possible to arrange. Work environments that simulate actual business enterprises—such as a fast-food restaurant, supermarket, flo-

Table 5-2.   Activities for Work-Related Programming by Developmental Stage

Age (years)	Activity
3–7	Elevating parents' expectation of child's vocational potential Sorting (large cue difference) Stacking Attending behavior Simple direction following
7–12	Working alone Working in small groups Higher rates of attending Sorting (small cue differences) Small assembly (hand and simple tool) Switching task upon command Starting to work on time Remaining at activity site until given permission to move

12–18	High rates of production on assigned tasks
	High rates of attention on high- and low-interest tasks
	Low error rates
	High rate of switch-task compliance
	Starting to work on time
	Returning from breaks promptly
	Remaining at work station
	Signaling supervisor when encountering difficulties
	Working alone
	Working in groups
	Working quietly
	Recognizing work defects
	Correcting work defects
	Using common tools
	  Hand tools
	  Power tools
	Work site safety behavior
	  Head protection
	  Uniform use
	  Eye protection
	  Recognition of and response to work site warning signs

From K. F. Lynch, W. E. Kiernan, and J. A. Stark (Eds.), *Prevocational and Vocational Education for Special Needs Youth: A Blueprint for the 1980s*. Baltimore: Paul H. Brookes, 1982.

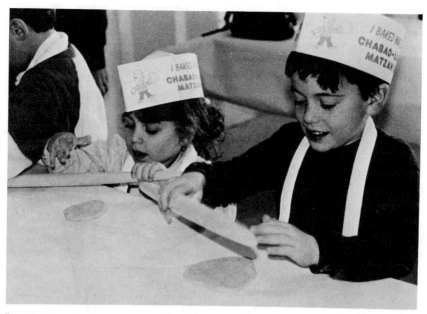

Figure 5-1.   Exposure to various types of jobs through school field trips. On one such trip, children had the opportunity to perform the tasks involved in making matzoh.

rist, bakery, or greeting card company—can be created in the school. Academic training can be easily integrated into this model through collaborative efforts of the occupational therapist and teacher. For example, simple arithmetic problems can be designed around the purchase of a week's groceries or a cheeseburger and fries, while allowing the children to practice work behaviors. To approximate actual industrial demands, training should move from the school to actual job sites as soon as possible.

TRANSITIONING

By the high school years, educational programming should have an increased focus on work, especially the opportunity to work in the community, which will assist in the transition process upon graduation from high school. In addition, transitioning is dependent on three "pillars" of successful community adjustment: residential environment, employment, and social and interpersonal networks (Figure 5-2) [4]. For the student with special needs, the transition process should begin at least two years prior to graduation.

Wheeler remarks, "Transition is both a *product* and a *process*. The product of effective transitioning should be successful community adjustment. The process of transitioning involves determining what types and levels of support are needed to assure individuals the most normalized lifestyle possible"[13].

According to Wehman, transitioning is a three-step process involving:

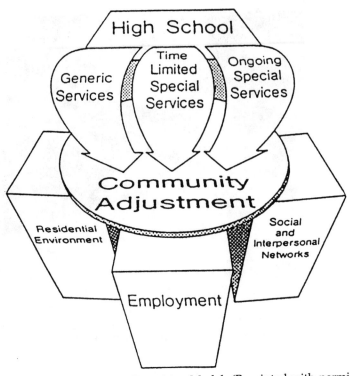

Figure 5-2.   Halpern's Transition Model. (Reprinted with permission from A.S. Halpern [4].

1. Input and foundation—the educational foundation acquired during the school years, particularly high school
2. Process—"the planning and implementation of formal individualized transition plans, the utilization of consumer input, and the development of interagency cooperation and coordination"[3, p. 10]
3. Outcome—vocational placements, residential environment, and social and interpersonal networks [12].

In this chapter a small sampling of occupational therapy work practice with various child and adolescent populations will be presented. Although the programs described do not reflect the entire spectrum of disabilities served by the occupational therapist, they together contain the elements necessary for developing programs for any group.

LITTLE PEOPLE'S SCHOOL

In 1970 the Little People's School was established as a private, nonprofit day school for students aged 3 1/2 to 15 years with severe learning difficulties and language and hearing problems. The school serves 85 communities in the Boston area. It is certified by the Department of Education of the Commonwealth of Massachusetts for special needs children, conforming with Massachusetts Public Law 766 and U.S. Public Law 94-142.

Since 1979 the Little People's School has provided work-related occupational therapy programming to a preadolescent and adolescent learning-disabled population.* The work-related program was established to meet the changing needs of the occupational therapy population. Because of these students' ages, the need had arisen to begin planning programs that would assist in developing the behaviors and skills important for future vocational tasks and job placement.

The first step in the process of program development was to assess students' level of functioning. As indicated in Chapter 4, no assessments were available that could be utilized with a learning-disabled adolescent population. Therefore an assessment had to be developed. I devised the JPSA to meet this need. This 15-task evaluation assesses the student's ability in a variety of work-related areas (see Chap. 4 for an in-depth look at this instrument).

After the student has completed the JPSA, an interest inventory is sent to his or her home to ascertain leisure skills and interests. Information gathered from the assessment, the interest inventory, classroom observations, and informal discussions with the student and staff was used in developing the occupational therapy programs at the Little People's School. These programs include an arts and crafts fair, assorted crafts (e.g., needlepoint), business skills, food service skills, horticulture, job simulation, leathercraft, leisure and life skills, and woodworking. This is not an all-inclusive list of available activities. For example, the Little People's School has established a work activity center (see Figure 5-19, p. 163). Many other activities can readily be adapted to a work-related skills focus.

Because of limited funds, in developing each activity I investigated community and school resources. For example, for the business skills activity we needed equipment and supplies to simulate an office environment—typewriters, office furniture. IBM Corporation was contacted for typewriters because it has a special needs program that provides renovated electric typewriters at a reduced cost to persons with physical disabilities. In addition, IBM provided, at a small cost, a spastic key guard, which is a shield that covers the keyboard and has holes cut out over the keys to prevent misstrikes. The key guards were not only useful for occupational therapy students who have cerebral palsy or motoric problems but were beneficial in some manner for the majority of students, by providing tactile input and making figure-ground distinctions easier. For more information on the IBM special needs program, contact your local office for eligibility criteria.

Stone & Webster Engineering Corporation was contacted for the donation of office furniture. The Corporation gladly gave us its obsolete

*There are four common types of learning disabilities: (1) reading disabilities, which usually indicate perceptual difficulties; (2) language and writing problems—difficulty reproducing written symbols or repeating sounds; (3) problems with concepts and abstractions—an inability to find commonalities in beings or subjects; and (4) behavior problems—distractibility, short attention span, inability to sit still, unwillingness to cooperate.

items—typing tables, secretaries' desks, time clocks, filing racks, metal stamps—which were received as treasures for our program. We have an ongoing relationship with Stone & Webster, which generously donates outdated equipment and material for our students.

Local copy shops were contacted for surplus paper items. One such company eagerly kept for us a box of assorted scrap paper, which we carted away weekly.

Theoretical Framework

In each occupational therapy program, activities are presented in sequential order based on the hierarchical stages of play specified in the occupational behavior approach. These three stages are as follows:

1. *Exploratory play* is the earliest kind of play behavior; the individual is motivated by curiosity and interest in novelty. He or she "plays" with the many aspects of an object. In this process, the individual learns not only about the objects, but about his or her own capabilities and limits.
2. *Competency behavior* is a skill-building stage. In this stage one practices newly acquired skills in an effort to achieve mastery.
3. In the *achievement* stage the individual is engaged in interacting with the environment with an emphasis on performance, using an external standard of excellence and taking risks.

The rationale for using this model is that play is the antecedent to work. Gayle Thompson has devised a clinical model of vocational development that has been most beneficial in formulating the program (Fig. 5-3).

To ensure continuity in the occupational therapy program between the school's divisions (elementary and secondary), all occupational therapy is now based on a work-related skills training model. What this means in fact is that along with the student's academic curriculum, the majority of learning experiences provided have a direct relationship to career or prevocational development. It is hoped that by infusing these basic work skills at an elementary and middle school age, we will have a longer period of time for reinforcement. The difficulty one finds in attempting to provide vocational programming originating at a secondary level will, it is hoped, be alleviated by initiating this early training.

Occupational Therapy
Arts and Crafts Fair

The goal of work-related occupational therapy programming is exemplified by our arts and crafts fair. The fair was created as an opportunity for students to make a transition into a work role, with exposure to other students, family, and the local community, within the confines of a safe, structured environment. This was all done within the milieu of the fair and its preparation (Fig. 5-4).

Preparation for the fair, which was originally held every spring, began after Christmas vacation. Students from this time on prepared items that would be sold, for example, cookbooks, belts, plants, needlepoint

Phase 1

INITIATION: AWARENESS, INTEREST, MOTIVATION

Models
Hershenson's social-amniotic and self-differentiation stages
Reilly's exploration stage
Mosey's individual interaction (pregroup) and parallel group

Goals
Client feels safe and supported, discovers interests, becomes motivated, and
    seeks to become identified with the group of "workers" in the setting

Climate
Supportive, relatively free, nonstressful
Planned variety and novelty in surroundings to invite interest and exploration
Opportunity to explore, repeat, imitate successful models
Observable models of involvement; workmanlike, craftsmanlike, sportsmanlike
    behavior
Group members accept person first as visitor, then new member

Therapist's Role
Provides for client dependence and establishment of trust
Assistive, moving to some independence
Encourages, supports efforts
Gives guidance, provides some basic instruction

Activity Attributes
Exploration and engagement
Short-term, allowing for experimentation with variety of materials and products
Controllable materials and predictable products
Minimal tool use—either common tools or a few specialized or new tools
Choices available within activity materials and products
Use of different processes or independence in repeated processes
Exploration of what can be done (or will work) with certain materials

Figure 5-3.   Clinical model of vocational development. (Courtesy of
Gayle Thompson, M.Ed., OTR.)

Phase 2

MEMBERSHIP: SKILL AND HABIT DEVELOPMENT

Models
Hershenson's competence stage
Reilly's competence stage
Mosey's parallel, project, and egocentric cooperative groups

Goals
Client learns work skills and develops work habits and interpersonal behaviors,
    e.g., appropriately seeks feedback, accepts supervision, works cooperatively;
    acquires identity as a worker; finds areas of abilities and skills

Climate
Teaching-learning
Activity viewed as important in adult world
Role models of workers in instructors (staff and volunteers) and in peer groups
Opportunity to compare own performance with that of others
Specific knowledge of results of performance (work, habits, interpersonal)

Therapist's Role
Gives systematic instruction in work skills, tool use, and tool care
Gives clear orientation as to expected habits
Structures group interaction, provides model for task and maintenance roles,
    reinforces client in assumption of group and partner roles
Moves toward supervisor role
Provides feedback on skill and habit development and interpersonal attributes
Assists in problem solving and encourages independent problem solving

Activity Attributes
Skill development and problem solving
Products perceived as valued by adults
Longer-term, requiring delay of gratification and problem solving
Projects require planning, calculation, and organization of production
Emphasis on accomplishing whole processes
Creative expression is modified by tools and nature of materials
Problems require detection, correction, and assessment of results

Figure 5-3.   (continued)

Phase Three

TRANSITION: EXPERIMENTATION AND CHOICE

Models
Hershenson's independence stage
Reilly's achievement stage
Mosey's cooperative and mature groups

Goals
Client seeks to meet standards of quality and production, identifies realistic
areas of aspiration and development, and moves toward making choice

Climate
In protective setting, client expected to meet standards of workmanship and
to demostrate work habits acceptable in true work environment
In trial work placements, client tests work skills and habits with those of other
workers
Independence and initiative are reinforced
Client participates in shop maintenance, assists others, or functions as a foreman

Therapist and Client Roles
Therapist as work supervisor; client as apprentice, sometimes foreman
Therapist as resource supporting independence in work and community job
experimentation

Activity Attributes
Recognizing and attempting to meet standards
Advanced performance in areas of interest and skill selected by client
Transference of developed skills to real work tasks
Experimentation in real worker roles
Groups focusing on community and vocational reentry

Figure 5-3.   (continued)

projects. As the date of the fair approached, students in the food service
program made their baked goods and other products. All aspects of the
fair—setting prices, placing price tags on items, establishing student
work schedules, advertising, setting up decorations, selling merchandise, and clean-up—were attended to by the students under the supervision of the therapist. In addition, there was an extra incentive for
students' participation in the fair, a salary. This money came directly
from the fair's proceeds.

The fair was such a success that we now hold it twice a year—before
Christmas and during the spring—and it is now a school-wide event.
We have encouraged local participation and have sold, on a limited
basis, craft projects from other community programs that serve special
needs persons, for example, Fernald State School (see Chap. 6).

Business Skills

The purpose of the business skills program is to expose students to
typing as a means of communication. In addition, the development of
typing skills strengthens fine motor and eye-hand coordination, visual
discrimination, and memory.

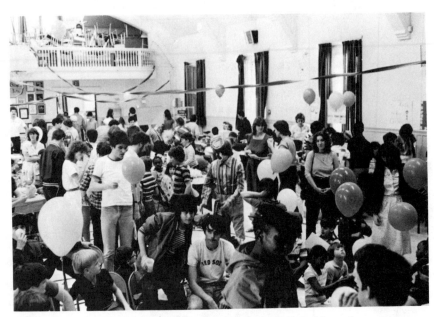

Figure 5-4.   Little People's School arts and crafts fair, held semi-annually.

Students are introduced to typing either individually or in groups of up to four. They are first allowed to explore the keyboard and are then instructed to type their own names. For the student who is unable to do this from memory, a typed representation of his or her name is shown as a guide. Next, the student types the alphabet in both capital and small letters.

Two texts were found particularly useful for these groups. The first, Jack Heller's *Typing for the Physically Handicapped: Methods and Keyboard Presentation Charts* is in two parts. The first part contains a discussion of effective methods of teaching typing to the handicapped. The second part contains 19 sets of keyboard presentation charts and drill lines for all possible combinations of missing fingers, for example, three fingers on the left hand and two on the right. Although this text is expensive ($100), the publisher has granted duplication rights for all illustrations [5]. The second text I found helpful was a linguistically oriented typing program called "Type It," developed by Joan Duffy, Learning Disabilities Supervisor for the Arlington Public Schools, Arlington, Massachusetts.*

When the student has gained some competency in typing and is beginning to use visual memory to find appropriate characters, he or she begins to type recipes for the school cookbook. This cookbook is subsequently duplicated and sold at the semiannual arts and crafts fair (Fig. 5-5).

In conjunction with typing, students are introduced to basic secretarial tasks: (1) the use of small office equipment such as photocopy machines, ditto machines, and electric staplers; (2) collating and sorting; (3) filing and retrieving; (4) dictionary use; and (5) use of the telephone directory.

*This program can be obtained from the author, c/o Arlington Public Schools, Arlington, Massachusetts 02174.

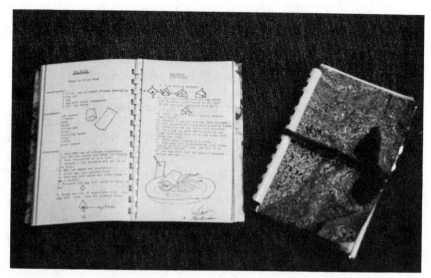

Figure 5-5.   Simple step-by-step cookbook developed by and for Little People's School students.

Food Service

Groups of two to three students are introduced to the kitchen by means of a simple step-by-step recipe book developed for these students (Fig. 5-5). The progression in the kitchen includes (1) safety and sanitation; (2) basic food preparation: spreading, pouring, opening, measuring and common abbreviations, and mixing; (3) knife skills; (4) basic kitchen appliance use: electric mixer, electric toaster oven, gas stove; (5) basic cooking: baking, frying and grilling, simmering, broiling; (6) setting a table; (7) serving meals; and (8) taking orders.

After the student has developed competence with the simple recipe book, he or she is introduced to regular step-by-step cookbooks and recipes cut off boxes or out of magazines. Finally he or she brings in a recipe that has been tested at home. Parents are encouraged to reinforce cooking skills at home with their children.

Role playing is an important aspect of these sessions. The roles of waiter or waitress, busboy or busgirl, salad maker, chef, host or hostess, and shortorder cook are introduced.

These student groups prepare all the baked goods for our semiannual arts and crafts fair and during the fair cook egg rolls, pizza, and tacos.

Horticulture Training

The horticulture training program has many purposes:

1. To expose the student to the fundamentals of greenhouse operation and processing; plant growth and identification; preparation of soil mixes; and seeding, potting, and planting techniques
2. To develop leisure interests
3. To develop vocational interests
4. To promote social skills such as working cooperatively, solving

problems and making decisions in groups, and organizing school tours of the center and field trips to local nurseries

Since space is limited, our horticulture center is composed of three metal wall shelves, each with a 4-foot plant light suspended over it. Despite all odds, we have been able to grow numerous varieties of flowering and foliage plants and vegetables from seeds. In addition, we have grown herbs and bean sprouts, which were used in our food service program. Students in the horticulture training program are also involved in the arts and crafts fair by selling their school-grown plants.

The following sample gradation of simple to complex horticulture activities may be found useful in planning this type of program:

1. Moving plants from one shelf to another
2. Carrying pots to shelves after they have been washed
3. Filling trays with pebbles
4. Arranging flats in stairs
5. Spraying plants with a flower sprayer
6. Filling and carrying watering cans and flower sprayer
7. Determining when pebble tray is dry and filling it with water; determining when individual potted plants are dry and watering them with watering can
8. Fertilizing individual potted plants
9. Washing pots and sorting them according to size
10. Removing dead leaves from plants
11. Weeding flats of seedlings and potted plants
12. Swabbing foliage to eradicate insects
13. Transplanting plants from small pots to larger ones
14. Noting when cuttings have roots and planting them
15. Measuring fertilizer and applying it to plants
16. Taking cuttings from plants
17. Dipping cuttings into root-promoting substance and putting them in sand
18. Staking individual plants
19. Planting bulbs in pebbles
20. Planting seedlings in flats
21. Writing one's own name, the date, and the type of seed for identification
22. Arranging cut flowers in suitable vases
23. Reading a thermometer
24. Measuring the distance from the top of the plant to the plant light
25. Identifying and naming plants with the help of a book
26. Deciding on plant prices for the arts and crafts fair
27. Giving a tour of the horticulture center to other students and staff.

Job Simulation

Job simulation is another method of reinforcing work skills and behaviors. Many jobs that simulate a work environment are available within the school, for example, office aide, maintenance assistant. The therapist uses these opportunities to have the student perform in a worker role under her supervision. In the case of the office aide, the student may run school errands or use the copy machine.

In addition, we frequently simulate the job of grocery store bagger, which is a realistic and age-appropriate job for some of our students. We have received support for this simulation from local supermarket chains that have given us supermarket supplies (e.g., a shopping cart) and have established programmed instructions on becoming a bagger.

Leather Craft

The rationale for using leather craft as a modality included (1) high student interest, (2) free access to equipment (I formerly had a leather business and lent all my equipment to the school), (3) limited cost or donation of supplies, and (4) the therapist's expertise. The occupational behavior model suggested the following sequence of activities:

1. The student is presented with a scrap piece of carving leather (6″ × 8″), a leather mallet, and 12 stamping tools and is allowed to explore this medium.
2. The therapist first demonstrates how to make a 3/4-inch-wide name wristband and then instructs the student to make one. This activity entails picking the correct letters for one's name from the alphabet stamping tools, stamping these letters in the correct sequence using a mallet, and returning them to their appropriate position in the alphabet.
3. The student is instructed to make a 1 1/2-inch-wide name belt.
4. The student chooses any appropriate project or one of the following projects: sun visor, wallet, coin purse, comb case.

Leisure and Life Skills

The occupational therapy department offered an eight-session leisure and life skills task group to four adolescent girls with the purpose of introducing options for using leisure time. This program evolved from the realization that a vast number of students spend their leisure time watching television or sitting at home with no concept of how to use unstructured time.

In this group the students were given the opportunity to decide on specific topics for each session. Each member, in addition to the therapist, was responsible for teaching topics. Briefly, these included naming the group and brainstorming for topics; a cooking project (Syrian bread); care of clothing—how to iron, fold, and hang clothing properly; making a leather name bracelet; grooming—use of makeup, nail care; babysitting; a needlepoint project; and gardening and flower arranging.

Woodworking

Students are exposed to basic woodworking activities by using prefabricated kits to make napkin holders, hot plates, key holders, and other items. The students learn to recognize and use tools and to handle them

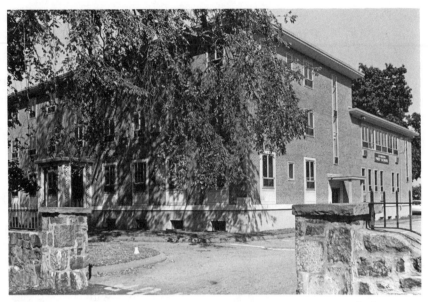

Figure 5-6.   Learning Prep School, located in West Newton, Massachusetts.

safely. They also learn sanding, gluing, staining, varnishing, and sawing.

LEARNING PREP SCHOOL

As the Little People's School administration realized the success of the
school's work-related occupational therapy program and the lack of a
similar secondary program in the area, the school was expanded in 1980
to include a secondary division. This division, called the Learning Prep
School, serves approximately 140 students 15 to 22 years old (Fig. 5-6).
It offers a language-based, life-centered curriculum designed to be flexible enough to meet the needs of the students. The program may lead
to a high school equivalency diploma.

In addition to functional academic education, the school offers several
work-related programs: a vocational program consisting of ten vocational training workshops; an occupational therapy program that provides both evaluations and treatment in the form of task groups; and a
work-study program that provides job placements in the community.
These three programs are described in the following sections.

Vocational Program

At the time the Learning Prep School was being developed, I was asked
to become its vocational coordinator and to develop and implement a
vocational program. Because of the success of the occupational therapy
program in the lower division, I used it as the basis for the vocational
program in the upper division.

The current and projected job market and the types of industry in
the local area assisted in determining the choices of vocational areas to

be offered in the program. Extensive research was performed by investigating regional vocational and technical schools and exploring the help wanted ads in the local newspapers. Other helpful resources included the Massachusetts Division of Employment Security, the Materials Development Center, Stout Vocational Rehabilitation Institute, University of Wisconsin-Stout (Menomonie, Wisconsin 54751), and the Jewish Vocational Services. After this in-depth search it became apparent that some of the original work-related occupational therapy programs could be expanded into vocational workshops. However, during the development of the programs, positive work behavior as the antecedent to specific skill development was recognized as equivalent in importance to job training. Therefore certain workshops that may not result in job placements were nevertheless included because they facilitate the development of interpersonal skills; responsibility to self, peers, and employers; and self-esteem. All the workshops operate on the premise that the development of work-related skills and behaviors is the basis for future job skills. This is reinforced by the school's system of grading, which reinforces workshop performance and behaviors such as arriving on time, organizing one's work area, attending to the task at hand, interacting positively with peers, and following directions (Fig. 5-7).

The original Learning Prep School workshops were business skills, carpentry, food service, graphic arts, horticulture, masonry, photography, and sewing. However, yearly research performed by the school to keep pace with the current and predicted job market revealed the need to expand or eliminate existing workshops and to develop new ones. Presently the school provides vocational training in the following fields: (1) automotive maintenance, (2) bicycle maintenance, (3) business skills, (4) carpentry, (5) child care, (6) food service, (7) graphic arts, (8) horticulture, (9) building maintenance, and (10) photography.

As with the work-related program for the lower division, the upper division vocational program was faced with limited funding. Once again I turned to the local community for support. For example, ADAP Discount Auto Parts stores donated supplies to begin the automotive maintenance program. Their interest in our school has continued, and in 1983 they donated a 1937 Plymouth, which was refurbished by the students and shortly afterward was sold at a school fund raiser (Fig. 5-8).

The vocational workshops are described below.

Automotive Maintenance

Training covers a variety of areas of automobile service, ranging from car washing and simple service-station-attendant functions to small-engine maintenance (Fig. 5-9).

Bicycle Maintenance

Students are trained in repairing and servicing bicycles and accessories. The assembly and inspection of parts is an integral part of the program. This workshop offers bicycle "tune-ups" to the staff at prices well below those in the community. With the proceeds the students are able to take periodic bicycle excursions (Fig. 5-10).

Student: _____   Teacher: _____
Workshop: *Graphic Arts*   Signature: _____
                                  Classes per Week: _____

FOCUS
(*indicates areas of concentration)

Illustrating
_____ Identifying, designing, and illustrating a logo
_____ Identifying and using basic typefaces in advertising
_____ Identifying, designing, laying out, and pasting up an ad
_____ Designing and illustrating an egg-shaped cartoon for advertising
_____ Designing and illustrating a fashion ad, a record album cover,
                 and a magazine cover

Printing
_____ Operating the platemaker (installing, checking, and cleaning
                 the electrostatic plates)
_____ Operating the plate processor
_____ Loading, operating, and maintaining the Gestetner Offset Press
                 (switchboard, panel controls, handwheel controls, and feed-
                 out board set-up)

SHOP PERFORMANCE AND BEHAVIOR
_____ Arrives on time
_____ Organizes work area
_____ Uses and cares for equipment properly
_____ Follows directions
_____ Attends to task
_____ Uses time efficiently
_____ Uses skills taught appropriately
_____ Completes a given task
_____ Interacts positively with peers
_____ Interacts positively with instructor

Comments

Figure 5-7.   Checklist used by graphic arts teacher Roger Tirrell at the Learning Prep School. Note the emphasis on work-related skills and behavior.

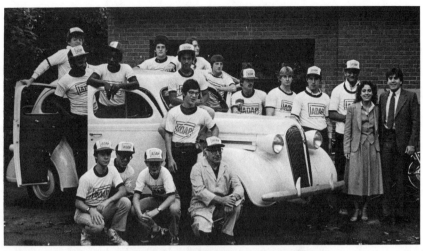

Figure 5-8.   Learning Prep School students with the 1937 Plymouth donated to the school's automotive workshop.

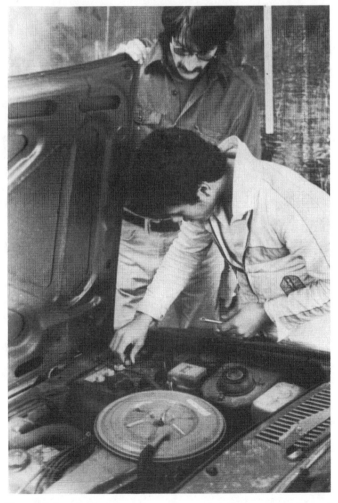

Figure 5-9.   A class in automotive maintenance at the Learning Prep School.

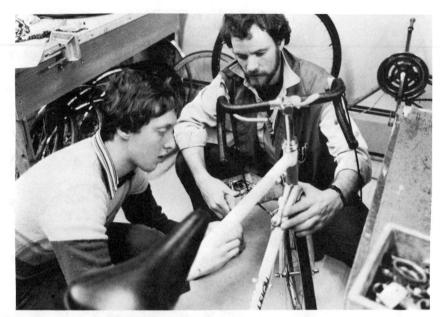

Figure 5-10.   Student learning bicycle maintenance and repair.

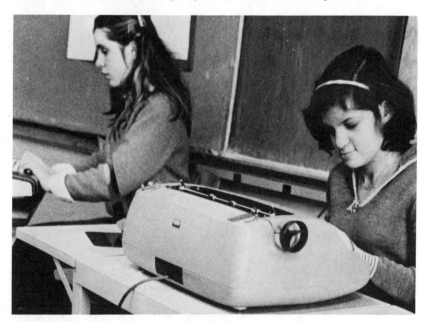

Figure 5-11.   Learning Prep School students practicing typing in their business skills workshop.

Business Skills

Activities in the business skills workshop primarily involve clerical tasks and distribution of information or messages by mail, by telephone, or in person. Students who enter this area may receive specialized training in typing, telephone use, and the operation of office machinery (Fig. 5-11). Integrated into the program is an emphasis on consumerism—checking and savings accounts, budgeting, credit application, charge accounts, and installment contracts.

Carpentry

The carpentry program has two levels: a basic course and more advanced apprentice training. Students are first trained in basic drafting, hand and machine skills, and measurements, which enables them to produce a variety of finished wooden projects (Fig. 5-12). The more advanced students have built a free-standing greenhouse and woodshed. The workshop has established a small business that sells its finished products to the public (Fig. 5-13).

Child Care

Students are trained to work as child care aides through on-site training at the school's child care center. These students are developing skills such as planning and implementing academic and nonacademic lessons and supervising children during play (Fig. 5-14).

Food Service

Students enrolled in the food service workshop are developing the basic skills of food preparation, safety and sanitation, equipment operation, nutritional standards, portion control, and customer service. These basic skills have enabled the students, under the instructors' auspices, to operate successfully a medium-scale federally certified lunch program and salad bar (Fig. 5-15).

Graphic Arts

The graphic arts program is designed to teach the fundamentals of printing and design. Students learn to operate a small offset press, an on-line typesetter, and a copy machine. The emphasis is on layout, paste-up, logo designing, and commercial illustration (Fig. 5-16).

Horticulture

The horticulture workshop is designed to train students in landscaping and greenhouse skills. Students learn the rudiments of lawn and tree care, landscape design, and proper use and care of mechanical equipment. The school's 14' × 22' free-standing greenhouse also affords students the opportunity to develop skills in plant propagation and care (Fig. 5-17).

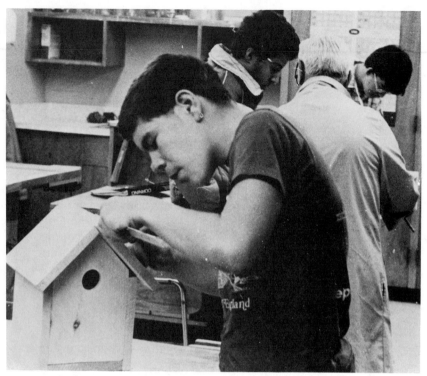

Figure 5-12.   A project in the carpentry workshop.

Building Maintenance

Students are trained in many aspects of building maintenance through on-site work. Dusting, sweeping, vacuuming, mopping, waxing floors, and washing windows are some of the activities in the curriculum. The student may also be trained to make minor repairs and become acquainted with cleaning equipment and cleaning agents.

Photography

In the photography workshop, students become familiar with basic photographic equipment, techniques, and vocabulary (Fig. 5-18). The development of good picture-taking and darkroom skills is an initial goal that serves as a foundation for a program encouraging creative self-expression and conceptual thinking. Projects include conventional documentary and studio photography in addition to exercises in multimedia work and special effects. In-house projects such as the yearbook and school-related publications are also an extension of the program. The students' work has been successfully displayed at the Carpenter Center for the Visual Arts at Harvard University.

Work Activity Center

According to a 1977 U.S. Department of Labor study, nearly half of all existing sheltered workshop programs are work activity centers [13]. Historically, such centers serve those who are not prepared to enter a sheltered workshop but who could benefit from exposure to work-oriented activities. Their purpose is to

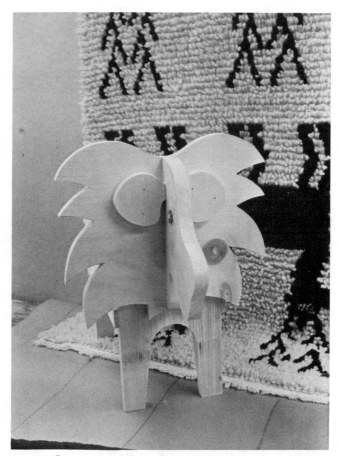

Figure 5-13.   Wood project constructed and for sale in the carpentry workshop.

provide appropriate and individualized developmental services to the whole person in order to build coping skills and abilities, enhance decision-making processes, foster independent or semi-independent living and develop vocational skills and related behaviors. The uniqueness of the individual will prevail in the program by recognition of strengths, weaknesses and individual personality traits.[1]

At the Little People's School we established a work activity center for the older students (10–16 years) to prepare them for the transition to secondary school; to stress work-related behaviors, skills, and habits such as problem solving, decision making, responsibility, perseverance, cooperative behavior, and quality control; and to provide training in the direction of sheltered work. Because of the success of this program, we have expanded the center to include secondary school students who can benefit from this experience.

During the developmental stages of our center, we approached many local sheltered workshops and work activity centers for tours and assistance. Through one of these contacts, we established a mutually helpful arrangement whereby our center became a satellite program of a large and active local workshop. For us, this arrangement was ideal:

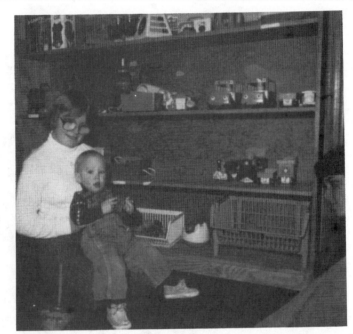

Figure 5-14.   Student learning child care in the Learning Prep School child care center.

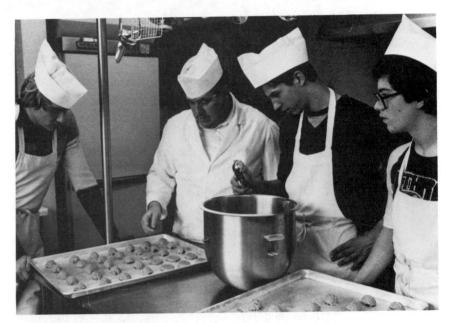

Figure 5-15.   Students learning food service.

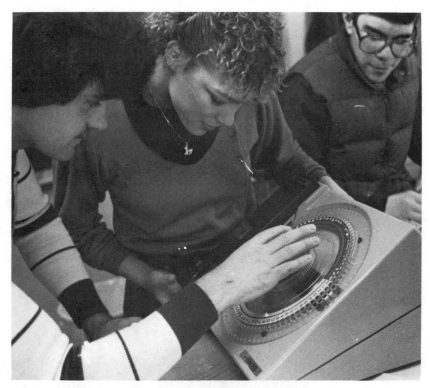

Figure 5-16.   A class in graphic arts.

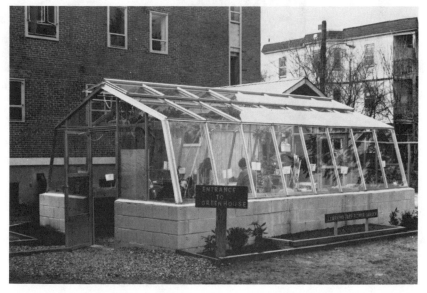

Figure 5-17.   Greenhouse constructed by students and staff at Learning Prep School and used in developing horticulture skills.

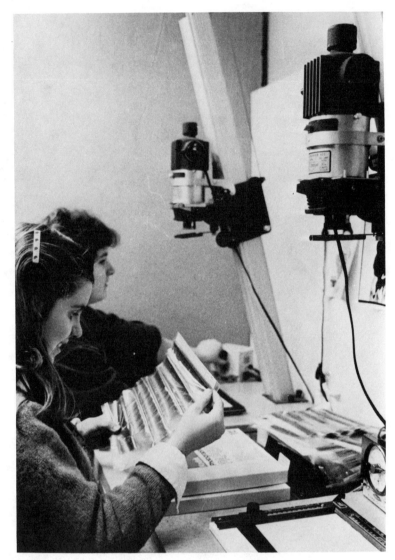

Figure 5-18.   The darkroom in the photography workshop.

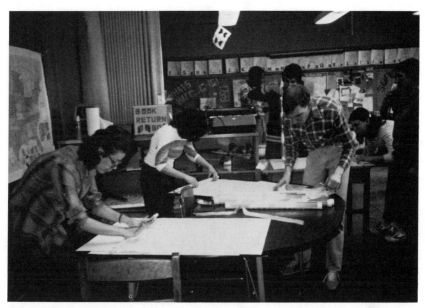

Figure 5-19.   Students doing piecework (rolling and packaging posters) at work activity center.

It not only eliminated the need for us to establish a certified program but also provided us with as much subcontract work as we can handle. During periods of contract overload, this local workshop provides us with subcontract work and the students receive remuneration for their production (Fig. 5-19). For periods when subcontract work is not available, the therapists have devised activities that simulate subcontract work, for example, collating, assembling, and packaging.

Occupational Therapy Program

Work-related occupational therapy is an integral link in Learning Prep School programming. The occupational therapist functions as the liaison between instructors and vocational and academic administrators. In this capacity the therapist acts as a consultant to personnel who may not have expertise in task and job analysis, adaptive and assistive equipment, techniques of work simplification, and activities of daily living. In addition, the therapist uses information from the JPSA to assist staff in developing teaching strategies based on the student's learning style. The therapist also functions as a role model, working side by side with several students or individually with one who may need extra attention. Various staff members including the psychologist, the nursing staff, the counseling staff, and physical and speech therapists collaborate with the occupational therapist to teach social skills through group discussion and modeling in such settings as sex education class, the lunchtime feeding program, and cardiopulmonary resuscitation (CPR) classes.

The occupational therapy department also provides evaluations and direct services to students who need remediation in specific work-related skill areas. A list of work-related behavioral objectives (Table 5-3 has been formulated for use as a guide in developing treatment plans

Table 5-3.   Work-Related Behavioral Objectives of Occupational Therapy

I.   Behavioral and Social
     The student
     A. Demonstrates oral and motor awareness
     B. Demonstrates oral and motor control
     C. Displays independence in performance of activities of daily living
     D. Displays awareness of appropriate repertoire of leisure activities
     E. Increases the frequency of appropriate informal social contacts
     F. Increases the frequency of appropriate social contacts with peers in a
         simulated work environment
     G. Controls disruptive behavior during therapy
     H. Controls frustration
II. Learning
     The student
     A. Performs matching and sorting tasks
     B. Performs classification tasks
     C. Performs alphabetizing tasks
     D. Demonstrates the ability to perform functional linear, liquid, and
         solid measurement
     E. Demonstrates the ability to perform functional money tasks
     F. Demonstrates the ability to perform one-to-one correspondence and
         number quantity tasks
III. Motor.
     The student uses compensatory strategies to
     A. Demonstrate fine motor coordination
     B. Demonstrate eye-hand coordination
     C. Demonstrate ocular motor control
     D. Demonstrate appropriate sitting posture
     E. Demonstrate the ability to use common tools, e.g., hammer, stapler
IV. Communication
     The student
     A. Demonstrates the ability to communicate basic needs appropriately
     B. Demonstrates the ability to follow
         1. two- to three-step visual directions
         2. two- to three-step verbal directions
         3. two- to three-step written directions
         4. two- to three-step visual and verbal directions
         5. two- to three-step visual and written directions
         6. two- to three-step verbal and written directions
         7. visual directions of three or more steps
         8. verbal directions of three or more steps
         9. written directions of three or more steps
         10. visual and verbal directions of three or more steps
         11. visual and written directions of three or more steps
         12. verbal and written directions of three or more steps
V.   Production
     The student
     A. Maintains task focus
     B. Carries out two- to three-step tasks in the proper sequence
     C. Carries out tasks of three or more steps in the proper sequence
     D. Adjusts work pace with supervision
     E. Adjusts work pace independently
     F. Accurately and consistently completes a specific task after having
         demonstrated the ability to perform the task
     G. Demonstrates flexibility in adapting to changes in the therapeutic
         program
     H. Independently maintains continuous work during a therapy session
     I. Monitors the quality of work produced in a therapy session

Table 5-3.   (continued)

VI.   Independence
       The student
       A.   Demonstrates the ability to use a model or sample to complete a task
       B.   Displays organizational skills
       C.   Develops and applies compensatory strategies to adapt activities for
             functional ability
       D.   Starts work independently
       E.   Begins work promptly upon receiving instructions
       F.   Solves problems in a simulated work setting
       G.   Makes decisions in a simulated work setting
VII.   Visual and perceptual
       The student uses compensatory strategies to perform activities involving
       A.   Figure-ground skills
       B.   Spatial relations
       C.   Directionality

and progress notes. Progress notes are written three times yearly with specific objectives selected and rated on a five-point scale. Fig. 5-20 shows a typical progress note.

The treatment offered by the occupational therapy department is in the form of occupational therapy task groups. Students are typically seen in task groups of two to five or six persons in two 45-minute sessions weekly. These group sessions provide a series of learning experiences that will enable the student to make appropriate vocational decisions and develop work habits necessary for eventual employment. Several of the task groups are described in the following paragraphs.

Babysitter Training

Social trends such as the trend toward more single-parent families, the increased number of families with both parents working outside the home, and the increased number of older siblings tending to younger family members have expanded the need for well-trained babysitters. For many adolescents, babysitting is one of the first opportunities to earn money and learn job responsibilities. Through the assistance of Laura Hollander, an occupational therapist from Faulkner Hospital in Jamaica Plain, Massachusetts, and the local chapter of the American Red Cross, we have developed a week-long intensive babysitter training program. This is open not only to the occupational therapy population, but to any Learning Prep School student, up to a maximum enrollment of 15.

In this training program, the students are guided through a sequence of hands-on exercises on topics such as telephone protocol, ethics and contracts, child development, accident prevention, diapering, mealtime, bedtime, discipline, mouth-to-mouth resuscitation and clearing of obstructed airways, fire safety (a local fire captain discusses what to do in case of fire), and safety (a local police sergeant discusses safety precautions, e.g., never leaving a child alone).

For those students interested in learning CPR, we schedule a certification course in the following weeks. Thus far 12 students have been CPR certified (Fig. 5-21).

Prevocational Occupational Therapy Progress Reports
April to June 1984

Name: Keith   Date of Birth: 2/5/65
I.D. #: 3340
Frequency of Treatment Sessions: Two per week
Modalities Used in Treatment: Craft and leisure activities, school yearbook,
                                             lunchroom cashiering
Tests Administered: Jacobs Prevocational Skills Assessment

Key

1 = Rarely (Student displayed this behavior 0–20% of the time in ther-
       apy.)
2 = Occasionally (Student displayed this behavior 21–40% of the time
       in therapy.)
3 = Approximately half the time (Student displayed this behavior 41–
       60% of the time in therapy.)
4 = Frequently (Student displayed this behavior 61–80% of the time
       in therapy.)
5 = Consistently (Student displayed this behavior 81–100% of the time
       in therapy.)

Therapy Goals Addressed This Term	1	2	3	4	5
Learning					
The student					
1. Performs alphabetizing tasks		x			
2. Demonstrates the ability to perform functional money tasks			x		
Motor					
The student uses compensatory strategies to					
1. Demonstrate fine motor coordination		x			
Communication					
The student					
1. Demonstrates the ability to communicate basic needs appropriately			x		
2. Demonstrates the ability to follow:			x		
a. two- to three-step verbal directions			x		
b. two- to three-step visual and written directions			x		

Figure 5-20.   Occupational therapy progress note.

Independence The student 1. Solves problems in a simulated work setting	x		
2. Makes decisions in a simulated work setting	x		
Visual and Perceptual The student uses compensatory strategies to perform activities involving 1. Figure-ground skills		x	

COMMENTS

Improvement has been noted in Keith's ability to assess accurately his personal strengths and weaknesses. Keith more frequently asks for assistance from both peers and supervisors in a simulated work setting and has responded to suggestions that he choose work tasks that emphasize his areas of strengths.

RECOMMENDATIONS

It is recommended that Keith's performance continue to be monitored by the occupational therapy department. A home program has been devised by the therapist and given to Keith's parents to be used by him over the summer vacation.

Figure 5-20. (continued)

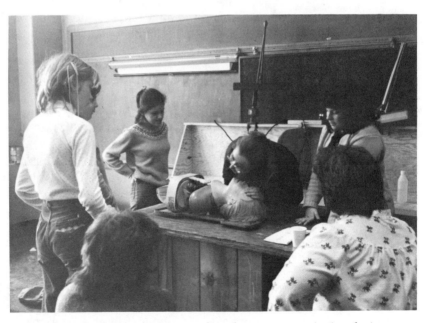

Figure 5-21.   Students practicing cardiopulmonary resuscitation during babysitter training class.

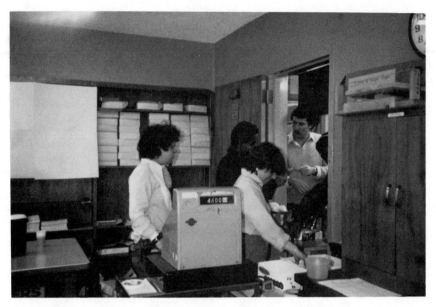

Figure 5-22.   Students working in the Learning Prep School store.

Library Group

The library group has set up and maintains the student library. Occupational therapy students perform tasks such as sorting books according to subject, labelling them (based on the Dewey Decimal System), and placing pockets containing cards inside the books. We hope this group will eventually become a functional pool of librarians.

School Store

Twice a week during class break, which lasts 20 minutes, two occupational therapy students operate a school store (Fig. 5-22). These students sell school supplies such as pencils and notebooks and refreshments such as fruit juice and cookies. Job responsibilities, which have been delineated by the students, include recording sales, checking inventory, tallying money, packaging items, and dealing with customers. A simulated banking system has been developed to monitor the store's profit, which I am happy to say is steady.

Yearbook

Occupational therapy produced the first school yearbook in 1982. Students serve as the production staff, determine the book's content, and schedule and monitor deadlines for various contributors such as the photography workshop and the printer. By selling advertising space in the yearbook, the students have been able to reduce the cost of the books and make this a financially independent venture.

Lunchroom Cashier

Before working in the lunchroom, students have the opportunity to practice in occupational therapy the job responsibilities of a lunchroom cashier—social interaction, money skills. Once the student feels ready, he or she enters the lunchroom setting to perform this job under the

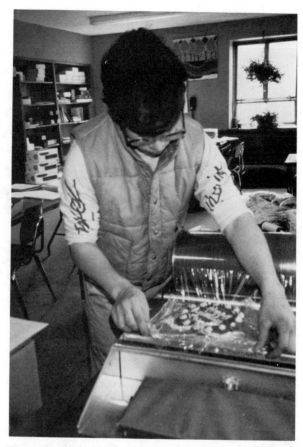

Figure 5-23.   Student shrink-wrapping a "cookie-gram."

therapist's supervision. This group has devised a system for keeping a record of those who owe lunch money, and it is the group's responsibility to dispense collection notices!

Cookie Group

Students were given the task of setting up a functional business enterprise. After many brainstorming sessions, they elected to establish a "cookie-gram" company, which bakes large (and delicious) chocolate-chip cookies and customizes them with frosting messsages (Fig. 5-23).

Students are responsible for all aspects of this business and learn to cope with working under pressure occasionally, for example, during a large-volume holiday season. This has been a very successful group; after only one year in business it is in the black.

Volunteer Program

Based on the transitional employment program model, the occupational therapist selected volunteer jobs (e.g., cafeteria aide) for appropriate occupational therapy students (Fig. 5-24). Once the job has been obtained, the following procedure is followed:

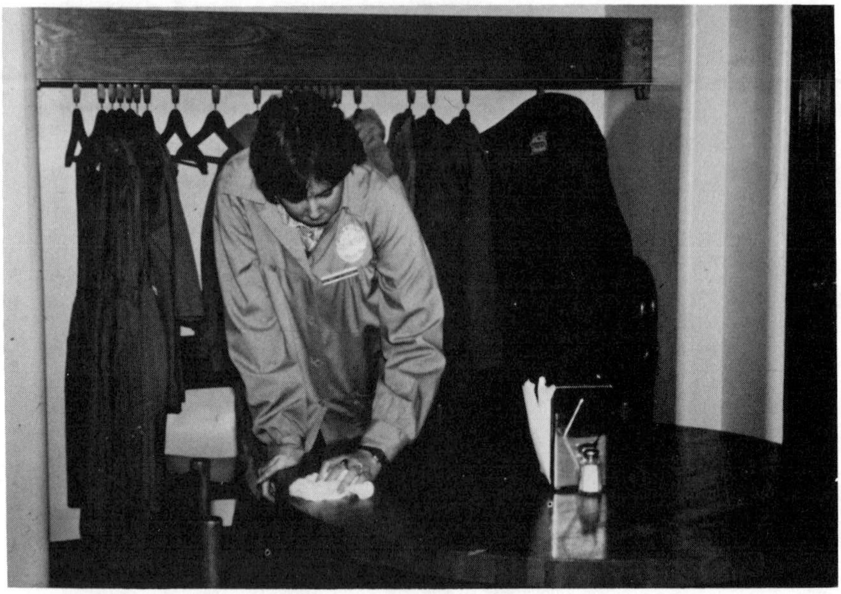

Figure 5-24.   Student working as a volunteer cafeteria aide at Newton-Wellesley Hospital, Newton, Massachusetts.

1. The therapist performs the job for a day or two to gain an understanding of what is required and what will be expected from the student.
2. The therapist performs the job side by side with the student.
3. The therapist watches the student perform the job.
4. The student performs the job without the therapist and eventually commutes to the job site independently.

Craft Group

The craft group is the lowest-level occupational therapy group. Group members engage in repetitive and structured craft and art activities, for example, leather craft, weaving, model assembly, sewing, and the traditional yearly construction of a colorful school banner, which is hung in the students' cafeteria. Typically the other items produced are sold at the semiannual arts and crafts fair.

Work-Study Program

In an additional administrative capacity as Job Placement and Development Coordinator, I have had the opportunity to apply my occupational therapy skills across the occupational choice process. The ultimate goal of our programs is to realize the greatest potential of all the students. When a student has learned the necessary prerequisite vocational skills and behaviors, he or she is eligible for the work-study program. This program has three components and may be viewed as a transition in the occupational choice process from career exploration to realistic career choice.

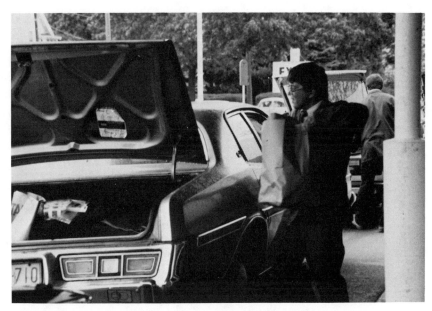

Figure 5-25.   Under the work-study program a student is a bundler-bagger at a local supermarket.

Volunteer Training

Volunteer training in the work-study program is an expanded version of the occupational therapy volunteer program (i.e., it involves more students and more time on the job). Volunteer positions are provided one or two days per week to expose students to various worker roles. Placement has been provided at local facilities such as hospitals and nursing homes and at the National Spinal Injury Foundation.

In-house Work-Study

In-house training in positions such as child care aide, office and maintenance assistant, and lunchroom cashier is provided on an alternate-week basis. The therapist consults with the staff at these job sites to assist them in developing programming that will facilitate the student's success in the "real" work world.

Work-Study

Students are placed in jobs appropriate to their skill levels and interests in their local communities on an alternate-week basis. Once placed in a job, the student may progress through the normal advancements of that position. Community response to hiring students has been excellent; many students are gainfully employed in the greater Boston area (Fig. 5-25).

Fund Raising

Common in education, particularly the private sector, is limited funding. I have been able to use small school fund raisers both to finance programs and equipment and to reinforce students' work-related behaviors and skills outside the school setting.

The Learning Prep School has fund-raising drives periodically to support, for example, the purchase of computers or recreational equipment. On these occasions we may raise funds by selling products such as cloth calendars, pot holders, beach towels, community theater tickets, and ads in our yearbook in the students' local communities. Participating students have the opportunity to practice social skills, by contacting persons in their communities; communication skills, by explaining what they are selling and why; and money skills. A prize program has been devised as a motivator so that students who sell the most receive a direct benefit from their efforts.

The Learning Prep School program has been nicely conceptualized by Nancy Mazonson in a model that also shows the parallel development of interests outside school and the occupational choice process (Fig. 5-26). The following case study will also assist in illustrating the occupational therapy program. The student, Stacey, was discussed in Chapter 4; her results on the JPSA were presented on pages 100–103. You may find it beneficial to refer to that section.

Case Study*
Name: Stacey
Chronological age: 17

Clinical Picture
Pregnancy was unremarkable. Stacey was born after a 12-hour labor, an Rh baby with jaundice. Postnatal developmental milestones were within normal limits: sitting up at 6 to 7 months, walking at 14 months, toileting at 3 years. Language development initially was within normal limits; however, vocabulary, phrasing, and sentence development delayed.

Medical History
No illnesses or hospitalizations. Stacey began to receive speech therapy at age 3. Therapy continued until age 5 1/2, when she entered kindergarten, at which time language and academic delays were noted and special school placement began. At age 13, Stacey entered the Little People's School.

Social Status
Stacey lives with her mother and two sisters.

Emotional Development
Stacey presently receives group and individual counseling at school to address feelings of low self-esteem. Stacey has used denial as a defense mechanism and has fabricated stories about her social life to appear normal to her peers. Stacey exhibits unrealistic expectations and denial of the limitations of her disability.

School Program
At present Individualized Educational Plan goals for Stacey are as follows:

Language
To improve receptive and expressive language, emphasizing vocabulary, understanding of concepts, grammar, and functional language.

Reading
To improve comprehension, vocabulary, and recognition of parts of speech.

*This case study was provided by Nancy Mazonson, M.S., OTR, Learning Prep School, West Newton, Massachusetts.

Occupational Choice Process	Fantasy and exploration stage	Tentative choice stage		Final stage
Learning Prep School Activities	Vocational workshops OT groups Cookie-gram group School store Library group Yearbook Craft group Cashier group Arts and crafts fair School fund raisers	Vocational Workshops In-house jobs Cashier Child care (volunteer) Office assistant Maintenance assistant Volunteer work Babysitter training	Narrower range of vocational workshops Child care ($) Maintenance ($) After-school job placement Summer job placement	Work/Study Job Apprentice training program
Parallel Development Outside School		Volunteer Work Babysitting Yard work Paper Route	After-school job Summer job	

Figure 5-26. Learning Prep School activities in relation to the process of occupational choice and nonschool activities. (Courtesy Nancy Mazonson, M.S., OTR.)

Math
To improve money, banking, and budgeting skills.

Study Skills
To improve dictionary skills, use of contextual clues to deduce word meanings, use of encyclopedia and reference pages, and letter-writing skills.

Career Awareness
To improve awareness of career options.

Vocational
Participation in three workshops: photography, food service, and child care.

Goals of Therapy

Speech Therapy
1. To discriminate between grammatical and nongrammatical sentences with 90-percent accuracy within a structured setting
2. To construct grammatical sentences in present and past tenses in conversation with 80-percent accuracy
3. To use self-monitoring skills to improve discrimination, identification, and correction of errors
4. To use turn-taking and listening skills in group conversation through the use of written and spoken sentences and paragraphs, role play, group discussion, and peer feedback.

Counseling
1. Individual—To improve expression of feelings and self-esteem
2. Group—To improve expression of feelings concerning the social stresses of adolescence and understanding and implementation of appropriate behavior in a variety of social settings

Occupational Therapy
1. To improve ability to assess strengths and weaknesses
2. To improve problem-solving and decision-making skills
3. To improve ability to use visual cues in following directions, sequencing, and memory
4. To improve ability to follow three-step directions
5. To improve fine motor skills
6. To improve functional money skills

Occupational Therapy Program
Stacey's occupational therapy activities are performed in a small group setting that simulates a work environment. Tasks involve measuring, manipulation of small objects, following written and oral directions, planning, decision making, and functional use of money.

Stacey's programming in occupational therapy has followed a progression of increasing difficulty. At ages 15 and 16 she participated in a variety of small task groups: cashiering group, production and craft work, girls club. By age 17 Stacey has developed the work skills and behaviors necessary for successful functioning in a highly supervised work environment. She has shown a particular interest in the child care vocational workshop and has expressed her desire to work in the area of human services in the future. As a result it has been recommended that Stacey become an assistant (apprentice) in the child care center, with expanded work hours. This placement is monitored by the occupational therapist, who provides consultation to the child care supervisors, so that programming and work responsibilities can be designed to foster growth in the areas of need assessed by the Jacobs Prevocational Skills Assessment.

In the child care setting Stacey can learn diapering, toileting, meal preparation, and clean-up procedures and how to maintain a time sheet. Supervision

Work Behavior Checklist

Name: _____

Date: _____

___	1. Attendance	Coming to work on the days you are supposed to
___	2. Punctuality	Coming to work on time
		Coming back from break on time
___	3. Starting work independently	Starting work by yourself without needing help
___	4. Independent work skills (initiative, follow-through)	Working on your own
		Finishing jobs you start
___	5. Attention span	Keeping your mind on your work
___	6. Use and care of tools and equpiment	Taking care of tools and equipment and using them correctly
___	7. Organizational work area	Keeping your work area neat and organized
___	8. Problem solving, judgment	Making good decisions if there is a problem
___	9. Quality of work	Always doing a good job
		Taking care of everything that needs to be done
		Being thorough
___	10. Work pace, work endurance	Working at a good speed—not too fast, not too slow
		Being energetic and staying with the job
___	11. Flexibility	Being able to make changes in the way you do the job
		Being able to do things in a new or different way
___	12. Meeting deadlines	Being able to have something finished or ready by a certain time
___	13. Safety rules	Remembering safety rules
___	14. General appearance	Dressing nicely for work
		Looking clean and neat for work
		Following the rules if there is a dress code
	Other:	

Figure 5-27.   Work behavior checklist. (Courtesy Nancy Mazonson, OTR.)

feedback on performance and self-assessment can be done on a weekly basis through the use of a work behavior checklist designed by the therapist (Fig. 5-27).

As implied by the variety of programs discussed in this book, the occupational therapist may assume many different roles in the context of work practice. In the following example, therapists have determined the need for additional evaluations and training of students to make an ongoing program more comprehensive.

MARGARET WALTERS SCHOOL

Located throughout the state of Colorado are Community Center Board programs, which provide services to low-functioning, developmentally disabled persons. The Margaret Walters School is one such program, addressing the needs of persons up to age 21 with IQs of 50 or below who have various diagnoses: Down's syndrome, developmental delays, mental retardation (etiology unknown), cerebral palsy, high-risk infancy. The school is actually just one arm of a larger organization called Jefferson County Community Center, a birth-to-death program consisting of several residential facilities, three workshops, two schools, and an intensive-care facility for those who would otherwise be in a nursing home.

The prevocational occupational therapy program, which was developed at the school by Sherry Olin and Mary Haldy, evolved from an ongoing Work Experience and Study (WES) program. The WES program, developed for students aged 18 to 21 years, involves a continuum of classroom study through in-house job placement to community job placement.

Therapists observing the WES program realized there was a need for an additional, more comprehensive evaluation to facilitate a better match between a student's strengths and an in-house or community job. Such an assessment was developed and became one of the major components of the current prevocational occupational therapy program. Other components include job task analysis, consultation, a decision-making group, and program planning.

Occupational Therapy Evaluation

Students' physical capacities, behavioral skills, interests, and tool use are evaluated to determine the students' strengths and weaknesses and to aid in making recommendations for job placement.

Physical Capacities

The department uses an adapted version of the Physical Capacities Evaluation developed by the Delaware Curative Workshop, Wilmington, Delaware, to determine ability and functional tolerances in standing, sitting, lifting, and repetitive work. The Purdue Pegboard, the Minnesota Rate of Manipulation Test, and the Bruininks-Oseretsky Test of Motor Proficiency are also given. Finally, range of motion testing and sensory testing are done.

Behavioral Skills

The Comprehensive Occupational Therapy Evaluation Scale (COTE scale) is used to assess behavior in various situations [2]. The scale defines 25 observable behaviors that "are particularly relevant to the practice of occupational therapy" [2]. These behaviors are divided into three categories: general behavior, interpersonal behavior, and task behavior. For example, under task behavior, decision making is evaluated in the following manner [2]:

Decision Making:
0—Makes own decisions
1—Makes decisions but occasionally seeks therapist approval
2—Makes decisions but often seeks therapist approval
3—Makes decision when given only two choices
4—Cannot make any decisions or refuses to make a decision

Each of the behaviors on the scale is rated from 0 to 4, with 0 representing normal function or an absence of problem behavior and 4 indicating a severe problem. Scores are totaled, and ratings can range from 0 to 100; higher scores indicate more severe problems. The COTE scale can be used to measure the student's progress in treatment programs.

Interests and Tool Use

An interest checklist is completed by each student. The student is also asked to perform workshop tasks, for example, hammering, bolting, stapling, punching holes, to determine his or her functional level of tool use.

Job Analysis

Before making a job placement, the therapist may arrange a visit to the proposed job site to analyze potential jobs, focusing on the following skill areas: (1) fine motor coordination, (2) gross motor coordination, (3) perceptual skills, (4) academic or cognitive skills, (5) social interactions, (6) tactile skills, and (7) tool use. For example, a day care aide job would be analyzed in the following manner:

Skill*	Job Requirement
S	Friendly and playful interaction skills
S	Giving directions, and keeping children involved in activity, finding new activities
S	Self-control and patience
S	Handling fights
S	Independence and decision-making skill
Tac	Tolerance for touching children appropriately
P	Finding toys and supplies on shelves and putting them away
P	Tolerating noise and confusion
P	Putting servings on plates and placing plates on table
A	Memory for names

A	Counting ability
FM	Fine motor ability (picking up small items, eg., puzzles)

---

*Key: S = social, Tac = tactile, P = perceptual, A = academic, FM = fine motor.

Through this process of job analysis, students have been appropriately placed in jobs such as cafeteria server, hotel and nursing home laundry helper, dishwasher, groundskeeper, day care aide, and maintenance assistant.

Consultation

The therapist may assume the role of consultant to the teaching staff to discuss such issues as appropriate job placement of students.

Decision-Making Group

Under the direction of a therapist, groups composed of several students who hold in-house or community jobs develop cooperative work habits, independence, and initiative. Students decide on an activity and then share the responsibility for its organization and implementation. In time the group becomes increasingly independent of the therapist. Eventually the therapist is able to determine which students will be successful candidates for different community or sheltered workshop jobs.

Program Planning

Therapists at the Margaret Walters School are involved in program planning to meet the long-term goal of extending the occupational therapy program to students aged 13 to 17, with the explicit purpose of developing or improving prevocational skills at an earlier age. It is hoped that earlier exposure will facilitate an easier transition into the WES program.

Case Study*
Name: David
Chronological age: 20 years

Reason for Referral
David was referred to occupational therapy for an assessment of strengths and weaknesses in fine and gross motor areas for current and future job placement.

Background Information
David has mental retardation, etiology unknown. He also had a ventricular heart defect and has undergone two heart catheterizations. He has a mild sensory hearing loss and usually wears a hearing aid in the left ear.

David was in special education programs from 1970 to 1975 before entering the Community Center Program.

Observations
David has participated in a weekly group meeting of several vocational students to increase independent decision-making skills. In this group David has dem-

*This case study was provided by Sherry Olin, OTR, and Mary Haldy, OTR, Margaret Walters School, Arvada, Colorado.

onstrated mature behaviors; he socializes appropriately with peers and staff, takes responsibility for his own actions, and is very cooperative. He is interested in most tasks and carries them to completion with few or no reminders. He is able to check his work and usually corrects his errors independently. David needs approval and guidance at times when making decisions or solving problems.

David's main interests are hiking and checkers. He usually listens to music and watches television after school. He has said that he would like to have more to do in his spare time.

Testing Results

Physical Capacities

The physical capacities test measures strength, endurance, balance, and ability to perform gross motor tasks. David demonstrated fairly good balance and endurance during the squatting and stooping activities, although he said his legs became a little tired. He climbed a stepladder easily and safely while carrying a paint can and maneuvered a fully loaded wheelbarrow with control.

David handled 35 pounds easily, both lifting and carrying. He lifted using good body mechanics. Grasp strength as measured by a dynamometer was 50 pounds with the right (125 lb is the norm) and 35 pounds with the left (117 lb norm). Pinch grasp was measured as 10 pounds with the right (22.5 lb norm) and 6 pounds with the left (21 lb norm). David has more strength in the larger muscles proximally (shoulders) than in the fine muscles distally (fingers). Also noted was a slight tremor in David's hands when he was placing and displacing small items on shelves.

Range of Motion

David has no joint limitations that would hinder his ability to perform gross motor tasks. He is not able to evert and invert his feet fully, but this is probably due to lack of body awareness of the ankle.

Sensory Testing

The sensory test measures stereognosis (tactile discrimination with eyes closed) and pain, temperature, and position sense. David completed all the tasks satisfactorily.

Right–Left Discrimination

David correctly identified the right and left sides of his body and of objects in his environment. He was not able correctly to determine right and left on another person, identifying them as opposite of what they were.

Hand and Office Tool Test

David used a stapler, scissors, hole punch, and paper clip satisfactorily. He had difficulty tearing tape from a tape dispenser at first but learned quickly after a demonstration. David knew how to use a screwdriver but demonstrated poor coordination when attempting to keep the tool in the screw slot. He knew how to use the pliers but it took him some time to make them do what he wanted. He also had trouble using two tools at once (e.g., screwdriver and wrench). He used a hammer satisfactorily.

Bruininks-Oseretsky Test of Motor Proficiency

The Bruininks-Oseretsky test measures speed, dexterity, and strength of limbs together with visual motor abilities. David scored at a 10 years 5 months level in upper limb coordination (target throwing and kinesthetic awareness of arms). Visual motor control fell at 7 years 11 months, upper limb speed and dexterity at 7 years 2 months, and speed of response at 5 years 8 months. These results indicate that David can plan how to use his arms but performs tasks at a slow rate. The visual motor tests indicate the presence of perceptual problems (especially shape reproduction) and some difficulty with fine motor control of a pencil.

Minnesota Rate of Manipulation Test, Purdue Pegboard and Grooved Pegboard
Tests of fine motor dexterity and manipulation indicate that David has average ability in this area. He was able to manipulate the test items satisfactorily at an average rate of speed.

Academic Skills
David demonstrated some difficulty discriminating between typewritten letters and numbers. His ability to match names and addresses is fair. During this task he looked over his work upon completion, found his own errors, and corrected them. David counted 20 items easily. He has learned safety words by rote but is unable to do any other reading.

Summary
David's areas of strength include gross motor endurance and functional strength, balance, and overall body awareness. Cooperation, ability to relate to others, and ability to learn from demonstrated tasks or his own mistakes are also positive traits. David's fine motor abilities are fair: His speed is average, and he has some tremoring.

Recommendations
David would be successful in a job requiring gross motor skills such as janitor, groundskeeper, or kennel worker. He could also learn jobs using fine motor skills such as packaging or other workshop tasks, but his slow working pace would affect his success. Because of his high social skills and ability to accept responsibility, it is felt that David could succeed at a community job.

HANDICAPPED EMPLOYMENT TRAINING ASSISTANCE UNIT

Another example of a program developed for physically disabled teenagers and young adults has a group emphasis. It is the Handicapped Employment Training Assistance (HETA) Unit, established in 1978 by the Crippled Children's Association of South Australia. HETA trainees "are carefully monitored through a group work/work assessment programme until they have the skills to make realistic job choices, gain employment and maintain themselves in the work force" [8].

The program consists of three units that have been devised in a developmental progression; successful completion of one unit allows for entry into the next [3]. The first unit involves *group sessions* that assist trainees in setting goals that can be achieved within a group discussion framework. For example, the trainee might set the goal of presenting himself or herself in a positive manner during a job interview. In the second unit, on *job assessment placements*, trainees have the opportunity to test out in actual work situations the work skills and behaviors they have gained through the group sessions. HETA has 325 employers to draw on for placement, and each trainee receives several two-week placements (an average of three placements per trainee). Finally, for trainees who have completed at least three successful job assessment placements but remain unemployed, the *future employment unit* offers a job-finding club. "Members are encouraged to actively seek work, develop meaningful recreation activities and maintain and develop new skills" [8].

In the HETA units, the occupational therapist plays a key role in the comprehensive evaluation of trainees, as a resource person, and in counseling. Modapts* (Modular Arrangement of Pre-determined Time Standards) are commonly used to evaluate work ability. In addition, general physical functioning is assessed.   As a resource person, the occupational therapist interprets medical information for the staff and helps the vocational coordinator to make appropriate job placements. The program's philosophy is to find positions that are appropriate to the trainee's abilities, but in some instances adaptations are required. In these cases the therapist makes simple adaptations to a job placement, for example, ramps, telephone head set, volume control phone.

The therapist has a small case load for counseling, which takes place in group sessions. "As an extension of this involvement in groups the occupational therapist is responsible for the development and cataloguing of the programme kits. Activities and games that have been developed to demonstrate concepts such as risk taking, consensus, confidence etc. are documented in kit form in order that the ideas and materials can be used more than once" [8].

HETA has had a high success rate with trainees. Approximately 65 percent of its trainees have been successfully placed in open employment [8].

CPRI PREVOCATIONAL PROGRAMS†

CPRI, formerly called the Children's Psychiatric Research Institute, is a children's mental health center located in southwestern Ontario, Canada. CPRI provides 118 residential beds and extensive outpatient service. Service is provided to children from 19 counties, an area that approximates the size of the state of Massachusetts. CPRI is funded through the Ontario government's Community and Social Services Ministry. Academic and research links exist between CPRI and the medical and health science faculties at the University of Western Ontario and numerous other teaching institutions throughout Ontario.

CPRI provides assessment and treatment to emotionally disturbed and developmentally handicapped children, using an interdisciplinary approach. Specialized programs exist for infants who are medically fragile, have genetic disorders (e.g., Down syndrome), autism, or multiple handicaps. A behavioral program for developmentally handicapped children and adolescents treats disturbed, aggressive, and often self-abusive children. Community-based programs, such as a home behavior training program and a specialized foster care plan (Homeshare), are also coordinated through CPRI.

The Madeleine Hardy School, operated by the Board of Education for the city of London, provides educational programs to CPRI residents and up to 10 children on day treatment. This segregated school has a staff-client ratio of one to six. School personnel are also members of the multidisciplinary team and are active in the goal setting and treatment programs of the residents.

*Information on Modapts can be obtained by writing to Australian Association of Predetermined Time Standards and Research, 525 Elizabeth Street, Sydney, N.S.W., Australia 2006.
†This section was written by Kathleen Murphy, OT(C).

In the early 1980s, a joint proposal was made to CPRI and the Madeleine Hardy School for the establishment of a prevocational program to be coordinated by an occupational therapist and a special education teacher. Initially the program was established for six adolescents. This provided the foundation for the development of cooperative programs between the two departments. Presently, these programs can serve up to 25 adolescents at any one time. The success and expansion of the program is felt to be the result of the leader's ability to provide functional activities for adolescents of widely varying intelligence and abilities.

Assessments

The most commonly used assessments are as follows:

The Work Skill Attainment Series*

This assessment provides 20 graded activities in the areas of discrimination, assembly, and packaging. The most basic activity involves sorting discs into containers by shape and color. The highest-level task involves packaging products by weight and heat-sealing the packages. Each task can be graded to form sequential training tasks for those unable to complete the standard task. The assembly and packaging tests are normed using the Methods Time Measurement (MTM) industrial norming system. Individualized goals can be established, measured, and achieved.

The Jacobs Prevocational Skills Assessment

Some components of the Jacobs Prevocational Skills Assessment (JPSA) are used more than others. Frequently used subtests include quality control, filing, carpentry assembly, office work, telephone directory, money concepts, and functional banking. Modifications were made to the carpentry assembly task by including a Robertson screw and screwdriver (with a square head), which decrease the possibility of slippage at the head of the screw. Food preparation was modified to make mini-pizzas (English muffin, prepared spaghetti sauce, and a slice of process cheese). This was done because honey butter is not a common food in this area and was unknown to the adolescents.

The Adaptive Functioning Index†

The Adaptive Functioning Index (AFI) is designed for use with adolescents and adults who are developmentally delayed. It has three components that assess a variety of basic skills deemed necessary for work, such as independence with community living skills, residential checklist (for persons who have a history of institutionalization), and work behaviors. Tasks range from completing a job application and defining common work terminology to discriminating objects by basic colors or

---

*The assessment retails for approximately $3000 and can be obtained from Attainment Company, P.O. Box 103, Oregon, Wisconsin 53575 (telephone 1-800-327-4269).
†This assessment, including scoring books and materials, can be purchased for under $100 through VRRI Research and Training Materials, 3304 33rd Street N.W. Calgary, Alberta T2L 2A6.

shapes. The subtest, the Social Education Test (most frequently used at CPRI) takes approximately 40 minutes to administer. Scoring for the assessment highlights areas that require further skill development.

Social and Prevocational Information Battery*

The Social and Prevocational Information Battery Assessment can be administered to a group of up to 20 at one time. A series of statements is read by the evaluator, with the respondents indicating whether the statement is true or false. Two subtests frequently used are "Work Related Behavior" and "Job Search Skills." Norms are based on an mentally retarded adolescent student population.

Programming:
Work Skills Groups

Four levels of student groups have been established as part of the prevocational program: low, basic, moderate, and advanced. Adolescents are initially assessed by their occupational therapist and their teacher to determine the appropriate group. Individual goals are set for each adolescent and are reviewed at least every three months. Progression from one group to another is usually initiated by the therapist, when she or he feels that the individual is ready for new challenges.

Low Level Group

This group is for adolescents who are severely retarded, have behavioral problems, and often have attended sheltered workshop programs. The emphasis is on learning a work task while maintaining acceptable behavior. The task is operating a shredding machine that has an adaptive protector so as to minimize the potential for any worker injuries (Fig 5-28). Directions are given simply and concisely, such as "begin" or "one at a time." The worker is taught to turn on the machine and feed each piece of paper into the paper guide. After completing a predetermined quota the worker receives an appropriate reinforcer, such as opportunity to look at a magazine or social praise. Adolescents can attend this group twice a week for up to 90 minutes. The instructor-client ratio is 1:2 due to the limited attention span and aggressive potential of the group members.

Basic Level Group

A group of four to six adolescents with mild to severe developmental disabilities gather twice a week for two hours to produce gift wrapping packages containing two sheets of wrapping paper and gift tags (Figs. 5-29, 5-30, 5-31, 5-32). Each member is trained to do one task in an assembly production. Tasks include measuring and cutting the paper from a large roll, folding the paper, punching holes and threading string into gift tags, packaging paper tags into clear bags and finally, stapling a label onto the package. Periodically group members have made decorative bags or produced gift bows. The staff-client ratio is two to six.

---

*The assessment is published by CTB/McGraw-Hill, Del Monte Research Park, Monterey, California 93940. A starter kit can be purchased for approximately $50.

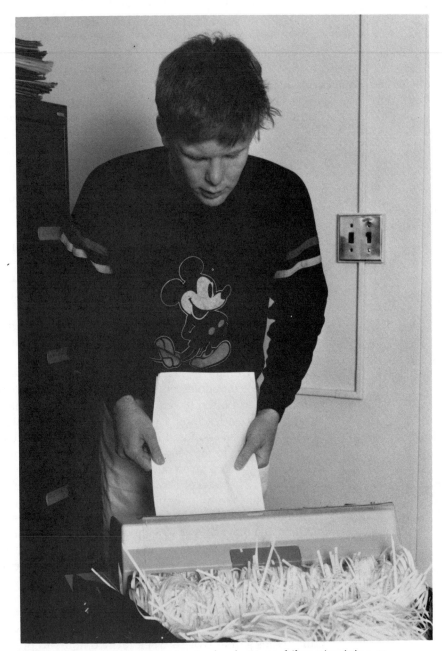

Figure 5-28.   A student learning to shred paper while maintaining acceptable behavior. (Photograph courtesy of Doug Sutherland, medical photographer, CPRI.)

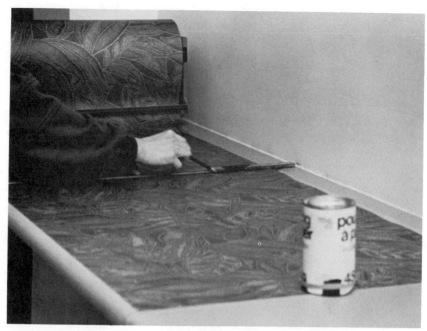

Figure 5-29.   Measuring wrapping paper.

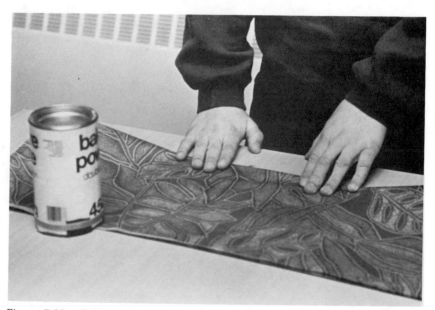

Figure 5-30.   Folding the paper.

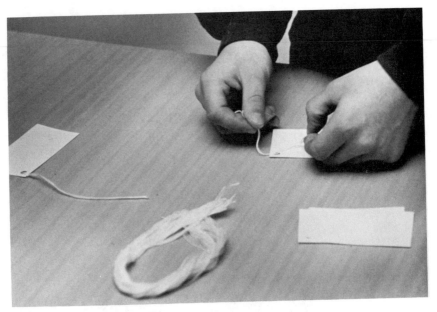

Figure 5-31.   Preparing gift tags.

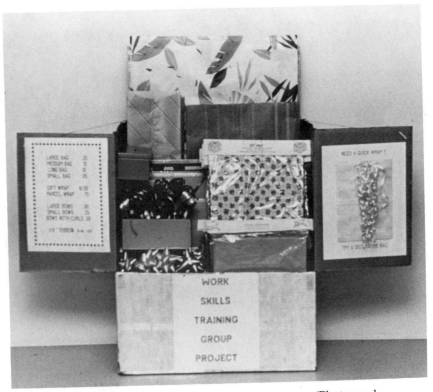

Figure 5-32.   The display stand for the wrapping paper. (Photograph courtesy of Doug Sutherland, medical photographer, CPRI.)

It can take some workers up to three months to become independent on their one task in the production. Finished products are sold in the CPRI lobby at a cost slightly above production costs. Workers receive a monthly honorarium which they spend as they choose.

Moderate Level Group

A local conservation group is conducting an experiment on bluebird nesting patterns. The group distributes unassembled wooden bird-houses for our work group (Fig. 5-33). The workers are expected to independently assemble six pieces of wood in a set sequence. The houses are constructed with square-headed Robertson screws, which are easier to manipulate than nails. After assembly, the birdhouses are painted.

Members of this group learn to work on a task independently and develop a sense of pride in their work. Monetary reinforcement is earned with the completion of every birdhouse.

Advanced Level Group

The highest level group challenges the workers through work skills, creativity, and socialization. Group members disassemble floral arrangements obtained from local funeral directors. With the flowers, they make small desk arrangements and deliver them to teachers and clinicians at no charge. Introducing oneself, making eye contact, and developing the ability to "small talk" with our customers are skills that are encouraged and praised. Recipients of the floral arrangements, always eager to see the delivery persons, provide much social praise (Fig. 5-34). The workers are also responsible for maintaining a list of recipients. The updated list is used to keep track of containers so that they can be picked up and reused for next work periods. When no flowers are available, the group assists in birdhouse assembling.

Work Placement Program

The occupational therapy department coordinates a work placement program for adolescents, which provides job experience along with individualized goals, which range from learning to follow instructions to increasing self-esteem. Most jobs are on site at CPRI and include work in the housekeeping, maintenance, dietary, clerical, and residential departments (Fig. 5-35). Some community-based placements have been established for retail and janitorial jobs. Adolescents receive an honorarium ranging from $1.00 per work period to a maximum of $15.00 per week, which comes from the occupational therapy department's operating budget. Other reinforcements, such as providing a uniform or including the adolescent in staff social gatherings, are as good a reinforcement as money.

Job School

In cooperation with the local office of the Canada Employment Centre, a monthly program on job search skills has been offered to adolescents. Six one-hour sessions cover topics such as determining one's strengths and/or interests, completing an application, using a job bank, finding a

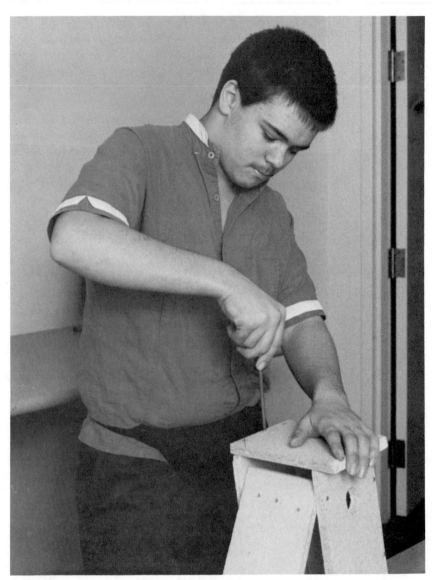

Figure 5-33.   The moderate level work skills group produces wooden bird houses. (Photograph courtesy of Doug Sutherland, medical photographer, CPRI.)

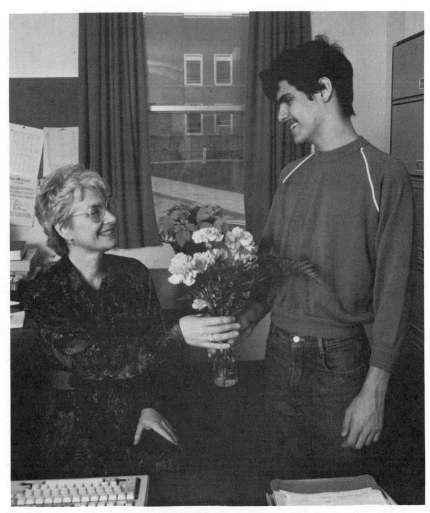

Figure 5-34.   Developing social skills are emphasized in the floral work program. (Photograph courtesy of Doug Sutherland, medical photographer, CPRI.)

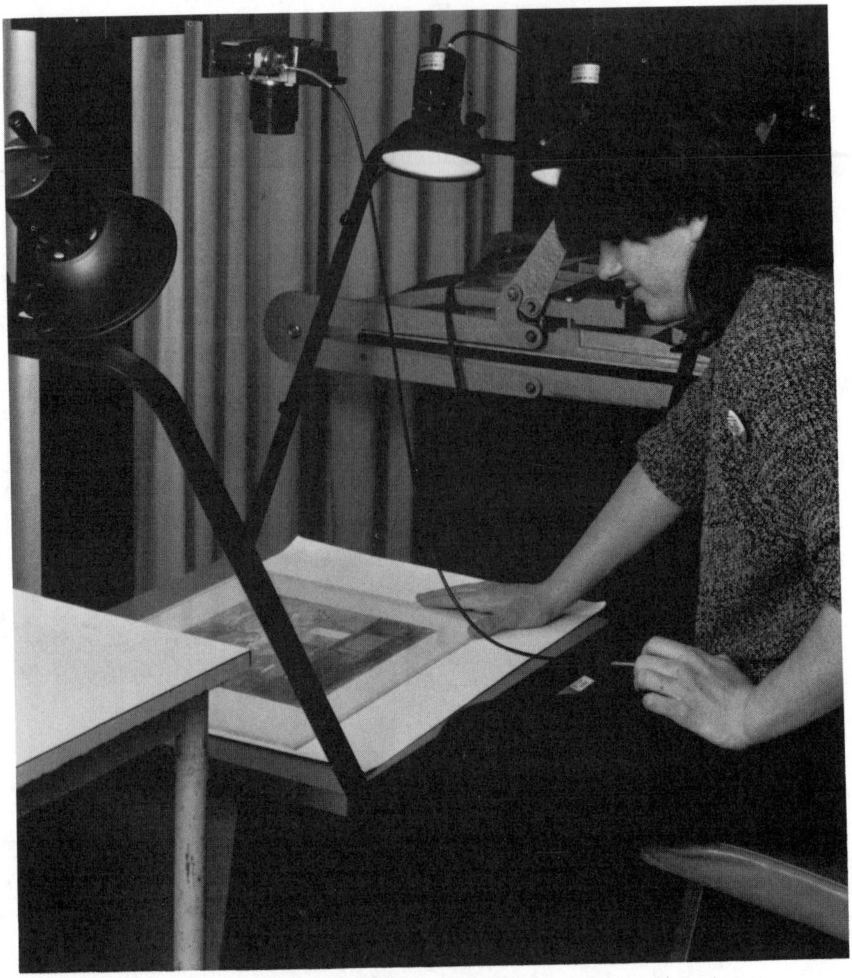

Figure 5-35.   A work placement in the photography department intro-
duces an adolescent to the specialized techniques needed to make
slides. (Photograph courtesy of Doug Sutherland, medical photographer, CPRI.)

job, preparing for an interview, and keeping a job. While the content of this program could be covered at CPRI, going to the Employment Centre is more interesting for the participants and also allows them to gain confidence in accessing community services.

Community Living Skills

Vocational success is dependent on a variety of other abilities, including getting to and from the job site using community transportation, spending earnings appropriately, and getting along with coworkers. Thus, a weekly living skills program was developed. The group, consisting of three to five adolescents, is led by an occupational therapist, who uses community facilities whenever possible. This assists in creating realistic settings and allows for practice of real life situations. Topics include hygiene and grooming, telephone and transportation skills, cooking and shopping, care of clothing, health and home safety, banking, leisure, and utilizing community resources.

Job Tours

Tours of various job sites in the community are an important part of the program. Our students have visited factories, gas stations, Pizza Hut, and the local ice cream vendor. These tours provide opportunities to ask what employers look for in applicants and to reinforce the importance of punctuality, quality, and quantity of work expected by the supervisor. Not only have the tours increased exposure to the work world for the adolescents, but they have helped employers gain a better perspective of the special needs worker. Following each tour, one member of the group is selected to write a thank you note on behalf of the group.

TERMINATION AND FOLLOW-UP

Treatment goals and discharge plans are set by the interdisciplinary team. Occasionally residents move from an inpatient status to day treatment, to ease the transition to the community. As the date of discharge approaches, a conference is held between the treatment team and representatives of community schools and/or vocational programs. A review of the resident's program, strengths, and areas requiring further development are highlighted. Appropriate vocational opportunities are established and graded. The occupational therapy department provides consultation with the adolescent for three months after discharge.

SUMMARY

The prevocational approach used at CPRI has developed over the last decade in combination with the Ontario government's philosophy of promoting supportive, individualized work opportunities. This is a change from past approaches which assumed large sheltered workshops were the best vocational placement for all special needs student. Assessing the adolescent's strengths and interests and providing practical work experiences assist in the transition between school and work.

REFERENCES

1. Bergman, A. *A Guide to Establishing an Activity Center for Mentally Retarded Persons.* Washington, D.C.: President's Committee on Employment of the Handicapped, 1977.
2. Brayman, S.J., Kirby, T.F., and Misenheimer, A.M. Comprehensive Occupational Therapy Evaluation Scale. *Am. J. Occup. Ther.* 30:94, 1976.
3. Crippled Children's Association of South Australia. *Handicapped Employment Training Assistance Unit Brochure.* Andrew T. Kyprianou, Programme Director, HETA, The Regency Park Rehabilitation Centre for the Disabled, Days Road, Regency Park, South Australia 5010.
4. Halpern, A.S. Transition: A look at the Foundation. *Exceptional Children* 51:481, 1985.
5. Heller, J. *Typing for the Physically Handicapped: Methods and Keyboard Presentation Charts.* New York: Gregg Division/McGraw-Hill, 1978.
6. Jacobs, K. It's Never Too Early . . . *CPRI Profile* 10:3, 1989.
7. Lynch, K.F., Kiernan, W.E., Stark, J.A. (Eds.) *Prevocational and Vocational Education for Special Needs Youth: A Blueprint for the 1980s.* Baltimore: Paul H. Brookes, 1982.
8. Lyons, T. HETA-A Groupwork Approach to Work Preparation for the Young Physically Handicapped. Presented at the Australian Association of Occupational Therapists Twelfth Federal Conference, August, 1982.
9. Maurer, P.A. Prevocational Activities and Evaluation for the Child and Adolescent. *Phys. Ther.* 48:771, 1968.
10. Maurer, P.A. Antecedents of Work Behavior. *Am. J. Occup. Ther.* 25:295, 1971.
11. Tash, P. A Case for Teaching Functional Skills. *TASH Newsletter,* Dec. 1987.
12. Wehman, P. Transition for handicapped youth from school to work. In J. Chadsey-Rusch (Ed.) *Enhancing Transition from School to the Workplace for Handicapped Youth.* Urbana-Champaign, IL: National Network for Professional Development in Vocational Special Education, University of Illinois, 1984.
13. Wheeler, J.D. Transitioning Persons with Moderate and Severe Disabilities from School to Adulthood: What Makes It Work? University of Wisconsin-Stout: Materials Development Center, 1987.

Appendix 5-1. Examples of Toys, Games, and Books with a Work Theme

Toys, games, puzzles, and books that have work themes are becoming more readily available at local stores. For example, some manufacturers have on the market many items that simulate foods, materials, and clothes from the major fast food stores.

The following is a modest listing of examples of some toys, games, puzzles and books with a work theme.

Books

Hey, Look At Me! I Can Be
by Merry Thomasson
(a book with windows to personalize the book with a child's photograph)
Source:
Merrybooks
Charlottesville, Virginia

The Berenstain Bears on the Job
by Stan and Jan Berenstain
Source:
Random House
New York

When I Grow Up
by Deborah Manley
Source:
Octopus Books Limited
Grolier Enterprises Corp.

Jack The Carpenter and His Friends
Tom The Grocer and His Friends
Anna The Doctor and Her Friends
Jill The Farmer and Her Friends
by Nick Butterworth
Source:
Discovery Toys
400 Ellinwood Way
Suite 300
Pleasant Hill, California

The Handy Girls Can Fix It!
by Peggy Kahn
Source:
Random House
New York

Puzzles

Things We Do
(7 pieces: teacher, fireman, doctor, nurse, policeman, farmer, mailman)
by Richard Scarry
Source:
Western Publishing Co., Inc.

Things That Go
(8 pieces for 2 years and up)
by Richard Scarry
Source:
Western Publishing Co., Inc.

People In Your Neighborhood—Sesame Street Muppets
(9 piece frame-tray puzzle)
Source:
Western Publishing Co., Inc.

Toys

Dress Me Up
Lacage: Professions
(2 dolls, male and female to dress up by sewing yarn, 32 pieces to make a fireperson, dancer, nurse, police, or gardener)
Source:
Maison Joseph Battat LTD
8440 Darnley Road
Montreal, Canada H4T1M4

I Can Fix It Tool Chest
(plastic tool kit, 3–8 years)
Source:
Toys to Grow On
P.O. Box 17
Long Beach, CA 90801

The Hollywood Prop Box
Personalized Doctor Outfit
The Doctor's Office
Super Star!
Kid's Business
(various dress-up materials)
Source:
Toys To Grow On
P.O. Box 17
Long Beach, CA. 90801

Games

The Allowance Game
(board game for ages 5–12 on earning allowance and spending it)
Source:
Toys to Grow On
P.O. Box 17
Long Beach, CA 90801

Hurry Home
(3 years and up; board game that identifies various people, places, and occupations in a community)
Source:
Discovery Toys
Early Discoveries
400 Ellinwood Way
Suite 300
Pleasant Hill, California

Employ Bingo: The Job Search Bingo Game
Source:
Media Materials, Inc.
Baltimore, Maryland 21211

Careers
(board game for ages 8 to adults)
Source:
Parker Brothers, Co.
P.O. Box 1012
Beverly, MA. 01915

Barbie: "We Girls Can Do Anything" Game
(board game on careers for ages 5 years and up)
Source:
Mattel, Inc.
Western Publishing Co., Inc.
Racine, Wisconsin 53404

Sesame Street—
My First Games™
Friends at Work™
(a matching and memory game, no reading necessary, for ages 3 to 6 years)
Source:
Milton Bradley Co.
Springfield, Massachusetts 01101

Work Programs for Adults with Psychosocial Problems

In our society, the twenties are a time of work preparation, job exploration, and settling in, while the thirties are years of work advancement.

—H. L. Hopkins and H. D. Smith

Many variables must be considered in planning and implementing a work program for adults with psychosocial problems. Because of their fear of failure, these clients often have difficulty making transitions and adapting to change. Often a therapist will notice that a client decompensates when a change in routine occurs, for example, entry into a "work" program. Other types of problems that are encountered by these clients with regard to work may involve their inability to organize, manage time requirements, get along with others (especially authority figures), and solve problems.

The therapist must continually be aware of inconsistencies in behavior and work performance evidenced by the client. Changes in medication or inconsistent use or even disuse may have a profound effect on the client.

Work assessments used should provide the opportunity for the client to work with other people. Unfortunately this ability is not always evaluated in these assessments and must be ascertained during therapy. At the New York Veterans Administration Medical Center, a portion of the Jacobs Prevocational Skills Assessment (see Chap. 4) has been adapted and found to be a useful instrument with a population of veterans with physical or psychiatric disabilities or both.

This chapter has been divided into two sections. In the first part, Rabin and Jeong present an in-depth look at work assessments and programs used with adult psychiatric clients. The second section includes additional programs used to illustrate the diversity in treatment facilities and program implementation. Not only are the traditional hospital and community mental health center discussed, but forensic psychiatry and correctional institutions are also included. Once again, it is hoped that you will gain insights from these program descriptions that will be useful in your own practice.

Work Programming for Psychiatric Clients*

There is no clear relationship between work capacity and degree of emotional recovery. . . . The ability to obtain a job and perform it does not require a certain degree of wellness. Some of the sickest and most disturbed people are able to work—some marginally, some with a high degree of competence. [24]

The current political and socioeconomic climate prompts important shifts in the treatment focus for psychiatric clients. Medicaid reimbursement standards continue to dictate the outcome requirements of reimbursements for psychiatric treatment. Current medical research has identified biological links to major mental disorders. There is movement towards a biological orientation in treating mental disease.

All this reaffirms the medical model, which is scientifically and biologically based. Palmer [28] describes this as the "medicalizaton of psychiatry." Although symptom reduction is still a priority, these outcome standards also make role dysfunction a treatment priority for providers. Schatzberg and Cole [29] assert that beneficial outcomes can only be attained by simultaneously reducing the symptoms and promoting the functional capacity of the individual.

Work programming for psychiatric clients is a new frontier for community mental health (CMH) centers. Mainstream mental health programs have a long history of separating CMH work activities from treatment. The recent use of the social rehabilitation and club house models has made it possible for work to be introduced into more traditional community mental health settings. A multidisciplinary approach to creating work opportunities for mental health clients, and the use of a new approach called vocational integration, have met with much success.

The term vocational integration will be used to describe changes in the CMH provider system that must take place concurrently with the rehabilitation of the individual [23]. A full range of work-related activities must be made available throughout CMH outpatient, day treatment, and residential programs which allow clients to build their skill levels as they move through treatment. Many clients may never be ready for referral to traditional vocational agencies. However, they still may want to work. Vocational integration accurately describes a process that encourages clients to maximize their potential as workers with the support of mental health staff. The goal is meaningful, purposeful work-related activity.

Mainstream CMH programs are ideal settings for vocational integration. Staff are already sensitive to the support clients need to engage in work-related activity. For example, occupational therapists in day treatment and inpatient settings are already skilled in evaluating, setting up, and coordinating work activities for individuals and groups. They can easily serve as role models for other staff who are interested in serving in similar capacities with their clients.

The vocational integration approach allows the greatest number of

---

*This section was written by Jack Rabin, M.S., L.C.S.W., and Glenda Jeong, M.A., O.T.R.

clients to participate in work. For example, CMH programs require maintenance and support services including food, janitorial, messenger, painting, gardening, clerical, peer counseling, and case management. A multitude of CMH clients can be hired to perform these services with the support and assistance of mental health staff.

Work readiness starts with a client's *desire* to work. It has been shown that clients who want to work have a much better chance of vocational success. Good predictors for success include completion of a training program, ability to get along with others, employment history, and motivation and enthusiasm for work. Psychiatric symptomatology, diagnostic categories, psychological tests, level of functioning in one environment, and most demographic data are not good indicators [3]. Mainstream CMH programs must be made better places for clients to acquire and build work skills. The vocational integration approach makes this possible.

A major barrier to the vocational integration approach lies in the psychodynamic and medical models that pervade CMH treatment programs. These models emphasize symptom reduction and maintenance modes of treatment [24]. They have little to say about how to engage clients in ways that have a greater potential for moving them through and beyond mainstream services. The vocational integration approach breaks this cycle of dependency. Clients are encouraged to experience themselves as clients who are workers.

ENVIRONMENTAL INFLUENCES

Several factors are influencing CMH centers to shift toward a social rehabilitation model of service delivery. These include the consumer empowerment movement, changes in sources of funding, and the value of work in American society as a whole.

Consumer Empowerment Movement

The consumer empowerment movement over the past decade has been led by many groups, including the Network Against Psychiatric Assault, the Alliance for the Mentally Ill, and the Mental Health Advisory Boards affiliated with CMH centers across the country. These groups have addressed numerous issues, including the rights of clients in voluntary and involuntary care. They have also promoted better ways of working with clients and their families, such as the psychoeducational approach. Most important, they have redefined the status of clients from "patients" to "consumers" of mental health services [7].

Funding Sources

The Medicaid requirements that CMH programs must meet for their continued funding are also influencing certain changes. Most CMH programs bill for on-site clinical services. In order to bill for these services, all clinical documentation must demonstrate medical necessity, behavioral goals, and behaviorally oriented interventions. Treatment plans must clearly document time-limited, measurable goals that lead to changes in a client's role functioning. Treatment objectives and interventions that document only observed behavior are not billable. Medicaid will pay only for a clinician's efforts at making measurable change in a client's life [14]. A client's involvement in work programming easily meets the objective of measurable, time-limited goals.

Medicaid funding also allows for reimbursement through an extended service plan called the rehabilitation option. This plan pays for both on-site clinical services and off-site socialization, training, and vocational services [11]. (However, clients cannot be involved in paid work.) Many states are applying to the Health Care Financing Administration for the rehabilitation option funding plan. This is an easy way for CMH programs to hire more specialty staff, including occupational therapists, to work in outpatient and day treatment programs. Here they can be assigned to make vocational assessments, provide job training to clients and staff, and coordinate vocational services in general.

The expansion of supported work funding is another resource that can be used to promote work activity. This funding pays for job coaches and placement services, which can be provided by CMH staff. However, clients involved in supported work must also be clients of the Department of Rehabilitation and be ready to work at least 20 hours/week [27]. While many CMH clients are not ready to work this much, this new funding source does encourage work-related goals.

The Work Ethic

The last decade was a time of fiscal austerity for social service programming, and the next decade promises more of the same. In this time of continual cut backs, work programming is an area of discussion that deserves wide-ranging support including support at the legislative levels. Because work goes to the heart of the American creed, efforts to engage more psychiatric clients in various work activities can only be viewed positively by potential funding sources.

OCCUPATIONAL THERAPY FRAMES OF REFERENCES/PHILOSOPHY OF PRACTICE

The two occupational therapy approaches that address function in relation to work programming for all levels of ability are Allen's cognitive disability frame of reference and Kielhofner's model of human occupation. Within the framework of these two models, a modality termed supported employment will be discussed.

There are clear differences in focus between Allen's and Kielhofner's theories. The former's is a neurobiologically based approach, whereas the latter's is a phenomenological approach. Their differences are as important to note as their similarities.

Allen [2] states that cognitive ability is a function of biological structure. Cognition functions as a major organizing factor in human performance [2]. Cognitive disability represents a physiological or biochemical restriction in sensorimotor actions, which produces observable, measurable limitations in routine task behavior [1]. According to Allen, the association made between sensory cues noticed and the resulting voluntary motor actions taken describe the degree of conscious awareness used to direct the sensorimotor performance [1]. Allen has devised six levels of cognitive function, which measure the complexity of sensorimotor associations formed during the activity process [24]. For example, cognitive level (ACL) 1 represents automatic actions that appear to be in response to internal or situational cues. Observed behavior is primarily reflexive and habitual. Level 1 is most commonly seen in individuals with severe dementia or recent head trauma. In contrast, at level 5, the individual spontaneously displays overt trial and error behavior while engaging in activity. At this level, there is the capacity for inductive reasoning. Level 5 can be often seen in individuals with remitting affective disorders, personality disorders, and schizophrenic disorders with good prognoses. The cognitive levels help identify realistic treatment expectations by clarifying the range of ability.

Kielhofner's occupational behaviors theory is concerned with the ability to competently perform daily life tasks/behaviors (work, play, and self care) and gain satisfaction from performance [19]. This model emphasizes motivation, sociocultural factors, and a developmental aspect to learning occupational roles within a temporal framework.

The individual is a human system. As an open cyclical system, it is dynamic and hierarchical in its interplay with the environment [20]. The human system simultaneously functions as a whole, with its own internal subsystems, and as a part of a larger system. The human system operates on four levels—the social system, symbolic system (conscious process), nervous system (brain), and musculoskeletal system [19]. Behavior is seen as a response to a gestalt image of the environment, rather than to any discrete stimulus. The image is defined as a network of information derived from the interpretation and reorganization of the environmental input [6]. Kielhofner states that one can "become through doing" because the human system has the capability for self-maintenance and change [19]; change is the process.

Allen [2], on the other hand, views change as occurring primarily as a result of external medical interventions, medication, and occupational therapy interventions upon the environment. Learning is also thought by Allen [2] to be clearly limited by disease. Since disorders of the brain can impede the ability to learn and remember, Allen asserts that learning cannot be assumed to be unrestricted or a given in the activity process. Allen identifies the need to distinguish between the process of *doing* a task and *learning to do* a task [2].

Kielhofner's model views learning as a continuous process within the human system. Learning occurs through experience via the system's ability to organize and integrate input information into an image. When this image is incorporated into the system, it changes the system, the system's interpretation of the information and the behavioral response [19].

Implementation

The sole use of just one of these approaches in practice often yields insufficient data regarding the individual as a whole. Using Allen's method of cognitive disabilities yields behavioral data on immediate cognitive status. However, the behavioral picture is obtained in a vacuum, without the individual's input regarding perceived needs, desires, and current life context. Hence, interpretation and scoring become problematic.

Kielhofner's occupational behavior approach relies upon the client's verbal and written communication skills to obtain data through inventories and self-reports. This becomes problematic if and when language or communication barriers exist, verbal and written communication skills are grossly impaired, or current mental status is questionable, because there is then no means to obtain behavioral data for identifying, comparing, and validating the self-reported abilities with the current skill capacity. As Allen [2] points out, there is often a discrepancy between verbal and sensorimotor performance; verbal ability often exceeds and masks the sensorimotor dysfunctions.

Empirically, complementary use of both approaches has in fact provided a balanced assessment and treatment approach in psychiatric day treatment programs, and current research supports the complementary use of the two [18]. Katz [17] delineates clear parallels that exist between the two approaches and identifies the common underlying theoretical principles. Integral to both constructs are the concepts of human adaptation, the individual as purposeful and self-directed, and the use of systems theory to organize components [17].

Given that both approaches are organized according to a systems framework, their relationship can be viewed according to systems theory which states that all levels of systems operations are interctive and interdependent. Both examine the dynamics of the same process of human adaptation within a larger sociocultural context but from differing levels of human systems operation including the neurosensory level (brain) and the symbolic level. The complementary use of both approaches demonstrates an integral link between the mind and the spirit.

The use of both approaches also allows the occupational therapist to shift treatment focus according to the client's functional status. The occupational therapy can plan intervention to elicit the client's highest adaptive response and to address the client's changing needs.

SUPPORTED EMPLOYMENT

Supported employment (SE) emphasizes a functional approach and increased client involvement. The philosophical basis for SE is psychosocial rehabilitation, the primary goal of which is to enable an individual to live, learn, and work in the community with the least possible amount of support [4]. This approach is often characterized as a "choose-get-keep" model. It is intended to be client driven throughout. Implementation entails working with a client to identify, search ("choose"), and develop the job slot of the client's choice. Once a job coach or developer makes the job match ("get"), the client is placed in that job. The client is then provided with ongoing job support ("keep") via a job coach and other support resources.

SE includes assessing the current level of skills function and the environmental support/constraints in relation to the environment in which the client wants to function. This is in agreement with occupational therapy's emphasis on functional assessment to ascertain both the actual skills present and the skills required to meet the environmental demands.

Intervention in SE involves training in job seeking skills and on the job training. Adapting the environment by accessing resources and making job modifications parallel the occupational therapy perspective of clinician being the monitor and orchestrator to adapt the parameters of the activity for successful participation. "Vocational maturity" is acquired through implementation of the appropriate developmental tasks during different life stages [5]. This perspective directly parallels the occupational behavior model, which describes a developmental process of role behavior acquisition within a temporal context, and recognizes the contribution made to self-esteem and wellbeing of work experiences that are personally relevant to the client.

In theory, SE is a completely client-driven approach. However, given the variability of behaviors with the psychiatric population, it is unclear if and to what extent this approach can be implemented in its true form. In practice, control over who determines the goal and direction of the work plan may be a major issue for client, clinician, and the support service providers. The roles and relationships must be renegotiated and clarified for all involved. This means major shifts in thinking and interaction, which may not be easily embraced by all [21]. Given the importance of ongoing support, how this support is to be actually provided will also need to be negotiated and structured according to what is feasible within the given system. Ongoing support is meant to be never-ending, while traditional treatment is clearly limited.

CURRENT USE OF ASSESSMENTS IN WORK PROGRAMMING

There is currently no consistency in perspective or approach for work programming in psychiatry. Programs vary greatly in their treatment emphasis, work assessments, and programming. The guidelines used for "assessing work readiness" range from verbal interviews to observed compliance with day treatment expectations to observed participation in work groups. Practitioners in programming agree that common terminology and definitions are needed.

"Work readiness" can be evaluated by looking at both the individual's history regarding work, education, and function and the individual's current work habits and skills [9]. Occupational therapy assessments are available to examine work readiness with psychiatric clients. The assessments all focus on the general areas of work habits, work skills, capacity for managing work relations, and work attitudes, but they differ in how they obtain the data. For example, the Jacobs Prevocational Skills Assessment [15] is a performance-based assessment, which looks at specific skill areas. Both Allen's [2] Work Performance Inventory and Ethridge's [8] Rating Scale focus on observed behavior. The Work Performance Subscale of the Role Activity Performance Scale [13] examines past work performance in an interview format.

For occupational therapists in psychiatry, program demands determine the type and extent of assessment. Given little time and resources, assessment occurs primarily through observation of a client in work groups or activity groups. Many clinicians utilize the setting's structure and resources to create opportunities for performance-based assessment of a client's work readiness.

THE SAN FRANCISCO EXPERIENCE: A MODEL PROGRAM

The San Francisco Community Mental Health (SF/CMH) system is a large system including many models of work programming practice. Reflecting a growing trend, SF/CMH has begun to encourage practitioners from differing perspectives to begin adopting a psychosocial rehabilitation approach. In order to encourage this shift, SF/CMH is using a vocational integration approach, which emphasizes change and the primacy of the client.

The SF/CMH has over 75 programs serving 14,000 adult clients annually. (There are 25 more programs that serve an additional 7,000 children, adolescents, and seniors annually). Twenty outpatient, nine day treatment, 20 residential, one inpatient, and three case management programs make up the adult system. These programs serve a rich diversity of multicultural groups including Black, Asian, and Hispanic clients. Over 49 percent of the total SF/CMH client population is nonwhite [26].

A group called Community Vocational Enterprises (CVE) has worked closely with the assistant director of Adult Community Services to develop paid work experiences for adult clients. CVE operates as a separate, non-profit organization and its staff are employees of another agency with which the city contracts. CVE was set up by an occupational therapist who is also a consultant to the program, in order to hire clients to work in various paid work projects, to procure contract work that can be distributed to SF/CMH programs, to start city-wide work projects, and to maintain program-based work crews involved in messenger, bulk mailing, food, and janitorial services.

Messenger Service

Several years ago, the CMH messenger mail service was under heavy criticism. This interoffice mail service for SF/CMH programs had broken down; the two Civil Service drivers who made up the service could no longer continue to sort and deliver mail to all 100 programs on a daily basis. CVE then made a proposal to hire and train clients to assist the drivers. The proposal was accepted, and clients were trained to:

1. sort the mail
2. ride with the drivers and run the mail between the mail car and programs (which is especially helpful in congested areas)
3. carry and deliver mail on foot to programs located within walking distance of the SF/CMH central administrative office, where the messenger service is based.

   Within two months, 10 clients had been hired, trained, and placed on the job. The mail service was back on its feet and ran better than ever.

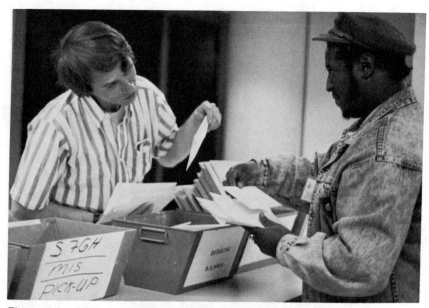

Figure 6-1.   Messenger service. (Photograph courtesy of Deborah Ralston, Director, Community Vocational Enterprises.) (continued)

Two years later, the service was re-evaluated and a decision was made to also hire clients to be drivers. CVE screened and hired four clients to work on a part-time basis. Each client has his or her own car, a valid driver's license, and personal auto insurance coverage. The CMH messenger service is now completely operated by clients (Fig. 6-1).

There are several points that can be made from this experience. First, CVE's proposal for an improved messenger service was a timely alternative to a deteriorating situation; the administration had never considered the use of clients as workers in this way before. Second, the clients hired were directly responsible for improving the service. The success of this project became a showpiece for what clients can do as workers.

Bulk Mailing

CVE also negotiates and procures contracts for bulk mailings of up to 20,000 copies from realty companies, retail stores, wineries, and various community groups, which are distributed to day treatment and residential programs (Fig. 6-2). The mental health programs that receive this work are given a deadline for their client crews to complete each project. The quality control of the crews is carefully monitored by program staff. This type of work fits in well with the day treatment and residential program structure, which involves a variety of group activities during the day. Clients are hired by CVE and paid according to their productivity. CVE has a sub-minimum wage certificate and carefully works out the standard for productivity.

Food Services

CVE operates a client-run refreshment concession (Fig. 6-3) located in the lunch room on the fifth floor of the SF/CMH central office building,

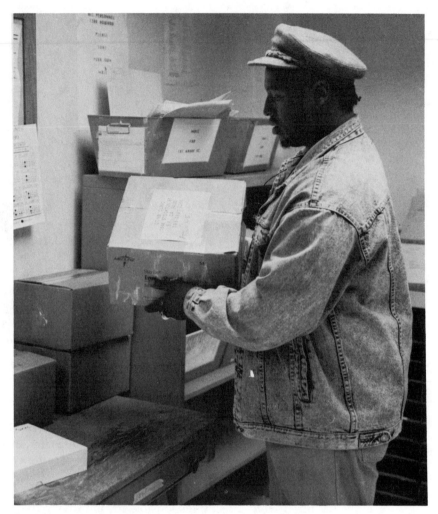

Figure 6-1.   (continued)

Monday through Friday between 8:00 AM—11:30 AM. Clients, who include the most fragile, the least job experienced, and the most motivated, operate a counter at which staff can choose from freshly ground
coffees, muffins, and donuts. Profits from the cafe have far exceeded
initial expectations.

Janitorial Services

Several years ago, the janitorial services provided to mental health sites
by independent contractors were re-evaluated. CVE made a proposal
to hire clients to do this work more efficiently and with greater care.
This proposal was accepted, and 20 clients were hired onto five janitorial
crews. Groups of two to four clients were hired to clean their own
program sites as well as other mental health sites located in other parts
of the city. Each site is cleaned two to five times a week. CVE contracts
with each site for the work to be performed. The benefits to clients are
both financial and social. They are paid minimum wage or better, they

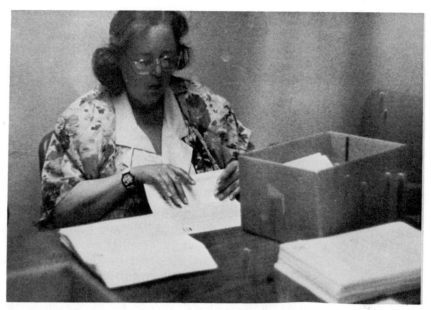

Figure 6-2. Bulk mailing service. (Photograph courtesy of Deborah Ralston, Director, Community Vocational Enterprises.)

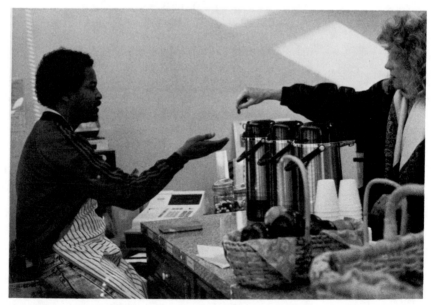

Figure 6-3. Community vocational enterprises cafe. (Photograph courtesy of Deborah Ralston, Director, Community Vocational Enterprises.)

gain the respect of their peers and counselors, and they get to work in different areas of the city and the CMH system.

Additional Work Programs at SF/CMH

The success of CVE has enabled more work opportunities to develop. Following is a discussion of these opportunities and the potential each represents.

Keystone Vocational Services

To fit in with required budget cuts, a proposal was made to close a day treatment program and open a vocational services program with some of the same staff. The new program, Keystone Vocational Services, was run by an occupational therapist.

Keystone fit well into the continuum of work activities CVE had begun to develop. CVE made it possible for clients to be hired for jobs of 10 hours or less per week. At Keystone, clients could be assessed with the possibility of being placed into a supported work situation, and clients could receive ongoing job support.

An agreement was developed for Keystone to be reimbursed for assessment, placement, and job coaching services. This funding was used to create four positions: a job coach, a job developer, and two job supervisors. Keystone also agreed to provide follow-up services to all clients after job placement.

Follow-up services are provided by the treatment team: the outpatient or day treatment therapist, residential counselor and case manager. The team provides continuous job support to each client, to prevent clients from falling into crises on the job.

The development of Keystone is an excellent example of how various organizations can join together, even in the face of ever-more-limited funding, to expand job opportunities for clients.

Use of Rule 34

Rule 34 designates Civil Service positions for the disabled, including the emotionally handicapped, in San Francisco. Clients who apply for a Rule 34 position need meet only the minimum qualifications of this position in order to be interviewed and hired. They do not have to engage in the usual testing process with other applicants or be ranked on a Civil Service list. This gives psychiatric clients priority in being hired for certain positions. This process also avoids confrontation with unions, since the unions were part of the negotiating team that established the Rule 34 classification. Keystone has already designated two support positions with this designation: a 20-hour/week clerical and a 20-hour/week custodial position (Fig. 6-4).

Income Disregard

The Department of Social Services (DSS) is considering an Income Disregard for general assistance recipients. This will allow CMH clients who receive general assistance to earn additional income. Up until now every dollar earned by a CMH client involved in paid work has been

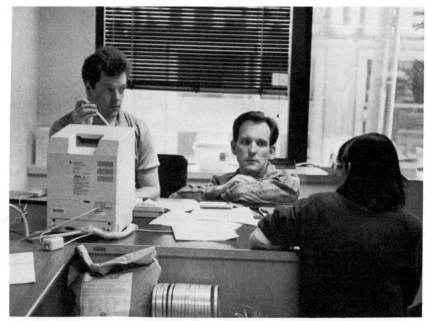

Figure 6-4. Effective use of a Rule 34 position. (Photograph courtesy of Deborah Ralston, Director, Community Vocational Enterprises.)

removed from the general assistance check. If this measure is passed, many CMH clients will have an added incentive to work.

Assessment and Referral Process

The Vocational Information Form (VIF) was developed by the occupational therapy consultant to CVE. The VIF can be used by all mental health staff to gather information about their clients' potential for work. The VIF assists clinicians in deciding how to include work experiences and/or training in overall treatment planning. The items in the VIF are factors known to be directly related to successful and gainful employment for psychiatric clients. These include interest in and motivation to work, employment history, and social interaction skills. Points are assigned to items on the form. The points are compiled to derive a total score. The preliminary criteria for cutoff points are based on minimal expected levels of performance.

The VIF also helps practitioners to identify potential areas of treatment focus, educates staff, and promotes discussion about work programming. These guidelines are the first step to establishing common terminology.

This one form provides three different vocational programs—Keystone, CVE and the Department of Rehabilitation—with valuable information. The VIF is used with all day treatment clients and all outpatient programs. This makes it possible for all primary care providers to gather consistent vocational information about their clients and thus make better referrals.

After receiving a referral, step-by-step coordination occurs between the occupational therapist, CVE, and the Department of Rehabilitation counselor. After the initial interview, efforts are made to identify each client's entry point for work programming. The client may be ready to work 20 hours or more per week, need to build up work experience (through work with CVE's small businesses), or need basic work adjustment experience (at Keystone). Once referred, the client is provided with ongoing support.

An interview and assessment format is used to collect basic data. This data provides the occupational therapist with the client's perceptions of his or her social interaction skills, observable task performance skills, and perceived personal strengths. The interview explores work and role history and client perception regarding previous work experiences (volition, habitual, performance). The self-assessment component assesses client perceptions regarding social interaction skills, work related skills, and personal assets. The tools used include the Bay Area Functional Performance Evaluation SIS self report [22], and the Katz Activity Checklist [16]. The performance component establishes the current level of treatment skills and areas needing more evaluation and provides baseline data for later comparative analyses. The tools used are the ACL, the Valpar General Clerical Work Sample (VCWS) #5, and a five-step work sample.

Other assessments are sometimes included to screen and rule out organic factors: the BaFPE floorplan component [22], the Frostig Developmental Test of Visual Motor Integration [10], the Neurological Soft Sign Exam [25], and the Screening Test for the Luria-Nebraska Battery [12]. The interview and assessment procedure can be conducted in one or two sessions.

Some components of various standardized and nonstandardized assessments are not being used as originally intended. Given this, the results derived from any one or combination of these tools cannot be assumed to provide a standardized assessment. However, consistent use of some components can be valuable in developing normative data for this population.

The Valpar Component Work Sample (VCWS) #5 is a standardized screening tool that measures worker characteristics found to be basic indicators of success across numerous job families. Its purpose is to measure 1) the ability to perform a variety of basic clerical tasks and 2) aptitude to learn these tasks. It can be administered to the individuals who have varying degrees of work experience. There is currently no normative data available specifically for psychiatric clients.

The Allen's Cognitive Level (ACL) provides an immediate measure of level of cognitive function to be considered in identifying work program goals for an individual. It is of interest to later review the ACL scores with client performance, work progress, and work outcomes.

With the data obtained, the occupational therapist can devise a plan of action with the client for work program goals in either the work adjustment component or supported employment component of vocational services. Regardless of where the client begins his or her vocational plans, support services, including health and education workshops and basic benefits counseling, will be available.

THE REHABILITATION COMMUNITY CENTER

The Rehabilitation Community Center (RCC) is a large day treatment and socialization program located in downtown San Francisco. A majority of the clients who come to RCC live in "board and care homes" for the chronically mentally ill in the area. Many clients have had long periods of institutionalization, receive SSI, and are generally thought to have little or no work potential.

The program is divided into occupational, vocational, and social-recreational areas:

1. *Occupational:* Twenty-five job descriptions have been written, which involve clients in a variety of jobs. Staff oversee these volunteer activities, which include coffee/snack bar sales, cooking, setup and cleanup, and supervision of workers in each job.
2. *Vocational:* Up to 25,000 boxes are delivered monthly for clients to assemble in work teams. Clients are involved in all capacities including quality control and assembly.
3. *Social-Recreational:* Clients participate in Special Olympics sports events scheduled throughout the year. Clients are also involved in organizing various social and recreational events on site.

Staff Involvement

Staff work with clients in all phases of activity on and off site. One staff member serves as the activity leader, and a second staff member doubles as a process observer. This minimizes the loss of important process issues that clients or staff may exhibit during an activity. Staff work together as a team, each taking responsibility for one or more major areas of the program structure. RCC is a good example of the use of the vocational integration model by an individual program. Work-related activities are well supported. Clients have an opportunity to engage in volunteer work, paid work on site, and supported work in the community.

Client Nightclub

Work programming can also be used to encourage clients to become involved recreationally. Some of the same skills used on the job—team work, planning, and preparation—can be used in play. Clients from throughout SF/CMH joined with a core group of day treatment staff to plan the first event. Clients ran planning meetings and discussed various possibilities for program, access, and security. They worked out the details of food preparation, set up, entertainment, transportation, and monitoring of activity during the evening. They also visited many programs and encouraged these clients to come. The Recreational and Parks Department donated a large space with a stage located at one of the neighborhood centers. Over two hundred clients and staff from all over the city came to the first event. The evening was filled with dancing, singing, plays, comedy, and poetry—all performed by clients. There were no incidents, and the evening was a success.

CONCLUSION

Many psychiatric clients desire to work and socialize just like everyone else. However, often they are afraid to engage in these activities. They need to be encouraged by people they can trust in safe, supportive settings. The CMH programs discussed in this chapter serve this purpose.

Meaningful, purposeful work activity is a right to which all individuals are entitled. The vocational integration approach makes work programming possible for all clients.

The ideas discussed here show what can be done with existing resources and little additional funding to develop a continuum of work activities that can be fully integrated into mainstream services.

The SF/CMH vocational integration approach uses the following guidelines:

1. Encourage all staff, especially occupational therapists, to participate in work activities. Involve staff who are already interested and/or knowledgeable.
2. Enlist the support of the administration and develop a strong administrative link.
3. Create graduated steps for client involvement in work. Avoid requiring clients to take steps for which they are not prepared.
4. Create a mechanism for hiring clients and consulting with staff.
5. Take advantage of all opportunities to hire clients. Use special designations like Rule 34 to facilitate this process.
6. Use the success of each new work project to promote more work opportunities.
7. Be alert for new funding sources on all levels to promote work programming.
8. Involve occupational therapists in developing work-related information and assessment tools that fit specific client populations and service systems.
9. Encourage clients to use their work skills to plan activities.
10. Use research techniques to demonstrate the value of work for clients.

Case Study

Paul is a 31-year-old man who was admitted to a San Francisco hospital in 1988 for a suicide attempt. His two-week hospital stay was followed by referral to a residential and day treatment program.

Paul was first hospitalized for his depressive episodes in 1986. At that time he was a college sophomore and was enmeshed in a chaotic marital relationship. From 1986 to 1988, he was admitted once a year for depression and suicide attempts. His brief hospitalizations reflected a lifelong pattern in which he never felt safe expressing himself and he would "stuff his feelings in." This "baggage" accumulated to a breaking point and he became severely depressed. He would then engage in escapist or self-abusive behavior such as drinking or hurting himself. After admission to the hospital, he would improve rapidly. Once discharged, he would return to work, do extremely well, and set very high expectations for himself. Without recognizing his stressors or communicating his feelings, he would once again find himself at a breaking point and "fall even deeper" into depression.

While in day treatment, Paul was consistently nonverbal and withdrawn. He regularly chose to sit on the periphery with his headset and sunglasses on. Only when engaged in work-related activities did he display any affect or interact with others.

His occupational therapy interview and assessment indicated he was bright and possessed strong problem-solving and organization skills. At ACL level 5+, Paul displayed trial and error behavior and was able to correct his mistakes. He had always done well academically and "loved school." In college he enjoyed his computer science classes, even though his grades reflected the chaos in his life. His work experiences had been primarily in manual labor; he had done mechanical work, plumbing, contracting, masonry, and farm work. The longest job he held (one year) was as a parking attendant.

Paul's interest inventory indicated strong interests in the clerical field. While in day treatment Paul began to participate in daily and weekly clerical work activities. Because of his interest and skills in food preparation, he also began to participate in one of the food crews. Paul began to slowly take on increasing responsibilities of his own choosing. The structure of the work program provided a non-threatening arena in which he could begin developing friendships, affirming his abilities to perform competently, and asserting his own basic needs and opinions. Over time, he became an extremely active participant in the program.

Concurrently, Paul also participated in the vocational component of his residential program. His involvement in both arenas allowed him to interact with different work demands and circumstances. Within eight months of admission Paul initiated steps to volunteer once a week, an action supported by both the occupational therapist and clinician.

At the time of his discharge, Paul stated he would like to do volunteer work and maintain his relationship with his private therapist. Paul was referred to both the Department of Rehabilitation (DR) and CVE. Paul contacted both agencies. A DR case was opened and a plan was coordinated between DR and CVE. Paul volunteered with CVE as a clerical assistant for 20 hours per week. The goal was for Paul to teach himself how to use the new computer, using only the manuals. He would then use the computer to start a citywide newsletter on work programming.

However, during this transition period, Paul experienced major stressors in his living situation, and shortly after beginning to volunteer, he readmitted himself to the hospital. He contacted CVE and his DR counselor and worked out an agreement; when he was ready he would call them and set up a return date. Upon his return to work, Paul shared the stressors with his supervisor and the occupational therapist. This incident gave Paul a chance to recognize his own warning signs and take the initiative in contacting his therapist and maintain contact with his support system.

Since returning to work Paul has performed consistently well in all phases of work. He is providing increasingly complex graphic work for both CVE and Keystone staff. The computer work he is doing also provides him with the opportunity to interact with other departments. Paul is also establishing positive working relationships. His work has even been commended by the Department's computer consultant; he said Paul's work is highly sophisticated, and he offered to refer Paul to a desktop publishing agency to do freelance work.

In November 1989, a decision was made to create a 20-hour Rule 34 position for Keystone Vocational Services. Paul was offered the job, and steps are being taken to coordinate this with his DR counselor, the occupational therapist at Keystone, his benefits counselor, and the CVE supervisor. While this is a difficult step for Paul, he feels more self-confidence than ever before. He attributes this to the friendships he has learned to make and keep, the excellent support system he has developed, and the insights he has developed. While awaiting the final steps of the civil service process, Paul has been busy doing both computer work and supervision and training of clients with the CVE cafe. He has also recruited a new volunteer whom he will train to use the computer.

REFERENCES

1. Allen, C. K. Occupational Therapy: Functional assessment of the severity of mental disorders. *Hosp. Commun. Psychiatry* 39:140–142, 1988.
2. Allen, C. K. *Occupational Therapy for Psychiatric Diseases—Measurement and Management of Cognitive Disabilities.* Boston: Little, Brown, 1985.
3. Anthony, W. A., and Jansen, M. A. Predicting the Vocational Capacity for the Chronically Mentally Ill. *Am. Psychol.* 39:537–544, 1984.
4. Anthony, W. A., Howell, J., and Danley, K. S. Vocational Rehabilitation of the Psychiatrically Disabled. In *The Chronically Mentally Ill: Research and Services.* Spectrum Publications, Inc. 1984, pp. 215–236.
5. Anthony, W. A., and Blanch, A. Supported Employment for Persons Who Are Psychiatrically Disabled: An Historical and Conceptual Perspective. *Psychosocial Rehab. J.,* 11 (2):5–23.
6. Boulding, K. General Systems Theory—The Skeleton of Science. In Buckley, W. (Ed.) *Modern Systems Research for the Behavioral Sciences.* Chicago: Aldine, 1968, p. 7–8.
7. Chamberlain, J. *On Our Own—Patient Controlled Alternatives to the Mental Health System.* New York: Hawthorn Books, 1978.
8. Ethridge, D. Pre-vocational Assessment of Rehabilitation Potential of Psychiatric Patients. *Am. J. Occup. Ther.* 22(3):161–167, 1968.
9. Fine, S. B. Assessing Work Performance and Cognitive Capacities in Mental Health Practice. *The AOTA Practice Symposium 1989—Program Guide.* Rockville, MD: American Occupational Therapy Association, 1989, pp. 48–49.
10. Frostig, M. L., Lefever, D. W., and Whittlesey, J. R. *Mary and Frostig Developmental Task of Visual Perception* (3rd ed.). Palo Alto: Consulting Psychologist Press, 1961.
11. Glenn, L. A Proposal for the Addition of the Rehabilitation Option to the Public Sector Mental Health System in California (in house handout), Jan. 1990.
12. Golden, C. *Screening Test for the Luria-Nebraska Neuro-Psychological Battery: Adult Form.* Western Psychological Services, 1987.
13. Good-Ellis, M., Fine, S. B., Spencer, J. H., and Divettis, A. Developing a Role Activity Performance Scale. *Am. J. Occup. Ther.* 22(3):161–167, 1987.
14. Health Care Financing Administration. Medicaid Program Review Report. Title XIX. 42 CFR, Section 435.3 (in house handout), Jan. 1990.
15. Jacobs, K. *Occupational Therapy: Work Related Programs and Assessment.* Boston: Little, Brown, 1985.
16. Katz, N. Interest Checklist: A Factor Analytical Study. *Occup. Ther. Mental Health* 8(1):45–55, 1988.
17. Katz, N. Introduction to the Collection. The Development of Standardized Clinical Evaluations in Mental Health. *Occup. Ther. Mental Health* (1):1–6, 1988.
18. Katz, N., Josman, N., and Steinmetz, N. Relationship Between Cognitive Disability Theory and the Model of Human Occupation in the Assessment of Psychiatric and Nonpsychiatric Adolescents. *Occup. Ther. Mental Health* 8(1):31–43, 1988.
19. Kielhofner, G. *Health Through Occupation—Theory and Practice in Occupational Therapy.* Philadelphia: F. A. Davis Co., 1983.
20. Kielhofner, G., Barris, R., and Watts, J. H. *Psychosocial Occupational Therapy: Practice in a Pluralistic Arena.* Maryland: RAMSCO Publishing Co., 1983.
21. Lang, S. K. Approaches to Vocational Integration for Psychiatric Clients.

The AOTA Practice Symposium—Program Guide. Rockville, MD: The American Occupational Therapy Association, 1989, pp. 82–86.

22. Lang, S. K., and Bloomer, J. *Bay Area Functional Performance Evaluation* (2nd ed.). Palo Alto: Consulting Psychologists Press, 1987.
23. Lang, S. K., and Cara, E. Vocational Integration for the Psychiatrically Disabled. *Hosp. Commun. Psychiatry* 40:9, 1989.
24. Mackota, C. B., and Lamb, L. H. Vocational Rehabilitation. *Psychiatr. Annals* 19(10):522–548, 1989.
25. Manschreck, T. C., and Ames, D. Neurologic Features and Psychopathology in Schizophrenic Disorders. *Biol. Psychiatr.*, 19(5):703–719, 1984.
26. Nguyen, T., and Marks J. Summary of Service Utilization during Fiscal Year 1988–89. San Francisco Community Mental Health Services (in house handout), Feb. 1990.
27. Noble, J. H., and Collignon, C. Systems Barriers to Supported Employment for Persons with Chronic Mental Illness. *Psychosoc. Rehab. J.* X1:2, 1987.
28. Palmer, F. The Present Context of Service Delivery. *Mental Health Forum: Skills for Assessment and Treatment.* Rockville, MD: The American Occupational Therapy Association, 1989, pp. 28–36.
29. Schatzberg, A. F., and Cole, J. O. *Manual of Clinical Psychopharmacology.* Washington: American Psychiatric Press, 1989.
30. Sue, S., and McKinney, H. Asian Americans in the Community Mental Health System. *Am. J. Orthopsychiatry* 45:1, 1975.

SUGGESTED READINGS

Stauffer, D. Predicting Successful Employment in the Community for People with a History of Chronic Mental Illness. *Occup. Thera. Mental Health* 6(2):31–49; 1986.

Manual for Valpar Component Work Sample 5: Clerical Comprehension and Aptitude. Tuscon: Valpar International Corporation, 1974.

Fabian, E., and Wiedefeld, M. E. Supported Employment for Severely Psychiatrically Disabled Persons: A Descriptive Study. *Psychosoc. Rehab. J.* 13(2):53–60, 1989.

Kirkland, M., and Robertson, S. The Evolution of Work Related Theory in Occupational Therapy. In *Planning and Implementing Vocation Readiness in Occupational Therapy (PIVOT).* Rockville, MD: American Occupational Therapy Association, 1986, pp. 17–25.

The Diversity of Psychosocial Work Treatment Programs

NEW YORK VETERANS ADMINISTRATION MEDICAL CENTER*

A prevocational program for veterans with psychiatric or physical disabilities (or both) has been developed at the New York Veterans Administration Medical enter. The program, which is open to both inpatients and outpatients, includes a daily workshop, a work incentive program, and community work alternatives.

The occupational therapy prevocational program involves four levels of care: screening, evaluation, treatment, and disposition. The program has helped veterans to explore vocational goals and to adapt to work (work adjustment).

---

*Most of the information presented on the New York Veterans Administration Medical Center was prepared by Lauren Kirson, OTR.

Occupational therapy, physical therapy, corrective therapy, and educational therapy are all sections of the rehabilitation medicine service (RMS) and are responsible to the chief of RMS, who is a physiatrist.

The occupational therapy department, headed by the chief occupational therapist, comprises an assistant chief occupational therapist; three psychosocial occupational therapists, each assigned to a separate pyschiatric inpatient ward; four physical dysfunction occupational therapists, three of whom are involved with general physical disabilities rehabilitation, the fourth being a hand therapist; and a prevocational occupational therapist. A case manager, who is responsible to the chief of RMS, assists patients with outside vocational and educational referrals and works closely with the prevocational occupational therapist.

Referrals to Prevocational Occupational Therapy

Referrals are made from the RMS through the physical dysfunction therapists and from the psychiatry service through the psychosocial therapists. Outside the RMS, referrals are made on a consultation basis and are usually a part of the medical team's treatment plan for the patient.

At the time of referral, the prevocational therapist requests medical background information about the patient from the occupational therapist making the referral or the staff member requesting the consultation. The patient's medical record is also used for initial data gathering. At the time of the referral the treatment team discusses the purpose and possible goals for the patient in prevocational treatment and the treatment team's probable discharge plans for the patient.

Before the initial prevocational evaluation, screening information is provided by the occupational therapist to the prevocational therapist. For physical disabilities patients, this information includes the initial occupational therapy evaluation, a functional summary, and, when available, a self-report. These items provide information about the following areas: (1) independent living and daily living skills and performance, (2) sensorimotor skills and performance, (3) cognitive skills and performance, (4) therapeutic adaptations, (5) leisure skills, and (6) any specialized evaluation results available. For psychosocial dysfunction patients the screening information includes the patient's history and course of hospitalization, present psychiatric status, and results of the following assessments: the Barth Time Construction*, Comprehensive Occupational Therapy Evaluation (COTE) scale scores [4], and a self-report.

The areas assessed in screening are:

1. self-care
2. homemaking and maintenance
3. work or school
4. leisure time and work-play balance
5. social interpersonal skills (group)

---

*Barth, T. The Barth Time Construction (©1978). Available from Health Related Consulting Services, 130 West 28th St., New York, New York 10001.

6. social relations
7. psychological intrapersonal skills (individual)
8. sensory motor and psychomotor functions

Prevocational Evaluation

As part of the prevocational evaluation, the patient is *interviewed* by using the screening sheet shown in Fig. 6-5 to obtain specific information about his or her educational, vocational, and leisure history and to aid in determining treatment goals. It is also important to find out if the patient is service connected, as service-connected veterans are eligible for more benefits. The veteran is also asked about his or her plans with regard to living situation, work, training, school, or volunteering.

In addition to the interview, a series of *structured tasks* is used to assess (1) sensorimotor skills, including gross and fine coordination, strength, endurance, sensory integrative skills (figure–ground discrimination, visual motor integration, and praxis); and (2) cognitive skills, including concentration, attention span, memory, and problem solving. The following tasks are administered:

1. The patient is presented with *a small box of screws* of various sizes. The therapist chooses one screw and asks the patient to pick a certain number of screws of the same size.
2. The patient is shown *pieces of colored paper* and is asked to identify one color at a time. Next the patient is given simple written directions to arrange the colored paper in a certain order.
3. The patient is given *12 cards*, each bearing a word starting with a different letter of the alphabet, and is asked to put the cards in alphabetical order. Then the patient is given another set of cards, this time with words all starting with the same letter, and again is asked to alphabetize them.

These assessment tasks are similar to those from the Jacobs Prevocational Skills Assessment.

4. The patient is also given a *tiled trivet assessment*. The following materials are required:

   8″ × 8″ piece of cardboard
   Box of tiles of assorted colors, sizes, and shades
   Glue
   Sample of a tiled trivet with light-against-dark of any hue

   The therapist sits on the patient's dominant side, about two feet away, and places the box of tiles in a position to encourage midline crossing. The therapist presents the sample trivet and asks the patient to "make a trivet with the same design and then glue the tiles in place."
5. A *prevocational assessment form* has been developed to rate the patient's work skills and habits, learning abilities, interpersonal relationships, and social and psychological adjustment after the interview and evaluation tasks (Fig. 6-6).

Prevocational Program Screening Sheet

PERSONAL DATA   Date _____ _____
  1. Name _____   6. Diagnosis _____
  2. Address _____   7. Ward (referring source) _____
  3. Social Security No. _____   8. Primary therapist _____
  4. Date of birth _____   9. Precautions _____
  5. Service connection _____   10. Source of income _____
    (percentage)

EDUCATIONAL DATA
11. What level of education did you reach? _____
12. Did you ever attend any special schools? _____
13. Have you ever received vocational training? (State where and when.) ___
_____
14. Do you have any degrees, licenses, or certificates? (Specify type, date,
and where received.) _____
15. What subjects did you like when you were in school? _____
16. What subjects did you dislike when you were in school? _____

VOCATIONAL DATA
17. What is the last job that you held? _____
18. When did you work there and for how long? _____
19. State your title and briefly describe your duties. _____
_____
20. What was your reason for leaving this job? _____
21. What other jobs have you held and how long? (Include service duties.) __
_____
_____
22. What was your favorite job, and why? _____
_____
23. What was your least favorite job, and why? _____
_____
24. How do you learn best on the job? _____
_____
25. In your work experience, did you have any conflicts with your supervisor
or other employees? (Please explain.) _____
_____
26. How do you spend your leisure time? (Special interests or hobbies?) ___
_____
27. What would you like to be doing a year from now? _____
_____

YOUR JOB INTERESTS, IN ORDER OF RANK
28. _____
29. _____
30. _____
31. _____

Figure 6-5.   Screening sheet used in interview for prevocational program at New York Veterans Administration Medical Center, Rehabilitation Medicine Service. (Courtesy Lauren Kirson, OTR.)

DOCUMENTATION RECEIVED
    Consult
    Doctor's order
    Self-report
    Functional summary (Phys. Dys.)

RECOMMENDATION
    Placement area:
    Starting time and date:

                                      Approved By:

Figure 6-5.   (continued)

Treatment Planning

After the initial prevocational evaluation is completed, a *treatment plan* is made, based on the patient's physical and functional status; work, educational, and leisure history; performance on the evaluation; attitude, motivation, interests, and goals; psychological and social characteristics; and, for inpatients, discharge data and probable discharge plans.

Patients *may be excluded* from the prevocational program if, when they are evaluated, they display two or more major deficits in the following performance components: motor, sensory integrative, cognitive, psychological, or social functioning. Patients may also be excluded if they are unable to satisfactorily complete a two-week comprehensive assessment in the prevocational workshop.

Prevocational Treatment

The *prevocational workshop,* which is supervised by the prevocational occupational therapist, provides patients with work samples in a variety of areas such as clerical work, piecework, mechanical and electrical work, and crafts. These work samples are used to assess a patient's interest and potential in different vocational areas and to improve work skills, work habits, learning abilities, interpersonal relationships, and social and psychological adjustment.

The workshop is open two hours daily, five days a week. Individual schedules are arranged based on the patient's availability (taking into account other scheduled treatment), need for daily structure, treatment plan, and endurance. Each patient's progress is updated once a month, and individual meetings are held with patients as needed to discuss their progress, treatment plans, and possible disposition. The prevocational assessment form (see Fig. 6-6) is used to evaluate the patient's workshop progress.

There are two levels in the workshop: The *ongoing assessment level* is for patients who need longer-term or ongoing comprehensive assessment and exploration of work-related goals. This level can be used to assess a patient's readiness for the monetary incentive program (MIP, discussed below) and to provide work training with ongoing supervision. This level is limited to approximately two weeks. The *skill practice level,* is for patients who, after the initial prevocational evaluation and

Prevocational Assessment

Name: Date:
                                                         Ward, Area:
SS#:   Supervisor:

Rating Scale: 5 = excellent or high; 1 = poor or low

I. WORK SKILLS AND HABITS	Excellent	Very Good	Good	Fair	Poor
1. Attendance	5	4	3	2	1
2. Punctuality	5	4	3	2	1
3. Responsibility	5	4	3	2	1
4. Neatness	5	4	3	2	1
5. Endurance	5	4	3	2	1
6. Organization	5	4	3	2	1
7. Initiative	5	4	3	2	1
8. Productivity	5	4	3	2	1
9. Works independently	5	4	3	2	1
10. Concentration	5	4	3	2	1
11. Manual dexterity	5	4	3	2	1
12. Work quality	5	4	3	2	1

II. LEARNING ABILITIES					
13. Verbal instructions	5	4	3	2	1
14. Written instructions	5	4	3	2	1
15. Demonstrative instructions	5	4	3	2	1
16. Memory, retention	5	4	3	2	1
17. Recognizes errors	5	4	3	2	1

III. INTERPERSONAL RELATIONSHIPS					
18. Accepts supervision	5	4	3	2	1
19. Works with others	5	4	3	2	1

IV. SOCIAL AND PSYCHOLOGICAL ADJUSTMENT					
20. Hygiene	5	4	3	2	1
21. Motivation	5	4	3	2	1
22. Confidence	5	4	3	2	1
23. Anxiety tolerance	5	4	3	2	1
24. Frustration tolerance	5	4	3	2	1
25. Independence	5	4	3	2	1
26. Attitude toward work	5	4	3	2	1
27. Self-esteem	5	4	3	2	1

DISPOSITION:

PLAN:

Figure 6-6.   Prevocational assessment form. (Courtesy New York Veterans Administration Medical Center.)

the two-week workshop assessment, need further treatment in the areas of work skill and habits and require a structured supportive setting with regular supervision. This level can be used to prepare patients for (1) further inpatient services, (2) outpatient referrals through the case manager, (3) the MIP, or (4) community alternatives. This level is limited to approximately six months.

The monetary incentive program (MIP), a program of jobs in various services throughout the hospital, gives patients first-hand job experience. The patient is given a choice of assignments and ranks them in order of preference. The prevocational occupational therapist secures the desired position by a visit or phone call to the area and then meets with the MIP area supervisor to brief him or her about the patient. Next, the therapist and patient meet to discuss the work assignment and possible hours of duty, which are finalized in a meeting of the patient, therapist, and MIP area supervisor in the MIP work area. A time card on which the patient records his or her work hours is kept in the MIP work area. The patient and therapist meet weekly to discuss the patient's progress. The therapist also contacts the MIP area supervisor to keep informed on the patient's progress. This program is limited to approximately three months.

Counseling about *work alternatives* such as volunteer or leisure activities in the community, stroke clubs, and senior citizen centers is provided for patients who have been in occupational therapy treatment. In most cases the patient is seen by the prevocational occupational therapist for an initial prevocational assessment. For these patients the stress is on their work history, the skills they still possess, their leisure interests, their community, the availability of transportation, and their ability to use it. In some cases phone calls may be made to obtain openings in community centers or to give patients information about specific community resources. Patients are advised to learn more about resources independently or with family members. Follow-up is provided through meetings with or phone calls to patients to see if they are able to make use of the referrals and to see if further intervention is needed.

Discharge and Disposition

When a patient has shown improvement in work skills and habits or has reached a baseline level in work functioning, he or she should be ready for discharge from the program. The patient should also have a better understanding of his or her assets and some acceptance of the limitations imposed by his or her disability. It is hoped that the patient will have more realistic and specific goals. These goals may take the form of referrals to various community resources. At this point the prevocational therapist works closely with the case manager to make appropriate referrals. Patients are most often referred to the following resources:

1. The Office of Vocational Rehabilitation of New York City, which has offices in the five boroughs, and provides counseling, referral to training centers, and placement

2. The Veterans' Upgrade Center, which provides counseling, testing, and job referrals
3. The VA regional office, which provides outpatient vocational counseling and rehabilitation and houses the Curative Workshop, a sheltered workshop open to service-connected veterans
4. The Job Service of the New York State Department of Labor, which provides testing, counseling, training, and placement
5. Federation, Employment and Guidance Service, which provides counseling, testing, and referral for training or placement
6. The Private Industry Council, which provides training and placement
7. The Employment Program for Recovering Alcoholics, which provides counseling, testing, and referral for training or placement
8. The Division of Substance Abuse Services of New York State, which provides vocational and educational training, testing, and counseling
9. The International Center for the Disabled, which provides counseling, evaluation, testing (TOWER System), prevocational and vocational training, and sheltered workshop training
10. The New York City Board of Education, which provides adult education programs and a directory of educational and leisure programs

---

*Case Study**

R. D. is a 50-year-old man who was separated from his wife before his admission to the inpatient psychiatric unit of the New York VA Medical Center in May 1982. He has a son aged 12 and a daughter aged 11. R. D. had been living with his family in an unfurnished apartment. The family slept on the floor in blankets. There were no cooking facilities in the apartment.

R. D. has had many psychiatric admissions as a result of marital difficulties and alcoholism. His provisional diagnosis on this admission was depressive reaction secondary to marital discord and alcoholism in a dependent personality.

After two months of treatment on the admissions unit, the patient was transferred to the intermediate unit for further treatment. He was referred for prevocational evaluation on July 19, 1982, by the occupational therapist on that unit. R. D. was seen initially in prevocational occupational therapy on July 23, 1982, when his educational and leisure history were obtained. His education was limited to the sixth grade. The patient's father apparently withdrew him from school after the patient had had to repeat a year because of failing grades.

Before his military service R. D. worked as a short-order cook for about two years. In 1950 he enlisted in the army and was stationed in Alaska, where he worked in communications and saw no military action. He received a rank of private E-2 and was honorably discharged in 1952.

After his discharge he worked as a furniture sprayer. He left this position after six years because he felt that the paint fumes were causing him health problems. For the next two to three years R. D. was either unemployed or worked at odd jobs.

From 1961 to 1965 he worked as an operations engineer at the Hess Refinery, checking temperature readings. During his time of employment at Hess, he became abusive of alcohol and eventually was fired from his position.

After 1965 R. D. worked at numerous odd jobs for short periods of time and

*This case study was prepared by Lauren Kirson, OTR, New York Veterans Administration Medical Center, New York, New York.

spent a great deal of time unemployed. Most recently he worked as a food preparer for four months in early 1982, before his admission to the medical center.

The patient's leisure time is spent watching television and occasionally fishing.

The patient was next given the prevocational structured tasks battery. The results were as follows:

1. Work skills and habits: Score 4—very good, with mild impairments noted in organization
2. Learning abilities: Score 3—good, with mild deficits noted in ability to comprehend written directions
3. Interpersonal relationships: Score 4—very good
4. Social and psychological adjustment: Score 3—good, with impairments noted in confidence, self-esteem, and anxiety tolerance.

R. D. expressed an interest working in the food service area. On the basis of the results of the prevocational assessment, he appeared ready and motivated for an MIP assignment in the food service area.

To assess further his ability to work with foods and to determine whether his skills were commensurate with an MIP assignment, R. D. was given a cooking evaluation, which was to make a simple salad and dressing. (The MIP assignment available to occupational therapy is in the ingredients control unit, which involves working with fruits and vegetables.) The cooking evaluation revealed that R. D. was able to work with foods independently, plan the preparation of food, and use utensils safely and effectively to produce a successful outcome.

The MIP assignment was used to improve the patient's deficit areas and to prepare him for possible future employment, perhaps in the food service area.

On August 3, 1982, R. D. began his assignment in dietetics, which was to work in the hospital kitchen three hours daily in the morning. R. D. worked in the ingredients control unit, chopping vegetables and making salad plates. He also had some stock duties. After a month, R. D. increased his assignment time to four hours daily and was willing to work during early morning hours. The patient's MIP area supervisor reported that his attendance and punctuality were excellent and that he was able to complete all assigned tasks well.

R. D. was also a member of the MIP discussion group, in which he participated actively, discussing work-related issues and plans for future employment. He also attended groups on the alcohol rehabilitation unit and was able to control his drinking.

During September the patient came to the prevocational occupational therapist asking for assistance in filling out an application for employment in dietetics at the medical center. The application was completed, and the patient submitted it to personnel. His MIP area supervisor had given the patient a letter of reference recommending him for the position. In October R. D. was notified that he had been accepted for part-time employment in dietetics. He began his part-time job in early November, while still hospitalized, and was then discharged from prevocational occupational therapy. Shortly thereafter, the patient found a furnished room to rent and was discharged from the medical center. The patient has been seen informally in the hospital and has remarked that his job is going well and that he plans to seek another part-time job.

PSYCHIATRIC REHABILITATION PROGRAMS
Fountain House

Fountain House is the first psychiatric rehabilitation program established in the United States for the purpose of facilitating the social and vocational adjustment of individuals into the community after psychiatric hospitalization [2]. At Fountain House, which is located in a home-like clubhouse in New York City, over 1,000 persons attend monthly as members of a club, not as "patients." The clubhouse is open seven days a week and provides a prevocational day program that includes six units: (1) thrift shop, (2) snack bar, (3) clerical office, (4) kitchen and dining room, (5) administration, and (6) education. The program is structured to include those activities essential to clubhouse function. Members select activities that are of interest to them and that will provide them with maximum success.

> Fountain House has arranged a world that cannot function unless its members are present and active. Members work on the switchboard and reception desk, and they do maintenance, research, member reachout, and clerical jobs (which include putting out a daily newspaper for members). They run the kitchen and large dining room; they shop for food, prepare and serve more than 250 midday meals, and clean up [13].

Approximately six staff workers are responsible for supervising each unit and providing rehabilitation to its members. In essence, each unit is a smaller Fountain House, having its own responsibilities for each of the services provided by the agency. These services include (1) the Transitional Employment Program (TEP); (2) a reachout program for dropouts and rehospitalized members; (3) an apartment program for members unable to obtain adequate housing; (4) High Point, a farm project located in New Jersey that enables members to learn to garden and care for farm animals; and (5) an evening and weekend social and recreational program.

It is the TEP that is of interest to us and that will provide an example to occupational therapy programs in other facilities.

Transitional Employment Program

Each weekday approximately 150 members work, on a half-time basis, in over 40 businesses in New York and New Jersey. Placement has been secured by staff workers who have approached commerce and industry for entry-level positions requiring little training or few skills. These jobs are usually subject to high turnover or absenteeism. Arrangements are made with the employer to fill jobs on a permanent basis, rotating employees every three to six months. Two members are placed on each job, one in the morning, the other in the afternoon; each receives the prevailing wage. The staff worker first performs the job for a few hours or days to understand its requirements thoroughly, and then works alongside the member during his or her first days.

TEP has a well-established success record, and agencies now contact Fountain House for employees. Eventually, some members progress from TEP to full-time employment. As Beard [2] has noted, "Transitional employment . . . is an example of a social device which circumvents a series of barriers which all too often prevent employment of many psychiatric patients who have the capacity to perform gainful employment."

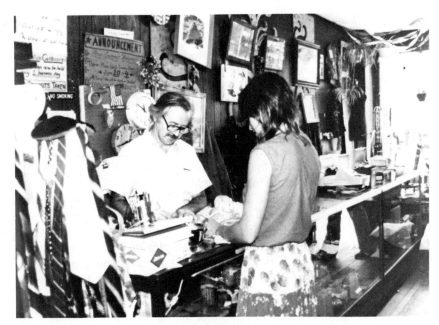

Figure 6-7. McLean Hospital's Open Door Thrift Shop, Belmont, Massachusetts. (Photograph courtesy of Matthew Gold.)

Fountain House serves as a model program, providing the impetus for the establishment of clubhouses and TEPs both nationally and internationally. In 1977 Fountain House initiated a national staff training program, which provides training opportunities "to stimulate the development of essential community services for the severely disabled psychiatric patient, and to significantly assist in the expansion of rehabilitation opportunities for this underserviced and most needful mentally disabled population" [13].

McLean Hospital Open Door Thrift Shop

McLean Hospital's Open Door Thrift Shop, a community-based retail program, is a derivation of the Fountain House model (Fig. 6-7). McLean is a private, nonprofit inpatient and outpatient facility for psychiatrically disabled clients. Within its rehabilitation services department, a variety of vocational rehabilitation programs, including a hospital-based clerical training program, food service training, and the Open Door Thrift Shop, are provided.

The shop was established in 1973 by an activity therapist as an integral part of the clinical vocational assessment program. It is an optional component in the training of McLean Hospital occupational therapy students. Donna Gatti, the program's coordinator, described the shop this way [8]: "The basic objectives of the program are twofold: to permit formal and informal evaluation of client's social, emotional and basic vocational functioning and to provide a transitional community setting for the habilitation or rehabilitation of work adjustment skills." In most cases the shop represents the first opportunity for clients to practice these skills outside the hospital. It has been effective in helping clients make the transition to more functional community roles.

The shop is located approximately one-half mile from the hospital, with a shuttle provided for the physically disabled. Over 60 patients participate in the program each year, for an average three-month period. This amount of time is in keeping with the 1975 Supreme Court decision on "patient worker wage and hour" legislation, which specifies a limit of 90 program hours for vocational evaluation and training of patients [8].

Shop tasks are analyzed, and clients are appropriately placed in jobs ranging from simple to complex. Clients work together on the truck that picks up donated merchandise, sort and price items, and, in the shop itself, sell directly to the public. Envelope stuffing, sorting, housekeeping, and activities of daily living such as vacuuming, dusting, and folding clothes are examples of highly structured, simple, one- or two-step repetitive tasks. Cashiering and preparing window and case displays are multistep, less structured tasks that require initiative and judgment.

Referral Process

Typically, after an inpatient has had various performance-related assessments, he or she can become eligible for referral to the shop by the rehabilitation counselor. Most clients referred are between the ages of 18 and 30 and have poor or nonexistent work histories; a large number have been hospitalized for more than 90 days.

Once referred, the client meets with the program coordinator for an interview, tours the shop, and is introduced to shop tasks. In the interview the client is asked to share both verbally and in written form his or her expectations and goals from participation in the shop and to discuss previous work history. At this time the coordinator discusses general program expectations such as dressing appropriately (in line with community standards), maintaining control over behavior disturbing to other workers and customers, recognizing impending loss of control and returning to hospital, being responsible for arranging appointments that are not in conflict with established work schedule and for making travel arrangements between the hospital and shop, following directions, maintaining a minimum level of verbal communication, and participating in weekly "employee" meetings. At the conclusion of the interview, clients who decide to begin placement complete a brief preemployment questionnaire and receive copies of the mutually arranged work schedule (Fig. 6-8).

Formal work evaluations are conducted monthly, with informal individual meetings held as necessary (Fig. 6-9). There is frequent communication among the program coordinator, the rehabilitation counselor, and hall (i.e., ward) treatment teams. On completion of the program the client is asked to fill out a program evaluation, which not only assists in synthesizing his or her work experience but also provides the coordinator with ongoing feedback on the entire program (Fig. 6-10).

Name _____ Date _____

1. What is your reason for wanting to work in the Thrift Shop?

_____

_____

_____

2. Do you think you could work on an "outside" job if one were available?

_____

3. Please rate yourself in comparison to people you have worked with before.

	Above Average	Average	Below Average
Attendance	____	____	____
Quality of work	____	____	____
Quantity of work	____	____	____
Ability to deal with co-workers	____	____	____
Ability to deal with supervisor	____	____	____

4. Please list, to the best of your recollection, all previous jobs held, and approximate length of time at each.

Figure 6-8. Questionnaire for McLean Hospital clients applying for work in the Open Door Thrift Shop.

FORENSIC PSYCHIATRY PROGRAMS

The forensic psychiatric institution presents a unique combination of goals and limitations for prevocational and vocational programs. By virtue of its patient population, it is usually a maximum security institution, not unlike a prison. However, it is also a hospital, with an emphasis on restoring the mental health of its patients and shaping them into responsible citizens. Work-related occupational therapy programs in two such institutions are described here.

Clifton T. Perkins Hospital Center*

Clifton T. Perkins Hospital Center in Jessup, Maryland, is a forensic psychiatric institution. It serves approximately 240 male patients, 25 percent of whom are "pretrial," that is, court-committed patients charged with major crimes. Before a pretrial patient goes to court, the patient is examined to determine his competency to stand trial (whether he understands the charges and is capable of cooperating with the court) and his responsibility (whether he was suffering from a mental disorder that caused him to lack substantial capacity to appreciate the criminality of his conduct and/or conform his conduct to the requirements of the law) at the time the crime was committed.

Fifteen percent of the population consists of penal transfers. These are patients who have become mentally ill while serving a jail or prison term. They remain institutionalized at the Center until their symptoms or behavior improve. Twenty percent of the patients come from other state hospitals. They are usually behavior or management problems,

*Most of this section was developed directly from information presented by Robin Klein, OTR.

Evaluation Form

	Needs improvement	Acceptable
PRODUCTION AND WORK SKILLS		
Concentrates on tasks		
Follows verbal directions		
Follows written directions		
Retains directions over time		
Accurate in written tasks		
Accurate in use of numbers		
Completes tasks in assigned time		
Paces own time		
Consistent in task performance		
Plans ahead in task assignments		
Establishes task priority		
Organizes two or more tasks		
Able to shift from task to task		
Able to learn new tasks		
Physically coordinated for task		
Physical tolerance (standing/ sitting)		
Can work in a noisy area		
Aware of consumer needs		
Uses tools/equipment properly		
Handles the unexpected		
COOPERATION		
Discusses work problems with supervisor		
Works with fellow workers		
Willing to redo tasks		

	Needs improvement	Acceptable
MOTIVATION		
When in doubt, asks questions		
Checks own work		
Attempts tasks until correct		
Avails self of suggestion to improve		
Uses independent judgment		
Sets own work goals		
Eager to learn		
Shares improvement ideas		
RESPONSIBILITY		
Attends regularly		
Arrives punctually		
Notifies work area when absent		
Takes breaks as scheduled		
Maintains organized work area		
Directs others in tasks		
Follows safety procedures		
Familiar with environment of area		
Accepts work standards		
WORK TRAITS		
Separates personal and work issues		
Appropriate dress/hygiene		
Use of verbal communication		
At ease in work setting		
Uses a sense of humor		
Pride in work completed		
Accepts praise		

Figure 6-9.   McLean Hospital Work Evaluation sheet, filled out monthly in conference between client and therapist.

Patient's Name _____ Hall _____ Date _____

Rehabilitation goal _____

Placement _____ Task _____ Rating _____

Current overall work strengths: _____

_____

_____

_____

_____

Areas needing improvement: _____

_____

_____

_____

Specific work goals: _____

_____

_____

_____

Patient's comment: _____

_____

_____

_____

Patient's signature _____ Hours per week _____

Accrued weeks _____ Counselor's signature _____

Staff signature _____

Name _____ Date _____

1. Please recall as clearly as you can your initial reason for coming to work in the Thrift Shop.
   _____

2. Has that goal been met? _____
   Why do you think this is so? _____

3. Please rate yourself in comparison with your co-workers.

	Above Average	Average	Below Average
Quantity of work	____	____	____
Ability to deal with customers	____	____	____
Attendance	____	____	____
Ability to deal with co-workers	____	____	____
Quality of work	____	____	____
Ability to deal with supervision	____	____	____

Do you think working in the Thrift Shop is: ____ similar to outside jobs
   ____ not at all like outside jobs

I feel ____ more able
   ____ less able
   to hold an "outside" job than before
   working at the Thrift Shop.

5. How do you account for this? _____
   _____

6. Please rate the Thrift Shop as you see it.

	High	Medium	Low
Amount of pressure on workers from customers	___	___	___
Amount of pressure on workers from supervisor	___	___	___
Amount of responsibility given to workers	___	___	___
Amount of criticism from supervisor	___	___	___
Amount of praise or support from supervisor	___	___	___
Amount of criticism from co-workers	___	___	___
General job satisfaction	___	___	___
Value of weekly meetings	___	___	___

7. What did you find most frustrating? _____
   Most fun? _____
   Most challenging? _____

8. What changes would you like to see in the Thrift Shop?

OTHER COMMENTS

Figure 6-10.   A program evaluation form, which McLean Hospital clients are requested to complete at the conclusion of their work experience program.

causing danger to themselves or others. Approximately 4 percent are at the Center for observation and treatment for competency before standing trial. The rest, about half of the Center's patients, have been declared insane by the courts (not guilty by reason of insanity) at the time of the commission of the crime; they are sent to Perkins until their behavior is no longer considered dangerous.

The average length of stay at the Center is 2½ years. Under the direct care of the hospital staff, patients are exposed to a multidisciplinary approach. They are seen regularly on their ward by a treatment team consisting of a psychiatrist, a clinical nurse, a nursing attendant, a social worker, a psychologist, and an occupational or activity therapist. This team evaluates the patient's strengths and weaknesses and attempts to coordinate a comprehensive program addressing those needs. Treatment includes drug therapy, verbal support groups, individual therapy, and activities. Occupational therapists screen patients, observing characteristics such as hygiene, physical disabilities, perceptual problems, time use, cognition, and interests, and assessing previous life situations. As a result further evaluation and treatment may be deemed appropriate.

The occupational therapy department is eclectic in its approach, taking into account the theories of Gail Fidler, Anne Cronin Mosey, Gary Kielhofner, and Claudia Allen [1]. The functional status of each patient is assessed in the hospital. Questions to be addressed include the following:

How does the patient cope with stress, relate to others and the environment, and take care of physical needs?

What does the patient attend to?

Can the patient follow written or verbal instructions? How complex?

Does the patient have special interests? How realistic are those interests?

What does the patient do during unstructured time?

Can the patient work in a group setting?

What are the patient's functional math skills?

Evaluation

All patients referred to the occupational therapy department undergo two hours of group testing. The first hour includes a questionnaire that assesses reality orientation, problem solving, time use, interests, perception, functional math skills, attention to written instructions, short-term memory, and leisure interests and identifies significant others. Reading and writing skills are also observed at this time. People who are functionally illiterate are questioned orally.

The second hour of the evaluation is task oriented. Patients are first given a model and instructed to reproduce it as closely as possible with the materials provided. This task addresses problem solving, sequencing, task organization, time management, fine motor skills, and the ability to follow verbal instructions. Patients are allowed 30 minutes to complete the project. Then a group task is presented. A large sheet of paper and several drawing media are placed on a table. The patients are instructed to plan, organize, and complete a mural as a group. They are allotted 30 minutes for the task. In this task each patient's ability to participate in a group is evaluated. The quantity and quality of contribution, the informal social interaction, the subject of the drawing, and its relation to the theme chosen by the group are all considered in this part of the evaluation.

The information extracted from the evaluation assists in developing a profile of the patient's functional abilities, interests, and values so that an individual treatment program can be formulated.

Occupational and Activity Therapy Programs

The hospital offers two interconnected departments: occupational therapy and activity therapy. The departments interface in patient treatment. However, the occupational therapist is solely responsible for evaluation and consults on activity therapy program development.

Patients are placed in an occupational therapy program according to their level of function. As skills develop and behavior changes, patients progress to the next higher level. The occupational therapy program's approach is similar to that of the hospital in that behavior and insight are the barometers of a patient's readiness to move to less restrictive and more privileged environments. This progression eventually leads to a work release ward and finally to the community, at which point the patient is placed in a halfway house. After placement in a halfway house, the patient is followed for five years and must meet specific conditions or be subject to legal action.

The various occupational therapy programs attempt to address patients at every level.

In the *one-to-one* program the goal is to assist the patient who demonstrates an attention span limited to about five minutes. The patient may exhibit severe disorganization of thought processes or may be unable to trust other patients or staff. The purpose of the therapy is to establish rapport through the introduction of simple familiar repetitive nonverbal tasks, such as playing cards, solving puzzles, drawing, listening to music, and playing ball.

In *dyadic skills* the patient is introduced to the group therapeutic setting, which is structured into periods of 30 minutes and accommodates six patients. Games and tasks continue to be familiar and repetitive, with the addition of verbal and nonverbal interactions between patients. Patients are paired, and activities are selected to elicit the sharing of materials. Verbalizing one's needs, decision making, and performance are encouraged.

The *project group* is task oriented. All craft activities and games are chosen by the therapist to maximize group participation and interaction. At this level the patient must be able to attend to an activity for an hour. Tasks are frequently novel, encouraging learning and exploration.

In *verbal problem and values clarification* patients are presented with verbal exercises and situations that stimulate discussion. Decision making, sharing ideas, and establishing personal norms are again encouraged. The emphasis here is on volitional development. Without this, interests and goals cannot exist since it motivates the pursuit of any vocation.

The *time management program* is for patients on the work release ward. One of the great difficulties for patients is the use of unstructured time. This problem often predates the patient's hospitalization. It continues throughout the course of hospitalization and can be exaggerated during the transition from a highly structured to an unstructured environment. Therefore, leisure planning and scheduling become an important focus. Simultaneously patients may attend a prerelease group centering on job hunting, interviews, money management, nutrition, grooming, apartment hunting, and homemaking. This group is continued when patients eventually move to the community halfway house.

In all groups activities are designed to be enjoyable, to stimulate self-activitation, and to foster "subcortical" learning.

Like occupational therapy programming, activity therapy programs are also on a grouped, graduated basis. Patients are initially placed in arts and crafts and gross motor activity groups and given on-ward cleanup duties. They progress to dining room cleanup and music therapy, then to custodial services. At this level emphasis is on janitorial work skills taught via classroom and practical experience. This program runs six hours a day, five days a week for six months. In addition, workshop programs, which consist of contract projects such as separating cotton batting and assembling bingo cards, are available. These are the only programs that offer a small monetary compensation. As patients progress to the less restrictive work release ward, they are assigned to various departments (eg., maintenance, dietary, and library services), where they learn different tasks through apprenticeship techniques. Patients are evaluated by staff members, who help determine readiness for working in the community. Most of the vocational programs are offered outside the hospital at other facilities. The emphasis within the hospital is on controlling behavior, improving insight, and developing the foundation skills necessary for survival in the community.

Limitations of the Forensic Environment

The forensic patient is often limited in what he can pursue prevocationally in the hospital. The security orientation of the hospital is extremely restrictive, with items made of materials such as glass, rope, metal, and wood often considered contraband or, if allowed, requiring close supervision. These restrictions narrow the variety of training that can be offered.

Cultural and educational considerations also play a part in vocational emphasis. The patient population at Perkins is of diverse origin (both rural and urban); many come from impoverished environments, and many are functionally illiterate. Other limiting factors are staffing and funding. (These limits are not exclusive to maximum security hospitals!)

A final limiting factor is the double stigma superimposed on all patients deemed "not guilty by reason of insanity." Not only are patients labelled "mentally ill," but they often have to cope with a "criminal" identification as well. Many of the patients are well known in the community because of media coverage of the criminal incident. This often interferes with obtaining work or entrance to training school. The occupational therapy department attempts to address this issue by role playing confrontations in groups.

Currently the occupational therapy department at the center is two years old. Patients who have been referred to the department are in either the early or late stage of their treatment course. Chronic patients require slow, steady incremental challenges to assimilate learning and build trust. Improvement is frequently minimal, and in some cases maintenance of present function is a realistic treatment goal.

Case Study*

L. D. is a 27-year-old single man who was admitted in 1980 on charges of assault with intent to rape. The offense was committed at another hospital.

When L. D. was 14 he was taken in to be raised by an aunt after the suicide of his father and the death of cancer of his mother. He was described as a poor student was was placed in special education classes from seventh through twelfth grade. He was active in sports and had many girl friends. At the age of 18 L. D. suffered a stroke, which resulted in right-upper-extremity hemiparesis with mild residual spasticity and atrophy, an ataxic gait, and some perceptual dysfunction. The patient was left dominant. He was hospitalized for one month at an acute-care hospital, then received outpatient therapy at a rehabilitation hospital. This therapy was discontinued after two months because of his irregular attendance. After his stroke his behavior changed dramatically. L. D. exposed himself in public, followed women soliciting sex, and was considered a nuisance by the neighborhood. He was employed for a short time but was fired because of his inability to concentrate on the job. Two weeks later he was persuaded by the family to go to a state hospital. At the hospital he attempted to rape a nurse.

After this offense, L. D. was sent to Clifton T. Perkins Hospital Center to be evaluated for competency and responsibility. He was diagnosed as having organic personality syndrome and was found competent to stand trial by all four state psychiatrists. He was adjudged not guilty by reason of insanity by the circuit court, which sent him back to Perkins for treatment.

The patient's course in the hospital was marked by emotional lability and impulsive agitated behavior. He was frequently observed pacing, talking to himself, using profanity toward staff, masturbating in the presence of female nurses, and provoking fights with other patients. Treatment with haloperidol (Haldol) and carbamazepine (Tegretol) was begun, with a resulting reduction in violent behavior.

The patient was referred to the occupational therapy department in 1981. Muscle testing revealed mild flexor spasticity in forearm, wrist, and fingers of the right upper extremity. Other motions in the right upper extremity were in the F+ to G− range. Mild sensory deficits were noted in sharp-dull discrimination on the volar surface of the forearm. The rest of his sensation was intact. No field cut was evident. Perceptual testing revealed mild deficits in figure–ground discrimination, constructional praxis, and position in space. The questionnaire revealed difficulty with written instructions, mathematics, short-term memory, spelling, and grammar. He was oriented to time, place, and person and completed the evaluation during the time allowed. In the tile coaster assembly task, the patient followed three-step verbal instructions correctly. He used his left (dominant) hand to manipulate the ¼-inch tiles and his right hand as a weak assist. The patient organized his project in a recognizable manner, and sequencing was accurate. He did not complete the task during the time

*This case study was provided by Robin Klein, OTR, Clifton T. Perkins Hospital Center, Jessup, Maryland.

allotted. L. D. performed on a parallel group level during the mural section of the evaluation. He did not contribute to the planning or implementation of the drawing. He observed others draw until most of the mural had been completed and then colored using broad strokes of a crayon in the area of the paper directly in front of him. Minimal verbal communication was noted.

L. D. reported that his employment history consisted of temporary janitorial work. He stated that his goals in the hospital are to "marry and get along with people on the outside." He listed his leisure interests as "games on the ward and baseball." The patient's description of a typical morning, afternoon, and evening outside the hospital was "I help take out laundry, bring back laundry, and sweep the floor," which was in actuality a description of his activities within the hospital. His response indicated deficits in reality testing and temporal awareness.

Treatment has been multifaceted, The patient exhibited psychological, organic, and motor deficits that impede skill, life role, and volitional development. The patient was initially placed in occupational therapy at the one-to-one level for one-half hour twice weekly. The goals were to maintain and improve right-upper-extremity function, increase compensation for perceptual deficits, improve written and oral communication skills, and increase leisure skill repertoire. His present role is as a patient rather than a worker (which is more age appropriate). His interests have been limited, and his day has been extrinsically structured (by the hospital). The primary occupational therapy used was card games, therapeutic exercises, Purdue Pegboard assembly, Frostig worksheets, programmed math and reading books, Nerf ball games, clerical tasks (collating and stapling), and strumming an autoharp. Treatment was slow and progressive. Initially the focus was on right-upper-extremity function with repetitive activities and exercises. As the patient learned to perform the tasks independently, he was advanced to writing exercises that incorporated reading and functional math problems. Exercises were then monitored periodically. Autoharp strumming and memorization of songs were added. Card games were used as a vehicle for learning new leisure skills and practicing communication skills by teaching the therapist new games. All tasks increased in complexity and challenge.

Six months after treatment began it was noted on the ward that the patient had ceased masturbating, was less "playful," and had stopped getting into altercations with the other patients. In the arts and crafts activity group it was observed that he was able to handle delicate ceramic greenware with his right hand. He was also able to follow two- or three-step verbal instructions and maintained a steady work pace without encouragement. However, the patient consistently worked alone.

L. D. was advanced to the dyadic skills group three months later. He continues to participate in arts and crafts, and a gross motor gym group has been added to his program. All tasks in dyadic skills require sharing verbal information and materials with a partner. L. D. has not been spontaneous in this area; frequent structuring and encouragement by the therapist are required. Once he can incorporate social interaction with task organization and completion, he will progress to higher-level groups until he is capable of working in a simulated hospital job. Assuming his behavior continues to improve, he will eventually be ready for community placement.

Calgary General Hospital Forensic Psychiatry Unit*

Calgary General Hospital, located in the city of Calgary, Alberta, Canada, offers another example of occupational therapy's involvement in forensic psychiatry. The psychiatric wing of the hospital consists of

*Most of this section was written directly from information presented by Robert C. Schneider, OTR.

three inpatient units (maximum 67 patients) and the forensic unit (maximum 20 patients). The patients are remanded to the forensic unit for up to 30 days for one of several purposes: (1) for pretrial assessment of fitness to stand trial, (2) for presentence assessment to recommend possible psychiatric facilities and treatment follow-up, (3) for assessment for parole, and (4) for acute treatment. At the end of the patient's stay, the assessment team submits a letter to the court indicating whether or not the patient is fit to stand trial, with recommendations for immediate or future placement and presentence reports.

Although the primary goal of this unit is assessment, patients also undergo treatment and therapeutic intervention in the form of therapy groups concerned with life skills training, basic communications, sexuality, alcohol, and psychodrama. The occupational therapist leads an assertiveness training program, an art therapy group, and a workshop program besides participating in daily community meetings.

As a member of the assessment team, the therapist evaluates the patient's functional level before and since admission to the unit, that is, how the patient copes with activities of daily living. Typically used is the standardized Bay Area Functional Performance Evaluation,* which consists of a task-oriented assessment, a social interaction scale, and a written functional assessment form. In addition, the workshop program described in the following section is an integral part of the assessment. Utilized in the workshop is the Activity Therapy Evaluation (Fig. 6-11).

The workshop is a daily 1½-hour program run in conjunction with the recreational therapist. It provides activities that serve as assessment tools and promote skill development. Patients construct toys that are distributed to needy children in the Calgary community (Fig. 6-12).

As an assessment instrument,

> [the] workshop functions as a means of patient assessment as observed through the activity process. This includes:
> 1. general task behaviors of frustration tolerance, level of concentration, motor coordination, decision making, judgment and problem solving;
> 2. interpersonal behaviors such as cooperation with others, level of independence, sociability or self assertion; and
> 3. work skills evaluation in areas of self responsibility, punctuality, motivation, initiative, dependability and quality of work produced, as well as some basic work history and attitudes towards the work [14].

As a skill development tool, the workshop encourages goal attainment and achievement. It develops in the patient a sense of responsibility for his or her own behavior through fulfillment of a work contract (Fig. 6-13) and active participation. It facilitates the daily interaction with others and awareness of their effect on the work environment through daily participation and weekly discussion. By means of weekly goal setting, group discussion, and the encouragement of independent decision making, the workshop develops independent planning and goal achievement. It develops basic woodworking skills through instruction and demonstration by therapists, and it fosters self-esteem through

*Consulting Psychologists Press, Inc., 577 College Ave., Palo Alto, CA 94306.

realization of accomplishment, achieved again through weekly group discussion, peer support of accomplishments, communication of the workshop achievements in community meetings, and positive feedback from therapists.

All patients meeting minimal criteria (able to tolerate a 45-minute structured group meeting and not actively suicidal or a threat to the security of the unit) are eligible for entrance into the program and are expected to attend an orientation session. In the orientation session the following information is provided:

I. Introduction to therapists
II. Explanation of workshop program
    A. Meeting time and days of workshop
    B. Break schedule
    C. Purpose of workshop
        1. An assessment tool
        2. A treatment group
        3. An enjoyable activity
III. Explanation of shop guidelines
    A. Tool use
    B. Cleanup of materials
    C. Arrival time
    D. Notification of therapists if late for appointment
    E. Explanation of contract
IV. Explanation of work history form
V. Tour of workshop

In addition, the patient is asked to perform a short, simple activity to provide the therapist with a preliminary skill assessment.

The workshop program includes a weekly 1½-hour meeting of all the patients involved in the program for the past week. The meeting is conducted by the workshop coordinator, who also writes notes on the meeting for the following week. This coordinator, who is selected by the therapists, is a patient who has been involved in the workshop program for at least one week and who demonstrates the capacity to coordinate the meeting.

The weekly meeting is an important aspect of the treatment process, providing for personal and group problem solving. It offers an opportunity to discuss achievement (or nonachievement) of goals. Patients develop awareness of others through sharing ideas and contributing project accomplishments to the group. During the meeting conflicts between patients and staff are worked out. Patients determine their personal goals for the following week and sign a contract for the following week (see Fig. 6-13). Other areas explored in the group include the patient's potential in the job market and possible avenues of career training while the patient is in prison (e.g., classes and training programs). The group may also help the patient understand his behavior and attitudes and their relationship to his ability to hold a job.

Low self-esteem, difficulties accepting authority, and alcohol addiction are major problems among the patients in the forensic unit at

Program/Date

1   Almost never
2   Occasionally
3   Half the time
4   Three-quarters of the time
5   Almost always
N/A Not applicable

A. LEVEL OF TASK DIFFICULTY

B. INTERPERSONAL/PSYCHOLOGICAL FUNCTION

1. Appropriate appearance in relation to role, social group situation, age, sex
2. Absence of nonproductive behaviors (rocking, playing with hands, repetitive movements, preoccupation)
3. Expression of affect (spontaneous, clear, appropriate)
4. Cooperative with group (verbal/nonverbal)
5. Demonstrates ability to initiate, respond to, sustain verbal interaction
6. Demonstrates ability to make own decisions
7. Accepts authority, yet can state own opinion without aggression
8. Demonstrates ability to compromise and negotiate
9. Recognizes and acts on strengths and weaknesses
10. Self-direction in unstructured setting and/or task
11. Demonstrates awareness of others' needs/feelings

Figure 6-11.   Activity therapy evaluation, Calgary General Hospital.

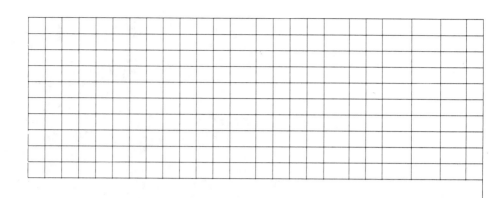

C. COGNITIVE/TASK SKILLS

1. Reality orientation (place, person, time, situation)
2. Attention span for activity duration
3. Demonstrates ability to engage in structured activity without staff encouragement
4. Follows oral directions
5. Follows written directions
6. Remembers instructions
7. Concentrates despite distraction
8. Appropriate pace in activity
9. Tolerates frustration
10. Able to organize task (plan, understand, perform)
11. Can solve problems
12. Assumes responsibility for own actions, thoughts, feelings

D. WORK BEHAVIOR

1. Punctuality
2. Neatness in activity
3. Reliability (adherence to expectations)
4. Demonstrates safety awareness

E. MOTOR SKILLS

1. Demonstrates spontaneous reactions and reflexes
2. Demonstrates adequate gross motor coordination for task (movement patterns, balance, proprioception)
3. Demonstrates adequate fine motor coordination for task (hand manipulative skills, eye-hand coordination, perceptual motor coordination)
4. Physical endurance for activity duration

F. ATTENDANCE

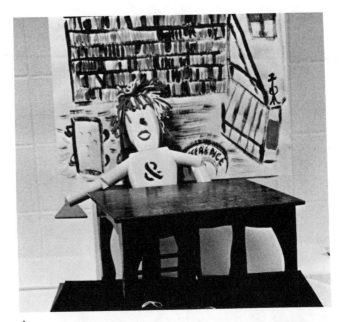

A

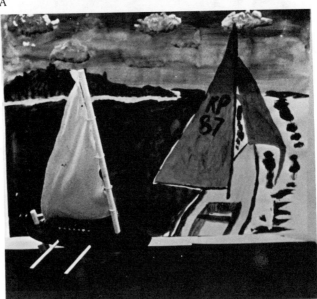

B

Figure 6-12.   Toys constructed by patients in the Calgary General Hospital workshop. A: Puppet. B: Sailboat.

```
WORKSHOP CONTRACT
Name: _____ Date: _____
Please think carefully about whether involvement in this program would be
helpful to you, and then fill in the appropriate space below:

(1) I agree to participate in the workshop and work for _____ of
    the five days of the week
or
(2) I would like to observe the program for one week _____
or
(3) I do not think it would be helpful for me because _____
    _____

Goal for the week: _____
    _____

[For next week...]
I achieved/did not achieve the above goal because _____
    _____
    _____

Signature _____
Witnessed _____
```

Figure 6-13.   Workshop contract used at Calgary General Hospital.

Calgary General. Participation in the workshop program has facilitated working through these issues.

Evaluation

The therapist assesses the patient's progress in the workshop program and all activity groups via the Activity Therapy Evaluation (Fig. 6-11). This evaluation is derived from the evaluation of the same name of the activity therapy department of Sheppard and Enoch Pratt Hospital, Towson, Maryland, as well as from Claudia Allen's work on cognitive disabilities [1].

The department uses Claudia Allen's hierarchy of cognitive *levels of task difficulty* (Table 6-1) to select and design activities that correspond to the patient's level of ability [1]. All activities have been analyzed using Allen's task analysis for cognitive disability (Table 6-2) and then graded on a scale of 1 to 5. These levels correspond directly to Allen's levels 2 to 6, that is, Calgary's level 1 corresponds to Allen's level 2, Calgary's level 2 corresponds to Allen's level 3, and so on. Allen's level 1 has been eliminated because the "reflexive" patient, that is, the patient who appears unaware of his external environment, would not attend occupational therapy but would be in constant nursing care. The following are examples of tasks for patients at the various levels:

In *Level 1* the patient sands and paints (with one color of his choice) a previously constructed toy. The toy is simple and without difficult corners. The patient works in a minimal-stimulation area.

In *Level 2* the patient does straight crosscut sawing. An example is a boat project, for which the patient cuts several blocks of wood, sands, and paints. The therapist shows the patient an unpainted sample, per-

Table 6-1.   Levels of cognitive disability

	Level 1: Reflexive	Level 2: Movement	Level 3: Repetitive actions
Attention	Patients do not seem to be able to focus their attention or screen out external stimuli	Patients attend to their own postural movements	Patients attend to the effects their own motor actions have on the environment
Goal Selection	Patients are conscious and reflexes are functional; they may or may not be able to eat and drink	Chance body movements create an interesting result, which patients attempt to repeat	Chance movements cause a perceived environmental result, which they repeat many times
Imitation	No imitation is observed	Patients can approximate gross body movements if they are familiar schemes; therapist may imitate patient's movement	Patients can imitate therapist when their own familiar schemes are demonstrated
Tangible Objectivity	Patients are subjective; do not seem to be aware of people or objects in the external environment	Patients watch with transient awareness people and objects that are moving	Objects and people are understood in terms of patient's own motor actions; external causes are not understood
Time	There is no behavior to indicate that patients can mark the passage of time	Attention is focused for a very limited period; patients require continual direction	Patients can focus their attention on tasks that have repetitive actions; can remember and anticipate a series of events based on their own actions

Level 4: End product	Level 5: Variations	Level 6: Tangible thought
Patients can focus their attention to complete a task; an end product that can be visually perceived; sustains attention	Patients seek novelty through variations in their actions and end products; perceptual cues are used to adjust motor actions	Patients begin to think about possibilities before physically testing the result; visual images guide motor actions
Patients can use several familiar schemes to achieve an end product	Overt trial and error is used to discover a new means of achieving the goal	Covert trial-and-error-problem solving occurs; images are used to test solutions to problems
Actions that expand their familiar schemes can be imitated, one scheme at a time; errors are not corrected	A series of schemes can be imitated and remembered; new schemes can be imitated and learned	Patients can imitate therapist when therapist is no longer present
When an object can be seen, patients are aware that it has its own movement, causing its own effect	Patients explore the potential of other objects and people	Patients begin to infer the cause of a change; they may need to validate the cause
Patients can anticipate future events based on an interpretation of signs, using the actions of others	Time is measured by the hours and days required to produce the novelty	Through the use of images, patients can separate themselves from the immediate present and project themselves into the past or future

Source: From C. Allen [1].

Table 6-2.   Task analysis for cognitive disability

	Level 1: Reflexive	Level 2: Movement	Level 3: Repetitive actions
Patient characteristics			
Attention to	Internal thoughts and feelings with little awareness of external stimuli	Patients enjoy planned postural movements	Energy is invested in doing simple tasks with repetitive actions
Attention span	Transient, generally less than 1 minute	Average 5–20 minutes; patients are distracted by movement and sound and need frequent redirection	Average 15–30 minutes; continuous refocusing of attention is required
Therapist's directions			
Imitation	Looks at demonstrated directions but does not imitate them	Gross body movements; you may need to guide the movement physically	Patients will follow demonstration when their familiar schemes are used
Verbalizations	May respond to one-word verbs such as "eat" or "chew"	Reinforce demonstration with a few simple nouns and verbs	Reinforce demonstration with repeated simple nouns and verbs
Number of directions	One direction, repeated	One direction, repeated	One direction, repeated
Task selection			
Structure of the activity	Most important tasks are eating and drinking	Familiar, repetitive gross body movements	Tasks with one repeated step or scheme
Predictability	Familiar foods and fluids	Familiar body movements	Repetitive actions with a uniform effect upon the environment
Choice provided	When possible, recognize individual food preferences	Therapist plans the movements and may respond to patients' suggestions or actions	Limited to two or three items to avoid distractions
Tools	Fingers and hands, rather than utensils	Objects that are associated with gross body movements, e.g., jump ropes, soft balls	Generally patients do better with their hands; some use of familiar tools
Storage of materials and projects	Obtained for the patients	Taken care of by therapist	Taken care of by therapist
Preparation by the therapist	Food packages and cartons may need to be opened for patients	Plan movements and obtain any needed equipment	Lay out supplies in advance; do any preliminary and/or finishing steps that are not repetitive or not familiar
Setting	Reduce the number of stimuli when possible	Open space	Clutter-free

Level 4: Goal directed	Level 5: Variations	Level 6: Tangible thought
Patients focus on visual sample of an end product	Overt trial-and-error problem solving; patients interested in similar tasks, which permit variations in their actions	Covert trial-and-error problem solving; energy is directed toward using images to plan an action
If interrupted, patients can refocus their own attention in order to achieve their goal; average task should be completed within 30–45 minutes	Attention may be sustained while external stimuli are present; tasks may take two or more sessions to complete	Within normal limits
Patients can imitate moderately novel demonstrations that expand familiar schemes	Patients can learn through serial imitation so that a number of steps may be demonstrated; unfamiliar steps may be introduced and through practice will be learned	Patients can learn through delayed imitation so that demonstrated directions may be retained over a period of time; through use of images, simple diagrams or familiar written directions may be followed
Use simple nouns and verbs, avoiding discussions or open-ended questions	Adjectives and prepositions may be used in explaining variations	Use of images may be encouraged when materials to be worked with are present
One direction for each step; wait until each step is completed before giving the next direction	Two or more directions may be given at one time	Two or more directions may be given at one time
Simple quick tasks with a visual end product, bright colors, and two-dimensional shapes; avoid childish connotations with adults	Activities that permit variation; the effects of one's actions can easily be seen and corrected	Activities that permit variation in selecting and planning steps
Potential errors should be easily corrected by the therapist	Patients must be able to physically perceive the effect their actions have on objects and end results	Patients must be able to predict the effect their actions will have on objects and end results
Avoid confusion by limiting the decisions and materials; provide opportunity for exact replication of sample	Several choices in materials, tools, and activity selection may be provided; demonstrate and clarify variations	Several choices in materials, tools, and tasks can be provided and discussed
Familiar objects; no power tools	Simple tools that are a linear extension of the hand or arm are the most successful	Patients can learn how to use unfamiliar machines and tools
Patients can place and/or find materials when clearly visible or very familiar	Patients can search for things in probable locations and can place or find things in labelled drawers or cabinets	Patients can follow verbal directions to place or find materials
Lay out supplies in advance, provide an exact sample of the finished product, and do the steps that require unfamiliar tools or schemes	Sample of the finished product need not be exact; patterns and procedures must be supplied by therapist	Materials, designs, and/or pictures must be present for covert problem solving
Other patients working on the same task	People, music, and clutter can be present	Free access to materials and supplies

forms some shaping of the hull, and assists the patient in stacking deck sections (see Fig. 6-12).

In *Level 3* a model stunt plane is an ideal project. The patient is shown a sample product, is given a pattern to trace, and performs rounded and angled cuts. The patient then shapes, sands, glues, and paints the airplane in a two-color scheme.

In *Level 4* the patient is given a choice of several simple patterns for a car. The patient performs all parts of the task except drilling holes for wheels, for which he may need assistance. Variations in color and other options are available.

In *Level 5* the patient may choose to draw an original plan for a toy. Limitations are set as to the size of the toy and the type of materials available.

Sections B through E of the evaluation (see Fig. 6-11) provide *other measures* of performance through the therapist's observations in the areas of interpersonal and psychological function, cognitive and task skills, work behavior, and motor skills. Progress is measured by an increased score within specific performance areas and by successful completion of increasingly difficult tasks.

Case Study*

A. A., a 61-year-old married male, was admitted to the forensic unit on transfer from a city court in Alberta, Canada, where he was facing several charges related to alleged sexual indiscretions with children. The charges leading to his admission to the forensic unit were his first contact with the legal system.

A. A. was at first quite wary of the unit and appeared overwhelmed by his situation. He initially appeared depressed, with social isolation, crying episodes, and a decreased appetite, but seemed to adjust to the unit in a few days.

A. A. is a farmer with an eighth-grade education. He appeared older than his stated age. He was oriented to time, person, and place, and he was not psychotic on initial contact.

On the third day after admission, the occupational therapist approached the patient to involve him in the workshop, explaining the program and its contribution to the forensic assessment. In the initial session, the patient demonstrated low self-esteem ("I can't do anything, I'm just a farmer") and stated that he had had minimal experience in working with wood. Nevertheless he was cooperative and agreed to "try" to attend the workshop.

In the following sessions it was evident that A. A. had had woodworking experience. With initial help from the therapist in deciding on a project, A. A. designed a doll chair. Although progressing successfully, he continued to voice self-deprecating comments and required reinforcement from the therapist for his short-term accomplishments. A. A. also experienced fine motor tremors and required occasional assistance in following a straight edge with a pencil. His goal for the following week was to have the pieces of the chair cut, glued, sanded, and ready for staining.

In the following week the patient consistently attended the workshop program. He became more bright and spontaneous. His self-esteem increased, as noted in his work independence and fewer self-defeating comments. The patient also became more definite in his decision making. In the weekly workshop meeting he stated that he had accomplished his goal from the previous week and gave others some woodworking suggestions.

Although continuing to exhibit a fine motor tremor, A. A. was able to handle

*This case study was prepared by Robert C. Schneider, OTR, Calgary General Hospital, Calgary, Alberta, Canada.

a saw effectively and cut a fine line. He continued with the project, sanded and stained it, and painted on two coats of varnish.

While waiting for the varnish to dry, A. A. designed a table to match the chair. He designed the table on paper, transferred the design on to x-ray paper to make a permanent pattern, and used the pattern effectively to cut pieces of wood for the table. He completed this table before discharge from the unit. His approach to the final product demonstrated forethought, constructive problem solving on detailed work, and a tolerance for dealing with the frustration that occurs daily in a workshop on a locked unit.

In early workshop sessions A. A. was demanding of the therapist's attention and demonstrated helplessness and inability to perform. However, this receded as the patient involved himself in his project. He grew less dependent and his skills became more noticeable. As his work progressed, he received encouragement and compliments from other workshop participants. They would ask A. A. for ideas, and he freely gave suggestions and demonstrated the use of various tools.

A. A. was involved in psychological testing for three days but attended 17 of 20 offered workshop sessions.

A. A. was found fit to stand trial by the forensic team. The occupational therapy workshop program provided the following information to assist in this decision:

1. The patient does not appear to be psychotic (i.e., no hallucinations or delusions noted).
2. Although he appeared depressed initially, his progress, increased socialization, increased motivation, and active involvement suggest that his mood would not affect his appreciation of the trial.
3. Although parkinsonian movements hinder his fine motor abilities, the tremors do not affect his functional performance.
4. The patient does not appear to have an organic brain condition or to be mentally retarded to a degree that would affect his comprehension of the trial.
5. The patient appears to possess adequate problem solving and decision making abilities and foresight to instruct counsel and assist in his own defense.
6. The patient seems to possess adequate frustration tolerance and control of his impulsiveness to tolerate the length of the trial and not to decompensate while awaiting trial.

Additional information on the patient's overall work and interpersonal skills in occupational performance was gained through observation.

The patient's discharge diagnosis (according to the format outlined in the Diagnostic and Statistical Manual*) was as follows:

Axis I. Paraphilia—pedophilia
Axis II. No diagnosis
Axis III. Questionable Parkinson's disorder
Axis IV. Psychosocial stressor moderate IV
Axis V. Adaptive functioning good III

A. A. was found guilty of his offenses and received a sentence of three months in the city jail system.

---

*American Psychiatric Association. *Diagnostic and Statistical Manual of Mental Disorders* (3rd ed.). Washington, D.C.: APA (1700 Eighteenth St., N.W., Washington, D.C. 20009), 1980.

CORRECTIONAL INSTITUTIONS

Work-related programs in correctional institutions are diverse, reflecting the goal ambiguity that exists in correctional philosophy. While rehabilitation is the avowed objective of incarceration, in reality funding priorities reveal a greater commitment to protecting the public from the offender and to maintaining order within the institution. For example, in 1979 only 1.5 percent of the total costs of incarceration in the United States went for work-related programs [5].

A brief review of the types of work-related programs will provide a framework for discussing occupational therapy's place in these facilities. There are two general categories of work-related programs: institutionally based and community-based.

Institutionally Based Programs

Most work-related programs in prisons are institutionally based. In most instances such programs are designed, implemented, and evaluated solely by correctional administration and staff. Others, however, involve community members in both curriculum design and instruction. The use of instructors from local educational institutions facilitates training that more closely resembles the type received in the community. In some instances, offenders released before completing such training may have the opportunity to do so when released. A third type of institutionally based program is designed to provide workers for the maintenance of the correctional facility or for prison industries. Historically, prison industries were created to offset the high cost of institutional operations and to provide job training while giving inmates opportunity to earn money while incarcerated. In reality, prison industries are often low paying and have little carry-over to community jobs. For example, it was not until recently that the manufacture of license plates, a common prison job, was also done commercially outside correctional facilities.

In 1975 the Law Enforcement Assistance Administration piloted the concept of combining realistic work opportunities with useful skill training. Entitled the Free-Venture Project, it required that

> representatives of industry be involved in the planning and implementation of the institutional industrial program. The project also requires that market surveys be conducted as a part of the planning process, equipment and training be comparable to that in industry, and job placement services be provided to offenders returning to the community. The program must replicate the community work environment as closely as possible. [5]

In one program inmates were trained as and became computer analysts for large firms while imprisoned. These inmates, upon discharge, were hired by the same firms [5, 7].

Another effort to provide institutionally based programs is the school district concept. Instructional services are designed and administered through collaborative agreements between correctional institutions and state or local education agencies [5].

Community-Based Programs

In community-based programs, which are less common, the inmates are released from the institution for a portion of the day to obtain on-the-job training or job-related training in a community facility. Work release and halfway house programs are two types of community-based programs.

Work Release Programs

Work release programs afford the inmate the opportunity to work outside the correctional setting. Although in the 1970s work release regarded as a promising reform, public resentment toward the presence of sentenced offenders in the community curtailed its expansion. Potter observes that except in a handful of states, work release has never really caught on: "Seldom are more than 10 percent of a state's inmates involved in work-release programs. Most often, the proportion is 1 or 2 percent" [7].

Halfway House Programs

Halfway house programs give inmates an opportunity to gain on-the-job training while residing in minimum-security institutions within the community, thus providing a gradual transition from institutional life to society. An inmate is typically eligible for placement in a halfway house within six months of release or when serving a sentence of less than a year.

Blackmore estimates that 2,200 prerelease or halflway houses are in operation in the United States, 600 of them housing adults. These centers house from 30,000 to 40,000 offenders. Fifty-one percent of all federal prisoners are released to these programs. These persons have lower unemployment rates, better job attendance records, and higher earnings than do those released directly from prisons into the community [5]. However, Penner [10] notes that "only those programs that combine realistic job-training with placement in worthwhile jobs appear to have any effect upon recidivism."

Occupational Therapy in Correctional Institutions

Gross, an occupational therapist who worked for two years with female inmates while doing her dissertation [7] notes,

> Prevocational programs for prisoners need to be based upon the type and needs of the population, which is mostly poor, urban, very inadequately educated, young and male. In order to enter the vocational system, they would need exposure to learn about vocational areas and skills, actual practice in social and vocational arenas and then the opportunity for this to be put into practice when they were discharged. Those programs where employers have a commitment to hiring them or where inmates work for wages and learn real job skills and requirements while incarcerated would be helpful.

Corrections is an area in which occupational therapy can provide a useful service, particularly in work-related programming. Although our profession's literature at present sparsely describes this role, I and others believe that this is an area of practice that may develop more fully in time [10, 11].

Correctional institutions typically have a number of security levels or classifications. These custodial and security policies may drastically affect the modalities of therapy and the extent to which occupational therapy services are provided. The therapist's role varies depending on the type of facility. Facilities for the juvenile offender may emphasize rehabilitation in areas such as activities of daily living, social skills, and the development of compensatory strategies. When appropriate, sensory integrative therapy may also be provided. In adult facilities, which are commonly segregated for men and women, occupational therapists can "assist in the maintenance of life-task performance; provide leisure-time activities; provide opportunities for social and cognitive development; and can work collaboratively with job training program personnel to assess and develop work habits and assist in the development of desired vocational and employability skills" [13].

It is essential for any therapist entering this area of practice to have a realistic set of expectations. In reviewing the literature on this subject, Penner [10] has formulated conclusions particularly relevant to the development of occupational therapy programs:

1. The conditions that seem to have the greatest correlation with avoidance of recidivism are availability of family or other social group support after release; stable job prospects; and aging.
2. Regardless of what occurs in the prison, programs are likely to have little effect on the conditions to which inmates return; some recidivism may be seen as inevitable.
3. Prisons exist primarily to punish. Inmates are not likely to view prisons as existing for their benefit, and are likely to reject anyone's claims that they do exist for their benefit.
4. It may be difficult if not impossible to ascertain the prisoner's desire for change, especially if there is any possibility that parole contingencies are attached to outcomes of the occupational therapy program.
5. Lasting behavioral change will occur only if the inmate truly desires to change.

Washington State Special Offender Center*

One of the few examples of occupational therapy's role in corrections is at the Washington State Special Offender Center, which is located 20 miles northeast of Seattle, Washington. It is a maximum-security prison housing 144 men. The typical offender comes from an impoverished population and has little or no work history and few or no work skills or positive work habits. The center comprises four 36-cell units with an occupational therapy clinic on each unit. There is one full-time occupational therapist. Occupational therapy plays an important role in evaluating the inmates and providing them with the opportunity to

---

*Most of this section was written directly from information provided by Sandra Palmer, OTR.

learn essential work-related behaviors and attitudes such as attention span and task tolerance, acceptance of and ability to follow instructions, and increased motivation before job placement.

Evaluation

Ideally each inmate is seen briefly within the first three days of admission. Evaluation, which lasts approximately one hour, occurs over the next few days. It is designed to assess several key areas of the individual's general functional and developmental levels: (1) basic living skills and activities of daily living, (2) cognitive and perceptual processing, (3) sensory integrative functioning, (4) work tolerance, (5) work-related skills, (6) avocational and leisure skills, (7) general coordination, (8) aptitudes, (9) hand dexterity, and (10) mental status.

The evaluation involves completing simple tasks such as writing, drawing, copying, following directions, and handling small objects, as well as gross motor and frustration tolerance tasks. In addition the therapist explores the inmate's self-care and homemaking abilities, decision making, interests, time management skill, and memory. Observations are made about the person's general behavior and interactions with the therapist.

Work-Related Programs

All work-related programs at the Special Offender Center are institutionally based, with three basic types of work stations: on-unit jobs, off-unit jobs, and "sheltered" jobs. Whenever possible, on- and off-unit jobs are arranged to simulate jobs in the community. The inmates are required to fill out applications, go through an interview process, complete written performance evaluations, receive training and supervision, await job openings, and cope with layoffs.

The emphasis of all the jobs is on building positive work habits and attitudes, self-esteem, community skills, and general job awareness. Participation in the work programs is required to advance within the treatment programs. In addition, practical training in job seeking—interviewing skills and job searching methods—is provided.

On-unit jobs are general operational tasks necessary to the maintenance of the unit. There are 20 to 25 jobs available on each unit, ranging from low-level janitorial tasks to more complex and independent work such as tier (unit) laundryman or porter. Other jobs include inmate meal server, bi-unit (two-tier) supervisor, recreation aide, and occupational therapy aide. Wages are variable up to a maximum of $30 per month. Inmates are allowed to hold more than one job; however, their maximum earnings remain fixed.

To be eligible for an *off-unit job*, the inmate must (1) require medium and/or high custody, (2) be active and successful in the unit programs, and (3) have no disciplinary infractions for a specified period. These jobs require higher functional abilities such as the ability to work independently, follow complex instructions, and accept supervision appropriately. Off-unit positions include laundry aide, maintenance aide, janitorial aide, plumber's aide, electrician's aide, and kitchen aide. At present there are 20 jobs; however, new ones are always being created.

Sheltered jobs at the Special Offender Center are similar to jobs in a sheltered workshop, although the center does not have a sheltered workshop per se. Investigations are being made into appropriate types of contracts and products suitable to the facility's limited space. Of interest are simple assembly and sorting tasks that can be graded for complexity.

Many of the inmates are transferred from the center to work-release facilities. These function like halfway houses and provide an opportunity for inmates to continue to learn and expand vocational skills.

In summary, Palmer [8] notes:

> Occupational therapy can play an active, contributing role to an individual's rehabilitation, adjustment and successful return to the community. Occupational therapy can provide a supportive, common link with community life by aiding in the personal growth and development of each individual, through guided activities. Individuals participating in occupational therapy have the opportunity to build needed experiential background to deal with the community and society in general.

Case Study*

Brett is a pleasant-looking, tall, blond young man of 23. He speaks in a quiet though clear voice and speaks calmly about most issues.

Brett has been involved with the social correctional systems of the state since age 8. At that time his parents were killed in an automobile accident, and Brett was placed in a foster home. He was able to remain at the same school in which he had started that year. His teachers repeatedly reported that Brett had difficulty paying attention in class and always seemed to be making up stories. He reportedly had no close friends and was most often alone at school and at home. Numerous referrals to the school district psychologists and communication specialists resulted in many confusing reports. No agreement was ever reached, but impressions included childhood schizophrenia, attention deficit disorder, traumatic adjustment reaction, and autism.

By the time Brett was 16, he was no longer in school. He had been suspended for creating disturbances in his classes several times and had finally been expelled. His foster parents (Brett's fourth placement) felt unequal to dealing with what they termed Brett's moodiness. On the recommendations of the school district, they attempted to enroll Brett in an alternative school for emotionally disturbed students. Brett refused to attend and withdrew further into himself. During this time he was on probation for numerous counts of drunkenness, disorderly conduct, and shoplifting.

Brett began staying out late and drinking quite heavily. He received money from a trust established from his parents' estates but was never able to make any budgeting decisions. He either gave his money away, bought alcohol, or made impulsive purchases.

The offense for which Brett is currently incarcerated is taking a motor vehicle without permission (joyriding). The charges were reduced from grand theft, auto, because of his close relationship to the car's owners, former foster parents. He had previously been in prison for two counts of burglary in the second degree and one count of indecent liberties. He served three years of a seven-year maximum sentence. Brett was on parole for about six months before being arrested for this current offense.

When Brett had served only six months of his current sentence (he was scheduled for release in less than eighteen months), he proved unable to remain within the general prison population at the Washington State Corrections and

*This case study was provided by Sandra L. Palmer, OTR, Washington State Special Offender Center, Monroe, Washington.

Training Center. He reportedly had been raped on numerous occasions and had been victimized in other ways. He was kept in protective custody.

During his final months at the corrections center, cell mates and staff reported Brett's ritualistic motions and habits. His cell walls were covered with drawings and patterns associated with satanic cults. He was periodically heard talking to himself in two different voices. Brett committed many infractions—having alcohol in his cell and being under the influence of intoxicants. Brett was observed to exhibit bizarre and self-mutilating behavior. After inflicting a three-inch laceration on his left leg that required stitching, he was transferred to the Washington State Special Offender Center (SOC) as a prisoner in need of immediate stabilization.

During the 30-day initial evaluation period, Brett was diagnosed by the members of the treatment team as being severely disturbed. He claimed to have two souls living within him: one Jesus the Savior, the other a warlock named Bodar. While he admitted that he drank a great deal and that he needed the alcohol, he stated that his drinking was not a problem and that he was not an alcoholic. He felt that alcoholics drink without reason, and he had a reason: "Bodar tells me to do awful things to people, and the booze keeps him quiet so I can hear the good things that Jesus is saying to me."

Brett agreed to take medications prescribed for him and to participate in the various aspects of programming offered on the admissions unit. He soon became involved in group therapy, individual therapy, therapeutic recreation, and occupational therapy.

The recreation staff was soon able to involve Brett in activities and continued to include him whenever possible. They attempted to increase his social skills, develop alternative leisure interests, and work on group belonging and cooperative play through sports and games.

In occupational therapy he was given a series of short-term tasks and crafts to establish reality orientation, provide success experiences, and increase his decision-making skills. His social skills were reinforced, his self-care was stressed, and a therapeutic trust relationship was established. The occupational therapist was able to extend Brett's group tolerance, attention span, and instruction following above minimum levels. Brett soon began showing more emotion and animation. He complained less often that Bodar and Jesus were bothering him.

Within six weeks of his admission, Brett was progressing well and the medications were controlling his delusions and hallucinations. At this point Brett had become motivated to change his behavior and stated that he felt happier without the two souls fighting over him. He was transferred to a long-term treatment unit.

In the new unit Brett became an active participant in his own treatment plan, showing rapid progress. He continued his involvement in occupational therapy and recreation with increasing goals and expectations. He began attending education classes to complete his GED requirements. He expressed more often his desire to plan for the future and learn skills to keep himself from decompensating badly again. He requested whatever job training could be offered him. He had already shown capability and was learning work habits as an on-unit janitorial aide. During his time on the treatment unit Brett had moved upward through the program privilege levels and was entitled to apply for off-unit work.

Brett made application to the classification committee for a change in his custody status—an advance from maximum security (his status since his commission to the department of corrections) to medium custody, which is required to leave the unit without escort or to work off-unit. Once his custody status was changed, he made application to work on the building's maintenance crew. He was interviewed and placed on a waiting list for the next available position. In about two weeks Brett was called to work with the building's plumber.

Brett proved to be an enthusiastic crew member and continued to improve in the areas of work habits, instruction following, and problem solving. Even though he was showing progress in these areas, he continued in occupational therapy groups to reinforce his existing skills, increase social skills, increase acceptance of female authority, and provide for continuing success experience. Within three months Brett was working three to four hours each afternoon; he received good evaluations from his job supervisor each month.

At about this time the occupational therapist and Brett's primary therapist both began noticing increasing anxiety and a quickness of temper not usually seen as Brett's behavior pattern on the treatment unit. Brett also began refusing to attend school and occupational therapy groups. His job supervisor reported that Brett was "almost working too hard, and is reluctant to return to the unit." In individual therapy sessions Brett's therapist uncovered several incidents of homosexual harassment of Brett by another inmate. Brett had been unwilling to report this because he felt it might affect the way staff saw his progress and placement alternatives. Once the investigations of these matters were concluded, Brett resumed active and progressive movement through the program's treatment objectives.

REFERENCES

1. Allen, C. Independence Through Activity: The Practice of Occupational Therapy (Psychiatry). *Am. J. Occup. Ther.* 36:731, 1982.
2. Beard, J. H. Psychiatric Rehabilitation at Fountain House. In Maislin, J. (Ed.) *Rehabilitation Medicine and Psychiatry.* Springfield, Ill.: Charles C. Thomas, 1976.
3. Blackmore, J. Community corrections. *Corrections Magazine,* October 1980, p. 4–15.
4. Brayman, S. J., Kirby, T. F., and Misenheimer, A. M. Comprehensive occupational therapy evaluation scale. *Am. J. Occup. Ther.* 30:94, 1976.
5. Day, S. R., and McCane, M. R., *Vocational Education in corrections.* Columbus, Ohio: Ohio State University National Center for Research in Vocational Education, 1982.
6. Gatti, D. Open Door Thrift Shop (handout for patients). Belmont, Massachusetts: McLean Hospital, 1982.
7. Gross, D. Personal communication, 1982.
8. Palmer, F., and Gatti, D. Transitional employment project. *Occup. Ther. Mental Health,* 2:23, 1982.
9. Palmer, S. Personal communication, 1983.
10. Penner, D. A. Correctional institutions: An overview. *Am. J. Occup. Ther.* 32:517, 1978.
11. Platt, N. P., Martell, D. L., and Clements, P. A. Level I field placement at a federal correctional institution. *Am. J. Occup. Ther.* 31:385, 1977.
12. Potter, J. Will work release ever fulfill its promise? *Corrections Magazine,* June 1979, p. 60.
13. Rehabilitation of the Mental Patient in the Community (application form and handout). New York: Fountain House National Training Program.
14. Schneider, R. Work Description and Proposal for Workshop Contract and Orientation Program. Calgary, Alberta, Canada: Calgary General Hospital, 1983.
15. Tiffany, E. G. Psychiatry and Mental Health. In Hopkins, H. L. and Smith, H. D. (Eds.). *Willard and Spackman's Occupational Therapy* (6th ed.) Philadelphia: Lippincott, 1983.

Work Programs for Adults with Neurophysiologic Problems

Occupational therapists working with persons with physical and/or neurologic disabilities may practice in a variety of facilities—inpatient and outpatient hospitals, rehabilitation centers, state institutions, independent private practice and industry. For these therapists, many variables must be addressed in planning work-related programs, including not only physical and neurologic ramifications of the disability, but also psychosocial impact, which is often overlooked. The person unable to pursue his or her present vocation or any vocation may become anxious and suffer a loss in self-esteem, self-image, motivation, and status within the family and society. When these issues arise, they must be addressed in therapy. When working with those with an acquired dysfunction, e.g., quadriplegia, right hemiplegia, head injury, back injury, or amputation, the therapist must be aware of the individual's feelings toward work before the insult or accident, as well as now.

This chapter describes innovative programming and assessment for clients with physical and/or neurologic disabilities, but first discusses some ramifications of specific dysfunctions related to work-related programming.

The employment potential of a person with a spinal cord injury "is not necessarily correlated with the injury and its residual manifestations. A person with a debilitating injury is able to return to work if he or she is motivated, possesses employable knowledge and skills, is offered reassurance from family and friends, and is able to find a job" [1]. It is important that in addition to finding a job the person be given a chance to be successful. For the hemiplegic "the effect on vocational potential can be serious, depending on skills previously attained and the impairment of intellectual functions. Return to previous vocation depends in large measure on the type of job the patient was doing, the patient's status in the company, the understanding of the employer, and the patient's ability to regain employable skills" [1].

The head-injured individual offers a challenge to developing work-related programs and assessments. They are more likely to be hindered by cognitive, behavioral, and social difficulties in performance than by physical deficits. "The level of pretrauma intellectual functioning and achieved educational level help in regaining vocational potential" [1]. Programming should provide head-injured patients with chances to work on familiar skills using multiple steps and repeating instructions. A time for practice and defined outcome criteria are also important [2].

The person with congenital neurophysiologic problems, for example, cerebral palsy or mental retardation, presents a different therapeutic picture. Many of these clients have had little or no exposure to work-related skills, behaviors, and habits. Thus, programming must be planned to facilitate acquisition of these abilities.

The therapeutic setting offers a wealth of in-house resources for evaluation. Equipment available to the therapist, such as computers, type-writers, carpentry power tools, and calculators, may serve a dual purpose in providing an evaluation and training tool to the clients. Whatever evaluation is used should provide information to facilitate the development of programs to teach clients new skills, behaviors, and habits; to train them in the use of adaptive equipment (when necessary); and to develop alternative job opportunities.

The first part of this chapter discusses chronic pain, disability, and rehabilitation of the injured worker. The second presents a functional assessment program of activities of daily living for brain injured individuals. The third describes innovative work programs for adults with neurophysiologic problems.

REFERENCES

1. Daub, M.M. The Human Development Process. In Hopkins, H., and Smith, H. (Eds.). Willard and Spackman's Occupational Therapy. Philadelphia: Lippincott, 1983.
2. Harris, P. The Role of Occupational Therapy in Cognitive Remediation and Prevocational Rehabilitation. Presented at New England Rehabilitation Hospital. Woburn, MA, 1983.

Chronic Back Pain, Disability, and Rehabilitation of the Injured Worker*

Industrial medicine is a division of occupational health that has evolved over the past decade. It is an area of importance for the health professional in terms of prevention, evaluation, rehabilitation, and research.

Statistics on chronic and acute pain are staggering. Approximately 75 million Americans suffer from chronic pain [5]. According to Bonica, the overall cost of pain in the U.S. is between $85 and $90 billion annually. The National Institute of Neurological and Communicative Disorders and Stroke estimates the total cost of managing chronic pain in the United States at approximately $60 billion annually. In 1977, disability payments by Social Security amounted to $11.6 billion. Less than 2 percent of the beneficiaries recovered enough to return to work [5]. Disabled beneficiaries of the Social Security Administration has

*This section was written by Carl M. Bettencourt, OTR/L.

grown from 2 million in 1971 to 5 million in 1980. This rate is 10 times faster than the growth rate of the general population. The disability costs for a single pain patient may run up to $24,000 annually [5]. Chronic pain is responsible for partial or total disability in 50 million individuals and causes the loss of 700 million work days annually [9]. These statistics certainly reflect the high cost associated with the treatment and management of chronic pain.

Low back injuries are the most prevalent and costly of all musculoskeletal injuries. Approximately 31 million Americans have backache, and in 60 percent of them the condition is severe enough to limit social and work functioning [3]. Back injuries account for $1 billion annually in disability costs and 20 percent of annual compensation payments. The national cost of low back pain treatment or compensation is an estimated $14 billion per year [3]. An estimated 2 percent of the U.S. industrial workforce suffers a compensable back injury every year [20].

The medical profession has determined that 80 percent of the population will experience back pain at some time; 70 percent of work-related low back injuries are caused by manual handling such as lifting, bending, and pulling [2,5]. These episodes are the most commonly reported injuries resulting in compensation claims [20].

THEORETICAL PAIN PERSPECTIVE

The pain experience is a highly personal, complex, and perplexing phenomenon. There have been many theories as to the causes and characteristics of pain. The "specificity theory" of pain is the traditional theory still taught in medical and graduate schools. It proposes that pain is a sensory experience and that its intensity is proportional to the extent of tissue damage. This theory implies a straight transmission system from the pain receptors to the pain centers in the brain. Based on this concept, neurosurgical techniques were developed to cut through pain pathways in order to alleviate pain. Unfortunately, the results have often been disappointing, particularly in surgery to reduce low back pain, neuralgias, and other chronic pain disorders. In some cases, pain not only returns to some degree, but new pains may develop as other iatrogenic complications occur [8, 16, 23].

The "pattern theory" postulates that pain is produced by coded patterns of nerve impulses. Unlike the specificity theory, the pattern theory proposes that all nerve fiber endings are alike and perception of pain is produced by marked stimulation of these nerve endings [8, 23].

Research supports the concept that pain is multidimensional. Current psychological evidence strongly points to the conclusion that pain is a complex perceptual and affective experience determined by several variables, including an individual's history, the meaning of the stimulus/situation, an individual's state of mind at that moment, and other sensory nerve patterns elicited by physical stimulation [11, 16, 23].

The "gate control theory" of pain, proposed by Melzack and Wall, presents pain as more than a sensory experience. This theory postulates that neural mechanisms in the spinal cord act like a gate and modulate the flow of nerve impulses between peripheral fibers and the brain [8, 11, 16, 21, 23]. After an injury, the stimulus travels through the spinal cord via neural pathways. These impulses are subjected to the modulating effects of the gate mechanisms in the spinal cord. The gate mechanisms are also influenced by descending nerve impulses from the brain, which may contain cognitive information about past experiences or cultural influences. In other words, pain impulses may be interpreted as mildly irritating or devastating, depending on a variety of factors.

Some degree of pain, whether physical or psychological, is inherent to all injuries. An understanding of physiological and psychological characteristics of pain, their ability to influence one another, and their implications for the injured worker is essential for effective interventions.

ACUTE VERSUS CHRONIC PAIN

Pain can be divided into acute and chronic. Acute pain is temporary. It often serves as a warning and is usually associated with a well-defined cause, such as burn or trauma. It may require analgesics or narcotics for a brief period of time, but usually stops after healing has occurred. It may require no medical intervention and usually does not involve significant sleep disturbances. There may be no psychological disturbances aside from anxiety associated with acute pain.

There are various autonomic responses that accompany acute pain, including increased cardiac rate, increased pupillary diameter, increased muscle tension, decreased gut motility, decreased salivary flow, and decreased superficial capillary flow [9, 16].

Chronic pain persists beyond the expected healing time for a particular injury or illness. Pain lasting longer than six months can usually be considered chronic [5, 9, 15]. Chronic pain is resistant to surgical interventions, and its prolonged course is associated with personality changes and psychological disturbances. These may include irritability, anxiety, insomnia, and social isolation. Psychosocial complications may develop, including depression, suicidal thoughts, relationship problems, sexual problems, narcotic and alcohol abuse, weight fluctuations, and feelings of helplessness and hopelessness related to a perceived loss of control.

Pain, whether acute or chronic, is *real*.

PSYCHOSOCIAL CHARACTERISTICS OF CHRONIC PAIN

Pilowsky and Spence found that chronic pain patients have difficulty verbally expressing their feelings, particularly anger [15, 16]. Blumer and Heilbronn stated that these individuals tend to be unable to recognize their feelings. Gentry, Shows, and Thomas noted that chronic pain patients' reports of emotionally moving experiences are minimal compared to their concerns with bodily functions and dysfunctions [15].

Another characteristic of chronic pain is an unusual concern and preoccupation with somatic processes and illness. Mitchell and Wallis reported that patients with chronic back pain demonstrate a significant preoccupation with disease and a marked somatic (as opposed to psychological) perception of illness. The American Psychiatric Association characterizes a person suffering from hypochondriasis as having a fear of disease, an illness conviction, a bodily preoccupation, and unsatisfactory pursuit of medical care. This person converts psychological stress into physical symptoms that may or may not be real. These real or fictitious restrictions are used to avoid emotionally difficult situations [15, 16].

The Minnesota Multiphasic Personality Inventory (MMPI) is a widely used psychological assessment. Researchers using the MMPI to assess pain [11] describe chronic pain patients as demonstrating denial and repression, as well as a strong desire for social acceptance, which they feel can be achieved only through denial of unpleasant characteristics. Blumer and Heilbronn reported that most chronic pain patients describe themselves as independent and solid citizens in their communities, deny any problems with interpersonal relationships or within the family system, and report a history of excessive activity and work performance [15].

Individuals with chronic pain appear sociable and outgoing, but they tend to be self-centered, demanding, and dependent. Gentry, Shows, and Thomas reviewed statistics on low back pain patients and noted the prevalence of limited education and blue collar manual or white collar clerical jobs. They also reported that many had a stable work history beginning at an early age, an early marriage, large families, and unmet dependency needs [15].

Individuals with chronic pain show depressive symptoms associated with delayed recovery [11, 15–17]. These symptoms include sleep disturbances, lack of initiative, inactivity, fatigue, inability to enjoy leisure, social, and sexual activities, helplessness, and hopelessness. Sternbach and co-workers reported that individuals with low back pain, with or without physical findings, showed elevated depression scale scores on the MMPI [8]. Faced with the inability to relieve pain following repeated attempts, the chronic pain patient views the situation as hopeless and becomes depressed. Some theorists report this lack of control as having an internal origin, and others report that pain patients attribute their lack of control to external factors [15].

Individuals with acute or chronic pain display behaviors to communicate to others that pain is being experienced. These pain behaviors include verbal complaints, crying, moaning, decreased activity, positional bracing, grimacing, rubbing and holding affected parts, and rigid guarded movements. When the individual demonstrates exaggerated and inconsistent pain behaviors, it is likely that these behaviors are attributable to conditioning and learning influences, rather than to organic pathology. Pain behaviors are subject to learning processes, including operant learning, habit, modeling, and association. Children who are raised in a cold and distant household but receive care and affection when they are ill or suffering will learn to associate illness with care and nurturing. If parents disapprove of care and nurturing behaviors, children may grow up associating illness with guilt and anxiety. Children also learn that certain behaviors can be used to influence and control others in their environment [8, 11, 15]. Pain as a learned behavior is further supported by research on pain in different ethnic groups and cultures; there is a strong relationship between ethnic background and an individual's beliefs and responses to pain [8, 14–16].

Derebery and Tullis reported that individuals who are receiving compensation for their illness might have a delayed recovery because of reinforcers from the injury. Sympathy, attention from family and community, income, escape from responsibility, and resolution of internal conflict are examples of reinforcers, also called secondary gains.

Family members might inadvertently play a role in prolonging an individual's illness. A wife who is forced to work for financial reasons might suddenly discover she enjoys her new role and unconsciously reinforce her spouse's sick role. Children might reinforce a parent's sick role because there is less fighting in a family following a parent's illness. A child who does not want to go to school might find the opportunity to stay home and care for the sick parent. The combinations and situations are endless. These are known as tertiary gains. They are incentives for family members or others to reinforce another's sick role [6, 8, 11, 15, 16].

A repertoire of behaviors for coping with pain and illness can be developed in a family system. Family members can serve as role models for the development of these behaviors or coping strategies. According to Blumer and Heilbronn, most chronic pain patients have a family history of depression and alcoholism, a disabled family member or relative that serves as role model for pain behavior [5, 15].

Learning theories have led to the implementation of behavior modification strategies in the treatment of chronic pain syndrome [15]. Behavior modification does not have to be an uncomfortable approach to treatment. Some clinicians do not fully realize they are applying basic behavior modification concepts to achieve their goals in treatment [5].

Chronic pain may be decreased or eliminated by introducing an incompatible behavior. For instance, standing and walking are incompatible with reclining; thus, these behaviors are introduced in a carefully monitored and paced reinforcement schedule which competes with reclining and eventually decreases the reclining behavior [16].

Traditional behavioral models have been based on the assumption that response-reward contingencies cause behavior change because of unconscious, automatic responses. Behaviorism has given way to cognitive theories, in which higher learning processes influence the development and maintenance of pain and disability. Through cognitive-behavioral techniques, individuals can be taught to identify and correct distorted conceptualizations and beliefs and thereby influence their degree of illness [5, 11, 15, 23].

ABNORMAL ILLNESS BEHAVIOR

The concept of abnormal illness behavior is Pilowsky's attempt to propose a more meaningful and comprehensive understanding of patients with physical complaints for which no adequate organic cause can be found [15–17]. Pilowsky states that a physician can determine illness behavior to be abnormal when the patient complains of symptoms in the absence of apparent pathology, or when the physician observes a reaction to pathology that appears inconsistent with the expected reaction.

Individuals react to aspects of their own dysfunction, which they evaluate in terms of "health" and "illness," based upon such factors as age, sex, ethnic background, social learning, position in the social group, and the importance of the individual's role for the group [15, 16]. For some, illness is characterized by dramatic emotional responses to symptoms in order to adopt the sick role. For others, the sick role is troublesome, awkward, and inconvenient. In this case illness behavior may consist of stoicism, despite the severity of the illness [15]. Pilowsky suggests that the presence of abnormal illness behavior be diagnosed through the identification of organic factors as well as psychosocial findings influencing illness and disability. He proposes the simultaneous evaluation of an individual's medical and physical status, including sociocultural factors and current sources of emotional conflict [17].

Symptom magnification syndrome is defined as "a conscious or unconscious self-destructive socially reinforced behavioral response pattern consisting of reports or displays of symptoms which function to control the life circumstances of the sufferer" [10, p, 257]. This theory involves three essential features: (1) "Non-negotiability of symptoms," or an individual's inability to control symptoms, leads to disability; (2) the symptoms control the environment, and (3) functional limitations are magnified by these symptoms.

Matheson identifies three types of symptom magnifiers: (1) the refugee, (2) the gameplayer, and (3) the identified patient [12, 15]. The refugee uses symptoms as an escape from conflict that is perceived as unresolvable. This type perceives him- or herself as irreplaceable in the family and community system. Health professionals are often involved in a "yes-but" scenario as they attempt to provide assistance for this person, and can observe helplessness and martyr-like qualities and behaviors. In the *DSM III*, this type is analogous to somatization disorder, conversion disorder, psychogenic pain disorder, and hypochondriasis [1].

The gameplayer is most similar to the traditional "malingerer." This type finds that symptoms can be used to provide the opportunity for financial gain and has a history of poor goal attainment. Goals tend to be unrealistic and extravagant. The gameplayer may act impulsive in a "heroic disregard" for the impairment and may thereby act irresponsible while appearing responsible. The gameplayer fails to take responsibility when things go wrong by saying, "It's not my fault, I told her/him that he/she should have done such and such."

For the "identified patient" the role of patient is primary, and symptoms serve to maintain this role. Goals, when they exist at all, are generally "grand" in nature, such as "to somehow provide for my family." The analog in the *DSM III* is chronic fictitious disorder with physical and/or psychological symptoms [1].

MEDICAL SYSTEM AND DISABILITY

Traditional medical practice for injured workers is primarily biological in nature. The search for an organic disorder to explain a patient's symptoms is the priority with traditional medical interventions. Common treatments include bed rest, physical therapy, medication, nerve blocks, and surgery. Efforts are rarely made to assess and quantify psychosocial factors and illness behaviors, despite the growing evidence from literature that these nonbiological factors contribute to pain, suffering, and disability as much as tissue pathology [3]. Patients are susceptible to attitudes, role expectations, and misunderstandings of a professional staff. Actions of staff members can increase frustration and alienation levels and promote a sense of helplessness and dependence [15]. Clear communication with patients regarding their disorders can be essential in facilitating an uncomplicated recovery. Deyo reports that assigning patients a diagnostic "label" without a clear explanation of symptoms and their implications can sometimes lead to an increase in sickness and self-limiting behavior. For example, diagnosing a patient with a backache as having a "back injury" can be translated into many frightening images that have the potential to influence a patient's recovery [7].

The speed at which individuals return to work is dependent on how they perceive their physical limitations. These physical limitations can be reinforced by a physician who reinforces disability messages by instructing the patient to avoid physical activities long after healing has occurred. Physicians can have a dramatic impact on how patients see themselves. The more a patient hears the message to take it easy, the greater the conviction that he or she is ill [5, 11].

Most chronic pain patients are committed to the notion that their pain is a result of damage to the body and that relief will come from external interventions from the health care system [16]. Waddell stated that rest "may be the most harmful treatment ever devised and a potent cause of iatrogenic disability. There is clear evidence that, despite general belief, activity is not harmful, and active rehabilitation not only restores function but also reduces pain." [15, p. 103]. Limited activity leads to additional complications including psychological distress, learning of avoidance behaviors, perception of pain as indicating tissue damage, loss of strength, endurance, flexibility, and adoption of the sick role [15]. Mayer described the major complication in individuals with chronic low back pain as a "deconditioning syndrome" caused by inactivity and prolonged disuse of muscles and joints [15]. Strang identified a "chronic disability syndrome" in individuals capable of working but "choosing" to be disabled. There is an absence of motivation to recover and a negative attitude about returning to work. The development of this syndrome often represents a failure to cope with life's disappointments in response to what may be a minor injury. Patients see themselves as disabled, and this allows for a solution to many non–work-related personal problems. They take the view that because they have been injured, they are unable to work. Brena and Chapman reported this cluster of symptoms to be inherent in chronic pain patients. There is a sequence of events that occurs in a significant number of chronic pain patients leading to the chronic disability syndrome. This process involves the development of chronic disability as a means of accepting the sick role and meeting underlying psychological needs. These needs are often dependency, depression, anxiety, job and family difficulties, and feelings of inadequacy [3]. Hirschfield and Behan found that certain internal conflicts can lead an individual in some cases to actually cause an accident and to hold on to the sustained injuries because the accident is a solution to current life problems. Such a person may actually seek a physician who will not cure him or her and reject others who appear capable [15].

DISABILITY, LITIGATION, AND COMPENSATION

Waddell reported that 15 percent of compensation surgical back patients undergo a second operation; 40 percent, a third; and 23 percent, a fourth. These statistics demonstrate progressively poorer results with successive operations [3]. McGill found that a lengthy period of disability predicted a low chance of ever returning to work: those out of work greater than six months had a 50-percent probability of returning, those for more than one year had a 25-percent chance of returning, and those out of work longer than two years were extremely unlikely to return to work [3].

Merskey reported that patients attending clinics for chronic pain have a higher incidence of unemployment and disability than those who do not. He proposed that those who remain at work may have less time to pursue additional therapies or medical investigations, even though they may still have pain [16]. Snook found that patients on Workers' Compensation for back injuries were less likely to have objective findings or a definite diagnosis than individuals with back injuries who were not receiving compensation [3].

Research indicates that back pain patients with pending litigation do not enjoy the same improvement in their conditions that nonlitigated back pain patients enjoy, until litigation is settled. After settlement, there is little difference in the improvement shown by the two groups [3, 7, 11, 16, 21]. An attorney may unintentionally encourage a client to prolong pain as a cautionary measure: "You don't want to settle until you're completely pain free." Such advice may be ethical and responsible legal practice, but does little to get injured workers back to work and is not always best from the medical and psychological points of view [21]. Exploitation of the disability system and abuse of the process to prolong the life of a claim is not uncommon. Indeed, the simple presence of an attorney in Workers' Compensation cases may be associated with failure to return to work following pain treatment [5, 15]. Unemployment, welfare benefits, and compensation have the potential to adversely influence return to work following a chronic disability [19].

The Workers' Compensation system is a morally just and humane system, however it has an undeniable potential for abuse [8, 21]. The system often refuses to continue financial support if physical illness is not readily observed. This is a definite source of stress for the injured worker [16]. Compensation boards and Workers' Compensation insurance plans can be damaging in encouraging persons to continue being in pain.

Tax-free income also may serve as a disincentive for returning to work. In a sense, patients are positively reinforced for disability and negatively reinforced for returning to work. Employers often contribute to the problem because they are unwilling to re-employ workers unless they are able to return to pre-injury activities [3, 5, 11, 15]. Even when injured workers show full recovery, employers are reluctant to re-employ them, since they are classified as impaired and may have recurrent back problems resulting in additional compensation costs [20].

This is certainly an inherent flaw in the compensation system. Instead of encouraging and motivating persons to return to work, the system rewards individuals for pain and disability and punishes them for feeling better.

TOOLS FOR IDENTIFICATION OF ABNORMAL ILLNESS BEHAVIOR (AIB)

There are several evaluation methods and tools to aid in identifying abnormal illness behavior and in developing treatment strategies that will most improve an injured worker's physical and emotional disposition.

A thorough intake interview during the initial meeting, including behavioral observations, is essential for gathering valuable clues about an individual's physical and emotional status and motivation for recovery. The initial interview can be structured to elicit responses regarding an individual's psychosocial and work history, including a history of the work injury. Lifestyle, habits, and activities and an assessment of social reinforcers for illness behavior can also be explored. This includes perceived expectations of the social support system and family members' secondary gain from the individual's disability. During this intake interview, an assessment can be made of an individual's functional tolerances, pain aggravants, alleviators, and response to symptoms. Signs of anxiety, depression, and other psychological and cognitive factors can be determined through asking questions about an individual's job. Finally, it is helpful to determine if there is pending litigation with regard to the present injury. This may provide information regarding any financial incentives or disincentives for returning to work [15, 17].

An anatomical pain drawing by the patient provides a subjective indication of pain location and characteristics that can be helpful in identifying abnormal illness behavior, especially with chronic low back pain patients. Mooney, Cairnes, and Robertson reported that "crisp and precise localization of pain" was associated with an acute onset of disc disease exhibiting classical signs and symptoms. "Expanded areas of pain localization, frequently with florid descriptions of intensities of pain" was associated with chronic pain, multiple surgeries, and unsuccessful medical interventions [15, p. 89].

Pain rating scales and questionnaires can be useful to document subjective changes in an individual's pain level over time and the effect of different activities, strategies, and interventions. Pain scales that are out of proportion to an individual's objective level of distress can be indicative of symptom magnification. A pain rating of 8, 9, or 10 should preclude normal ambulation and conversation [15].

The Minnesota Multiphasic Personality Inventory (MMPI) is an established screening tool for identifying and analyzing disabling psychophysiological abnormalities with back pain; however, there are several drawbacks to its use. A license psychologist must be available to administer and interpret the test, and the number of questions may make it too lengthy and impractical to use in some programs. The test also may be threatening to some individuals, who may decide that the clinician thinks "it's all in my head." Also, administration of the MMPI may be discouraged by referral sources and third party payers because its use could lead to a claim of a work-related psychological injury [15, 17].

Self-reporting scales can yield information regarding an individual's perception of his or her illness disposition, emotional state, functional limitations, and attitudes regarding pain and illness. Noting inconsistencies between scores on several similar scales and responses that appear exaggerated or inconsistent with observed distress and activity levels can be helpful in screening for abnormal illness behavior (AIB) [15].

The clinical examination provides the opportunity to collect objective information regarding an individual's strength, flexibility, sensation, capacities, and problem areas consistent and/or inconsistent with a particular diagnosis.

Waddel and colleagues developed an approach to the clinical examination for use with chronic low back pain patients [15, 24] that can be used to detect the presence of "non-organic physical signs."

1. Tenderness related to physical disease is usually localized to a specific skeletal or neuromuscular structure. Non-organic tenderness may include superficial tenderness to light pinching over a wide area on the lower back or tenderness to deep palpation that is broadly distributed and not isolated to certain anatomical structures.

2. In a standing position, the individual reports increased low back pain when the evaluating clinician applies a light downward pressure to the skull or passively rotates the shoulders and pelvis simultaneously.

3. Distraction tests involve manual muscle testing or flexibility testing and watching for inconsistencies. Findings that are consistently present are likely to be physically based. Findings that are present only on formal testing and disappear at other times may have a non-organic component.

4. Weakness or sensory disturbances in an entire extremity, a quarter, or half the body ("regional disturbances") do not relate to localized neuroanatomy and correspond to a positive score for non-organic signs.

5. Overreaction to the physical examination such as disproportion-

ate facial expressions, verbalizations, sweating, collapsing, and muscle tremors and tension all indicate possible non-organic pain.

The presence of three or more of these signs is clinically significant for an AIB pattern.

Testing for consistency of effort or maximum voluntary effort (MVE) can be used as an additional screening tool for abnormal illness behavior. The rationale for MVE testing is based on three assumptions. First, it is presumed that, given an inherently reliable procedure where anatomical posture, joint angles, and muscles are carefully controlled, an individual giving MVE during a strength evaluation will demonstrate a high level of reliability and a low variance in closely spaced consecutive trials. Second, an individual who is consciously or unconsciously magnifying dysfunction will not demonstrate maximal effort during testing. Third, submaximal effort is associated with inconsistent or unreliable performance. These three assumptions are loosely supported by observations of behavioral performance regarding the degree of effort with the consistency of performance. Observations include sweating, grimacing, increased respiratory rate, increased pulse or heart rate, recruitment of adjacent musculature, and red face [15].

There are several tests to assess the presence of submaximal voluntary effort. Several isometric strength testing units are commercially available for assessing lifting capacity and consistency of effort. An example of this type of test is the Force Gauge Platform devised by Blankenship. An individual's consistency of effort is determined over three to five consecutive trials by calculating the coefficient of variation (CV). A CV greater than 15 percent is significant for the presence of submaximal effort [15].

Static strength testing does have its drawbacks. Its safety for back injured clients has been questioned; muscle strains, soreness, and other injuries have been reported. Khalil reports that since injured workers are cautioned to use discomfort that is unacceptable as a criteria for stopping the test, these tests must be considered to be tests of "acceptable maximum effort." Because of this fact, the use of CV data from normal individuals may not be valid. Harber and Soohoo found that the CV for static strength testing in a pre-employment screening protocol with a back injured population was higher than that of normal subjects. Also, static tests that are conducted in only one position are not adequate for the assessment of the stresses inherent in dynamic lifting activities, which are performed through the body's full range of motion [15].

Cybex isokinetic equipment is available to determine maximum effort using dynamic strength testing protocols. This equipment is designed to test trunk, limb, and whole body dynamic lifting strength; and is capable of graphing force output against degrees of torque, or distance from the floor. The consistency and rate of the force output over repeated trials were indications of maximal effort [15].

Stokes reported an objective, reproducible method of documenting submaximal effort in hand injuries using the Jamar Dynomometer. Subjects are instructed to apply maximal force with each of the five handle positions, first with the uninjured hand. Readings are recorded and graphed. This should produce a bell curve with the lower readings at the extremes of the handle positions and the higher readings in the midposition. Individuals who are voluntarily exerting submaximal effort demonstrate a straight line on the graph. These readings are based on the fact that different gripping positions will require the use of different muscles in the hand. This variability in muscle recruitment will yield different gripping strengths [18].

Measurements of torque can be taken using the BTE Work Simulator. Three trials of static supination and pronation with each hand for four different handles, and three trials of upward pull and downward push on a lever with each upper extremity are done by the individual being tested. In this test, the shoulder is in a neutral position and the elbow is flexed to 90 degrees. A CV is calculated for each set of three trials. Consistency of effort is assessed by the number of CVs that exceed the experimentally derived cut-off points of 12 percent. This test has been determined to be safe to administer to persons with back injuries. Abnormal illness behavior will permeate all areas of performance. This test is not valid with an upper extremity impairment [13, 15].

It is significant to note that testing for maximal voluntary effort is not synonymous with testing for malingering. A positive score in any of these tests may be attributed to several factors. These can include an unidentified impairment, low endurance, fear of reinjury, pain, anxiety about testing, and symptom magnification. The sole use of effort testing in evaluating injured workers can result in inaccurate assessments and documentation [15].

Most researchers report that true malingering, the voluntary process of falsely or grossly exaggerating physical and psychological symptoms in pursuit of an objective that is obvious, is a relatively rare phenomenon [10, 15]. Gentry, Shows, and Thomas based this conclusion on a high incidence of "faking good" scores on the MMPI. (Malingerers exhibit low scores.)

WORK HARDENING MODELS

Work hardening is one component of an industrial rehabilitation program. A comprehensive industrial rehabilitation program model is designed to promote, maintain, and prevent work-related injuries and, when they occur, attempt to rehabilitate the injured workers and return them to work efficiently and safely. There are several components to an industrial rehabilitation program: employee injury prevention programs, worksite evaluations, pre-employment screenings, back schools, physical capacity evaluations, work capacity evaluations, vocational assessments and rehabilitation, ergonomics, industrial health programs, occupational medicine examinations, and work hardening programs.

Work hardening is an integral component of a comprehensive industrial rehabilitation program. Programs can be hospital based; freestanding units affiliated with a hospital or rehabilitation facility; or independent programs. A variety of these programs throughout the United States were reviewed for similarities and differences. The following information is based on a review of 21 programs [15].

Staffing patterns vary in terms of disciplines used in these programs. Occupational therapy and physical therapy are used most often in nearly all work hardening programs. A variety of disciplines are used in different programs. A multidisciplinary staff appears to be most commonly found in these work hardening programs. These include physicians, nurses, movement therapists, rehabilitation counselors, athletic trainers, recreational therapists, psychiatrists, psychologists, employers, insurance carriers, attorneys, technicians, and rehabilitation engineers. These disciplines are fulltime and part-time program staff members or consultants.

Program duration varies from 2 to 12 weeks, however the average length is four to six weeks, and each session ranges from two to eight hours long. Work hardening programs admit a variety of injured workers. The most prevalent injuries are back injuries, which include cervical, thoracic, lumbar, and sacral regions. In addition to back injuries, many other subacute, chronic, and post-surgical musculoskeletal conditions respond well to work hardening services. Other common injuries include hand injuries, amputations, fractures, nerve injuries, and other orthopedic injuries. The average staff to patient ratio is 1:5. These programs occupy 500 to 5,000 square feet and may have additional space shared with other programs and disciplines.

Work hardening programs are usually held in a group. This group structure or therapeutic milieu can be a powerful force in motivating injured employees to improve their physical and emotional status and ultimately return to work. The group structure offers support and camaraderie for individuals working together toward a common goal. A group atmosphere obviously simulates the worker environment in many cases. Group situations allow group processes such as cohesiveness, trust, identification, and self-disclosure. Another important function of a group is that it allows members to share common experiences and learn from one another. Group members are more apt to take advice from each other than from a staff member [3, 10, 11, 22, 23]. An understanding of group dynamics and the encouragement and facilitation of the above processes can greatly influence the success of a work hardening program.

Many programs have eclectic approaches, utilizing occupational and physical therapists' clinical experience, sports medicine approaches, models of human occupation, vocational rehabilitation, and cognitive-behavioral approaches. Program components can include musculoskeletal conditioning, stress and pain management, cardiovascular conditioning, vocational services, education, and work hardening/simulation activities. Most work hardening programs utilize work-related activity as a treatment medium. These activities range from simple lifting tasks using weighted milk crates to intricate programs using sophisticated computer hardware. A variety of tools, equipment, and work samples are available commercially for work hardening programs. The reader is referred to a resource list appendix in *Work Hardening: State of the Art* [15, p. 434]. The choice of work-related activities is also determined by the types of clients and specific job demands.

Work P.R.E.P.

The Billerica Ambulatory Care center is an outpatient facility affiliated with New England Rehabilitation Hospital in Woburn, MA. It serves a variety of disabilities and includes several specialized programs (young stroke, hands, pediatrics, sports medicine, and work hardening).

Work P.R.E.P. (Progressive Resistive Exercise Program) is a work hardening program designed to provide clients with the opportunity to increase their competence in performing work-related tasks.* A supervised routine of graduated work simulation, including body mechanics, postural awareness, general conditioning, and reinjury prevention, is fundamental to this program. The overall objective of Work P.R.E.P. is to maximize a client's work potential and to assist with a successful return to work.

The program utilizes a variety of specialized disciplines. A physiatrist, a physician who specializes in rehabilitation medicine, is available to provide initial evaluations and follow clients throughout the program as necessary. Vocational rehabilitation is an integral component of the program. Expert vocational direction is essential to focus clients, coordinate with employers, and identify obstacles and incentives in the return to work process. Licensed physical and occupational therapists with specialized training in industrial rehabilitation evaluate and supervise clients in activities including conditioning (Fig. 7-1), work hardening (Fig. 7-2), and simulation. Clients meet in group sessions, although individualized attention is available within the group structure. Stress/pain management specialists guide sessions in relaxation and stress management. This serves to help identify and deal with stress on and off the job (Fig. 7-3). Programs are tailored to each client's needs and job demands.

All admissions require a physician's written request. If a client does not have a referring physician, an examination by the program physiatrist is necessary. All clients are evaluated and followed by a vocational specialist, on staff or outside the facility, who coordinates with the Work P.R.E.P. team. Progress on each client is regularly communicated to the appropriate referral source.

A comprehensive multidisciplinary approach is the key to successful return to employment and is consistent with the philosophy of New England Rehabilitation Hospital.

SUMMARY/FUTURE TRENDS

Industrial rehabilitation is a growing field of intervention for the health professional. Back pain is a significant and growing problem in the United States at this time. Pain, especially chronic pain, represents a

---

*Work P.R.E.P. was designed and implemented in 1988 by Carl M. Bettencourt, OTR/L.

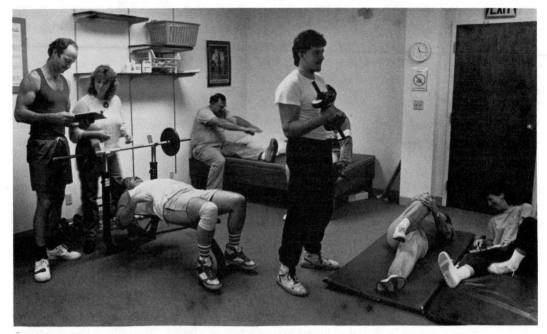

Figure 7-1.   One aspect of programming is individualized conditioning activities. (Photograph courtesy of New England Rehabilitation Hospital.)

multi-billion dollar cost to the medical system and exerts a tremendous toll on workers in terms of lost work days and disability. Pain is a perplexing facet of disease and illness with many characteristics, and its perception and affect on disability can be significantly influenced by a number of variables. Of significance is the impact of the medical, legal, and compensation systems on the injured worker in terms of degree of recovery or disability. Early intervention and mobilization appear to be critical in returning injured employees back to the work force in a timely, efficient, and cost-effective manner. This timely transition requires the cooperation of all those involved in working with the injured employee.

Work hardening, introduced as a component of a comprehensive industrial rehabilitation program, provides injured workers with the opportunity to develop and improve their physical and emotional capacities, including redeveloping and reinforcing the work ethic to optimal levels, in order to return to work.

Occupational therapists, by virtue of their knowledge, skill, and training, are key professionals in the industrial movement. They have a unique and creative perspective to contribute to the rehabilitation team, and can be instrumental to the development, implementation, and success of work hardening programs in the upcoming decade.

Case Study

John Smith is a 45-year-old truck driver who was referred for work hardening services at the Billerica Ambulatory Care Center. He is married, has three small children, and lives in a house purchased two years ago.

John was injured at work when he attempted to lift a 70-pound carton during

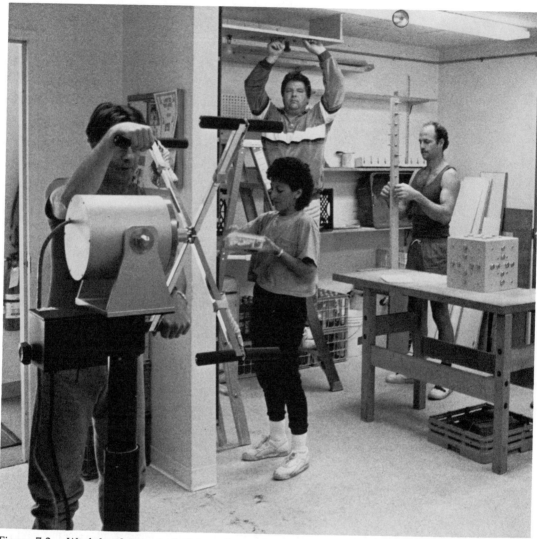

Figure 7-2.   Work hardening includes work simulation activities. (Photograph courtesy of New England Rehabilitation Hospital.)

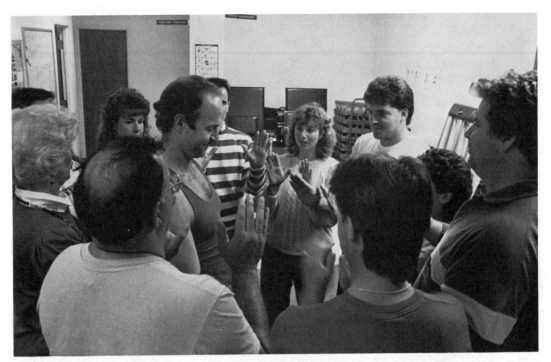

Figure 7-3.   A relaxation and stress management class. (Photograph courtesy of New England Rehabilitation Hospital.)

a delivery. His attending physician prescribed bed rest and analgesics. When symptoms worsened over the next two weeks, he was referred to an orthopedic surgeon. He underwent a diagnostic workup, including x-rays and a CT scan, which revealed a herniated L3–4 disc.

John was referred for physical therapy, where he was treated with hotpacks, ultrasound, electrical stimulation, deep massage, and exercises for the next six weeks. Although he reported considerable relief, he had lost a significant amount of strength and was quite fearful of returning to his previous job.

Following this acute intervention, he was referred by the orthopedist to a work hardening program to increase his overall work tolerances. He was initially evaluated by a physical therapist, occupational therapist, movement therapist, and vocational counselor. John's work hardening program addressed a variety of areas. He participated in a group program involving progressive exercises to improve strength, flexibility, endurance, and posture. His program also involved work-simulated activities specific to his job—lifting, carrying, pushing, and pulling. He was involved in a pain/stress management group. Low-impact aerobic sessions were held twice a week for the first two weeks to address endurance and cardiovascular conditioning. Weekly group educational sessions were also offered to teach and review principles in body mechanics, posture, return to work issues, and injury prevention. A vocational counselor met with John on a regular basis, providing direction regarding return to work. John was periodically evaluated by his orthopedic surgeon, who was regularly updated on John's progress.

John was involved in the work hardening program five days per week, 3–5 hours per day. He attended the program for six weeks. Upon discharge, John had progressed in all areas. He had gained considerable strength and was able to tolerate 3–5 hours of continuous activity without an increase in symptoms. This increased activity level included 1–2 hours of resistive activity, a target level determined upon admission, and a good understanding of symptom control strategies and their integration into his work day to improve his work performance. He had no difficulty with the driving aspect of his job, so this was not addressed during his program. Vocational rehabilitation had also communicated with his employer, insurance company, and other team members to coordinate a smooth transition back to work following discharge.

REFERENCES

1. American Psychiatric Association. *Diagnostic and Statistical Manual of Mental Disorders*, 3rd edition. Washington, D.C.: APA, 1980.
2. Anderson, L. Educational Approaches to Management of Low Back Pain. *Orthopaedic Nursing* 8(1):43–46, 1989.
3. Aronoff, G. M. Pain Centers: A Revolution in Health Care. New York: Raven Press, 1988.
4. Blankenship, K. Work Capacity Evaluation. Industrial Rehabilitation, American Therapeutics conference lecture notes, 1984.
5. Caplan, B. *Rehabilitation Psychology Desk Reference*. Rockville, Maryland. Aspen Publications, 1987.
6. Chapman, R. C. New Dimensions in the Understanding and Management of Pain. *Social Science Medicine* 19(12):1261–1277, 1984.
7. Deyo, R. A. The Role of the Primary Care Physician in Reducing Work Absenteeism and Costs Due to Back Pain. *Occupational Medicine: State of the Art Reviews* Vol 3(1):17–30, 1988.
8. Fordyce, W. *Behavioral Methods for Chronic Pain and Illness*. Saint Louis: C.V. Mosby, 1976.
9. France, R. D. Psychiatric Aspects of Pain. *Clin. J. Pain* 5:35–42, 1989.
10. Isernhagen, S. J. *Work Injury: Management and Prevention*. Rockville, MD: Aspen Publishers, 1988.
11. Loeser, J. D., and Egan, K. J. Managing the Chronic Pain Patient. New York: Raven Press, 1989.
12. Matheson, L. N. Work Capacity Evaluation: 1987. Anaheim, CA: E.R.I.C., 1987.
13. Matheson, L. N. Use of the BTE Work Simulator to Screen for Symptom Magnification Syndrome. *Industr. Rehab. Q.* 2(2):15–17, 1989.
14. Menges, L. J. Pain: Still An Intriguing Puzzle. *Soc. Sci. Med.* 19(12):1257–1260, 1984.
15. Niemeyer, L. O., and Jacobs, K. *Work Hardening: State of the Art*, Thorofare, NJ: Slack Incorporated, 1989.
16. Sternbach, R. A. *The Psychology of Pain*, Second edition. New York: Raven Press, 1986.
17. Sternbach, R. A. (1974). *Pain Patients: Traits and Treatments*. New York: Academic Press, 1974.
18. Stokes, H. M. The Seriously Injured Hand—*Weakness of Grip. J. Occup. Med.* 25(9):683–684, 1983.
19. Sheikh, K. Occupational Injury, Chronic Low Back Pain and Return to Work. *Public Health*, 101:417–425, 1987.
20. Taylor, M. E. Return to Work Following Back Surgery: A Review. *Am. J. Industr. Med.*, 16:79–88, 1989.
21. Tollison, C. D. *Relief From Back Pain: The Tollison Program*, New York: Gardner Press, 1987.
22. Tramposh, A. K. Work-Related Therapy for the Injured Reduces Return-to-Work Barriers. *Occup. Health and Safety*, April:55–56, 82, 1988.
23. Turk, D. C., Meichenbaum, D., and Genest, M. *Pain and Behavioral Medicine*. New York: Guilford Press, 1983.
24. Waddell, G., McCullock, J. A., Kummel, E., and Venner, R. M. Nonorganic Physical Signs in Low Back Pain. *Spine* 5(2):117–125, 1980.

A Functional Assessment Program of Activities of Daily Living for Brain-Injured Individuals*

A comprehensive assessment, program, and discharge planning tool known as GROWS is used at the Devereux Foundation Center for Head Trauma. The purpose of GROWS is to help to reintegrate brain-injured individuals not only back into the community but into the "working world." Each client is involved in an ongoing program of evaluation to determine his or her ability to participate in the vocational program. This program encompasses a hierarchy ranging from prevocational skills (work training) to competitive employment.

The Devereux Foundation Center for Head Trauma (CHT) is a post-acute rehabilitation program serving traumatically brain-injured persons who have completed acute rehabilitation but still lack the necessary skills to live successfully within the community. Clients are usually admitted within two years of their injury, although in certain cases, they may be admitted a number of years after the injury. These clients are referred to CHT through various insurance companies, school districts, rehabilitation hospitals, parents, and clinicians.

The location of CHT is vital to its success as a community re-entry program. Located in a growing county with a rapidly expanding business community affords many occupational opportunities. Residential services are located in an upper-middle class suburban neighborhood and are within a quarter mile of convenience and grocery stores, banks, and restaurants. Train and bus line services leading to a metropolitan area are located within two blocks.

CHT is accredited by the Joint Commission on Accreditation of Healthcare Organizations, the International Association of Counseling Services, the Commission on Accreditation of Rehabilitation Facilities, and the American Psychological Association. In addition, this facility is licensed by the Pennsylvania Department of Education as a private academic school and by the Pennsylvania Department of Public Welfare. It is a member of the National and Keystone Head Injury Foundations.

The philosophy at CHT is to help each client achieve his or her highest level of independent functioning. Toward this goal, treatment is offered in the least restrictive setting, ranging from structured residential treatment to community-based apartments with support services.

Since brain-injured individuals often have difficulty generalizing new information, the model of the program is functional and experiential, utilizing "hands-on" therapies and classes at the facility and in the community.

CHT employs a transdisciplinary team approach consisting of:

Neuropsychology
Psychiatry
Psychology
Medicine/nursing

*This section was written by Deborah L. Maloney, OTR/L, B.A., Nancy R. Feldman, CCC Sp., M.S, and Maria M. Foschi, M.Ed.

Education
Occupational therapy
Physical therapy
Speech-language therapy
Movement therapy
Vocational services
Recreational therapy
Equestrian therapy
Recreational and instructional swimming program for head trauma at
    the YMCA
Social service coordination

All services are integrated through an individualized treatment plan
developed within the first 72 hours of admission and revised within 30
days, following comprehensive assessments by all disciplines. Due to
the small size of the program, it is highly individualized and outcome
oriented.

CHT has two components of program delivery. The initial program
provides 24-hour supervision and can treat up to 22 clients in a dormitory. All clients begin their program on the residential campus. The
second component of program delivery supports clients in transitional
apártment living. These clients either attend an educational placement
program or are involved in part-time competitive employment.

Treatment at CHT is based upon the philosophy that all members of
the clinical, educational, and vocational team will work together toward
the goal of vocational placement. An estimated length of stay and a
tentative discharge goal are set for each client during the first 30 days
after admission.

Goals for the clients range from placement in a sheltered workshop
to fulltime competitive placement, with or without a job coach. Experience with this population has shown that prevocational skills are
important to obtaining and maintaining a job.

GROWS is divided into five different levels, differentiated by colors,
which make up the acronym GROWS:

Green level is a 30-day initial assessment period, composed of work
    training and vocational readiness classes.
Red level addresses basic low-level ADL skills.
Orange level encompasses basic skills that include community re-
    entry.
White level involves the transition from dormitory or restricted living
    to apartment or semi-independent living skills.
Silver level is reserved for independent living and work skills such
    as doing one's income tax, handling apartment problems, cooking
    for others, and managing home and clothing appropriately.

Each area can be worked on within the occupational therapy department but more commonly is addressed by a combination of team members.

As clients progress from one level to another, they are also placed in work training, vocational readiness, and job maintenance groups to improve specific skills related to a future job placement.

Failing to see their successes is a common problem with head trauma clients. GROWS has attempted to alleviate this problem by listing necessary prevocational components in small increments so that clients can see even a minimal improvement in a specific area (e.g., taking the bus to a work site).

ASSESSMENTS

The CHT developed the GROWS program to fill the need for a higher-level assessment of daily living skills than is commonly available in acute care settings. This program includes the following ten areas:

Communication skills
Community skills
Dressing and grooming
Health and safety/sex education
Home management
Meal planning and meal preparation
Money management
Shopping skills
Restaurant skills
Vocational planning and work assessment

Emphasis in the vocational component is on communication skills, community skills, dressing and grooming, health and safety, money management, and vocational planning and work assessment. A client moves to a new level when 90 percent of the items on a skill level have been completed.

Individual assessment sheets are kept in clients' memory books, so that any staff member working with a client can mark items as they are accomplished. The date, performance, and time needed to complete a skill are recorded.

PROGRAMMING

The Educational/Vocational Team has direct responsibility for implementing GROWS. Team members work in transdisciplinary groups with each other and with unit psychologists.

CHT's day program, operating Monday through Friday from 8:30 A.M. to 4:30 P.M., assists clients in the ten previously listed activities of daily living. Two afternoons per week are devoted to these ADLs. Clients are heterogeneously grouped into small units of three or four for one of five sections:

1. Meal planning and preparation and home management with the occupational therapist
2. Restaurant skills and communication skills with the speech/language therapist

3. Shopping and community skills dressing and grooming with the cognitive therapist
4. Health and safety/sex education with the physical education teacher
5. Money management/vocational planning and work assessment with the vocational counselor

Clients rotate through each of these sections, and each section lasts six weeks.

Prior to placement into one of these groups, a client on the Green level works on becoming familiar with GROWS and samples the various sections with the assistance of a senior residential counselor.

The evening and weekend residential counselors engage clients in activities designed to aid in carryover of skills to community living.

All team members have a dual role. Each counselor is both part of the staff focusing on activities of daily living using GROWS and works within his or her own discipline of vocational counseling. Vocational services at CHT include vocational assessments, vocational readiness classes, transitional evaluation and employment, career counseling, job placement, job coaching, and follow-up.

Formal assessments are available through the Vocational Rehabilitation Center. Here an individualized test battery might include interest, aptitude and work behavior measures (e.g., the Work-Related Interest Opinion Test). Measures such as structured behavioral observation techniques, in conjunction with performance on work samples (e.g., Singer-Graflex sample) are utilized to observe and assess style of work, attention to task, frustration tolerance, and ability to follow directions.

Devereux's Vocational Rehabilitation Center, a day program, operates a state-certified automotive repair center, a horticultural program, a manufacturing business of pewter figurines, and a silk-screening business. There are numerous job placements within Devereux in maintenance, child care, housekeeping, word processing, and data entry. All of these transitional evaluation and employment placements are paid work experiences.

Job development and job placement are performed on an individual basis. Assessment results are shared with the client and potential job goals are identified, explored, and discussed. For the majority of clients, the rehabilitation counselor is directly involved in the job procurement process and actively assists the client in securing and maintaining employment.

SUMMARY

GROWS has proven to be an effective discharge planning tool for the staff at CHT. It has been found that by using GROWS, clients can maintain maximum levels of independence and confidence in adapting to their home and community environments. "Hands on" experiences have enabled clients to apply skills and synthesize information while working closely with direct care, professional staff, and family members in structured, positive learning situations. A copy of the GROWS manual is sent to the family or aftercare placement facility to share information about a client's already achieved functional level.

Case Study
Miss Smith sustained a closed-head injury on January 15, 1987, when she was hit by a car while jaywalking to catch a bus. She lapsed into a coma for ten days. She sustained fractures of the pelvis and right femur. She returned home in November, 1987. At this point, home tutoring began.

In January, 1988, she exhibited verbal and physical aggression in addition to substance abuse. She was admitted to a psychiatric hospital in her local area. In August of 1988, she was transferred to a nursing home. She continued to exhibit physical and verbal aggression towards others and was transferred on September 30, 1988, to a psychiatric hospital with a neurobehavioral unit. During this hospitalization, Miss Smith's behavior improved and she was transferred to the Devereux Center for Head Trauma on January 24, 1989. However, her condition deteriorated rapidly, and she was readmitted to a psychiatric hospital on February 1, 1989.

After intensive treatment and stabilization at this facility, she returned to CHT in April, 1989, to begin community-based rehabilitation.

Rehabilitation Treatment
Initial Programming
Miss Smith was reintegrated into the CHT program gradually. During the first two weeks, she progressed from a one-hour visit to a full day at the program. As she was able to manage these visits successfully, Miss Smith was reenrolled into the CHT program on a permanent basis.

At this juncture, the program was modified to accommodate her needs. The following changes were implemented:

Programming was restricted to her private room, the living room, and dining room of her residence.
Each therapist came to Miss Smith's residence to carry out therapy.
She was not involved in any group activities.
She was restricted to campus.

These modifications lasted for approximately three weeks. Gradually, Miss Smith was integrated into various group therapies. By the end of six weeks, she was involved in full programming.
Her initial programming consisted of the following therapies:

Individual career counseling
Work training sessions
Activities of daily living
Problem solving group
Language pragmatics group
Occupational therapy group
Head injury group
Individual occupational therapy
Individual cognitive therapy
Individual speech therapy
Individual physical therapy
Individual psychotherapy

During this phase, various assessments were administered to determine her functional level (Fig. 7-4A & B). After these were completed, the treatment plan was revised. The treatment plan focused on improving her coping skills, memory, reasoning ability, balance, strength, and work tolerance.

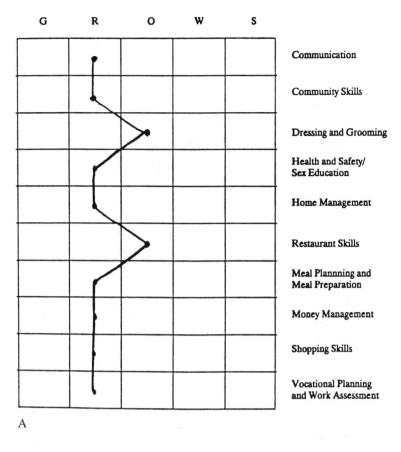

A

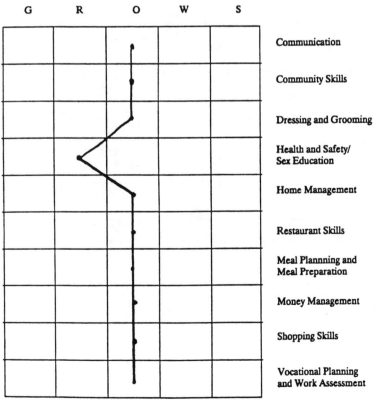

B
Figure 7-4.

DRESSING AND GROOMING

	Initial			Ongoing			Discharge		
1. What is your daily routine for maintaining body and hair cleanliness?									
* 2. Maintain a schedule of body and hair cleanliness.									
3. Show how to use a toothbrush, dental floss, toothpaste and mouthwash.									
* 4. Maintain an oral hygiene regime.									
5. Describe the steps for A. cleaning one's hair B. cleaning ears C. cleaning nails									
6. Describe the following nail care products: A. nail clippers B. cuticle remover C. nail polish D. nail polish remover									
7. Demonstrate how to care for fingernails and toenails.									
8. A. Name and describe commonly used menstrual aids such as tampons, pads and belts. B. Tell why menstrual aids are used.									
9. Explain how to use the above menstrual aids.									
10. Describe procedures for cleanliness during menstruation.									
11. What is the reason for using deodorant?									
* 12. Use deodorant properly.									
13. A. Describe the most important reasons for choosing and wearing certain clothes. Include reasons such as conditions, cleanliness and the activity chosen. B. Demonstrate wearing the above clothing.									
	P	T	D	P	T	D	P	T	D

Figure 7-5.   Red Level of Dressing and Grooming from GROWS.

Name: _____   *Grows • Red Level*

	Initial			Ongoing			Discharge		

14. Choose clothing for three different days:
  A. day at a beach
  B. snowy, winter day
  C. going out to dinner at a fancy restaurant									

15. A. How do you know when you need to wash your hair? **B.** What will happen if you do not wash your hair often enough?									
16. Follow appropriate hair grooming practices daily.									
	P	T	D	P	T	D	P	T	D

Figure 7-5.   (continued)

Name: _____   *Grows • Orange Level*

COMMUNICATIONS

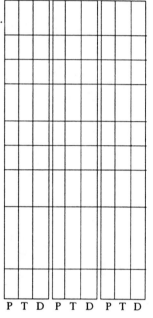

	Initial			Ongoing			Discharge		
* 1. Give clear and concise information during a conversation.									
2. Take six written phone messages.									
3. Write a letter independently.									
4. A. Write a letter and a postcard. B. Address and stamp a letter and a postcard.									
5. Acquire and fill out an individual address book.									
6. Demonstrate speaker/listener turn-taking.									
7. Demonstrate the ability to actively listen and respond in conversations.									
8. Use these parts of a telephone directory: A. white pages B. blue pages C. yellow pages (business, dentist and doctor)									
9. Introduce yourself and others appropriately.									
	P	T	D	P	T	D	P	T	D

Figure 7-6.   Orange Level of Communications from GROWS.

At the Red Level (Fig. 7-5), Miss Smith was able to carry out a daily routine for maintaining body and hair cleanliness, caring for nails, and following an oral hygiene routine. In addition, Miss Smith demonstrated her ability to choose appropriate clothing depending on the cleanliness of the clothing, activity chosen, and the weather conditions.

She progressed through the ADL areas and obtained the Orange Level in August. At the Orange Level (Fig. 7-6) Miss Smith was able to communicate effectively with co-workers and supervisors in terms of giving and taking information. She was able to use "help wanted" ads in the newspaper to contact an employer by telephone, and to fill out a resume and a job application (Fig. 7-7). On-going therapy included assistance in identifying three types of appropriate interpersonal interactions on the job. In addition, she advanced to the Vocational Readiness Group. At this level, the focus was on resumes, job applications, job interviews, and interpersonal communications with co-workers and supervisors. In conjunction with this vocational advancement, Miss Smith began an "in-house" vocational placement as an assistant to the unit secretary. Her job duties included collating, copying, answering telephones, and distributing mail. She had some difficulties with the tasks due to her organizational skills. However, when the job was modified to decrease the organizational aspects, she was successful.

When she moved to the White Level (Fig. 7-8), Miss Smith practiced drawing maps of frequently visited community areas so that she would be able to recognize road signs and landmarks. Although she is currently being transported to her job by staff, completion of this level will enable her to travel independently to her job using public transportation. In October, 1989, Miss Smith's clinical treatment plan review took place. At this meeting, the clinical treatment team discussed her progress and planned for her future programming. The possibility of Miss Smith obtaining a part-time job in the community as a secretarial assistant was discussed. The team encouraged this placement, and delineated the steps needed to be taken that would assure the success of this placement. It was recommended that the cognitive therapist, the vocational counselor, and the job coach would do an on-site task analysis of Miss Smith's potential job. Various strategies were put into place, including consultation with the occupational therapist regarding adaptive equipment.

Vocational Placement

Miss Smith's job placement consisted of the following:

1. removing memos from 65 mail slots
2. folding memos so they could be placed in envelopes
3. placing memos in appropriate envelopes (three sizes)
4. placing mailing labels on envelopes
5. weighing envelopes to determine postage due
6. putting envelopes through a postage machine

When a review of these job duties was discussed, the following changes needed to be made to assure a successful job placement.

1. *Removing memos from 65 mail slots.* The mailbox was situated on the left-hand corner of the wall, extending from the ceiling to the floor. A few changes were implemented to aid Miss Smith with organization. The mailboxes were color coded in sequential order according to the alphabet. Each color contained 8 to 11 different mail slots. For example, the white color code corresponded to the executive mail, the red color code corresponded to the A and B cities, etc. There were a total of six colors. In addition, a stool with a handle was provided so Miss Smith could easily access mail from the top of the mail boxes.

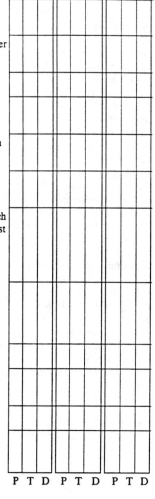

Name: _____   *Grows • Orange Level*

VOCATIONAL PLANNING AND WORK ASSESSMENT

	Initial			Ongoing			Discharge		
	P	T	D	P	T	D	P	T	D
1. State the difference between a job and a career.									
* 2. List the three most important personal factors to consider when making a career choice.									
* 3. Identify three jobs you are capable of performing now.									
* 4. List three resources that are typically used for finding a job.									
5. Identify the most commonly used abbreviations found in help-wanted ads.									
6. What is the most common information found in help-wanted ads?									
7. Find two help-wanted ads in the local newspaper for each of the three jobs you named in #3 above. (Each job must be located under a different heading, e.g., *dishwasher* may also be found under *restaurant help, food services, part-time*, etc.									
* 8. A. List three types of appropriate interpersonal interactions on the job. B. List three types of inappropriate interpersonal interactions on the job.									
* 9. What is your social security number?									
10. Describe five mistakes people commonly make when completing a job application.									
* 11. Complete a mock job application.									
12. A. How are a resume and a job application similar? B. How are they different?									

Figure 7-7.   Orange Level of Vocational Planning and Work Assessment from GROWS.

Name: _____   *Grows • Orange Level*

	Initial			Ongoing			Discharge		

13. A. Describe how to acquire relevant information about a job prior to the initial telephone contact.
   B. Explain why you should acquire this information prior to initial telephone contact.

14. What information is exchanged during a telephone contact to set up a job interview?

* 15. Describe the potential consequences of being late for an interview.

* 16. A. Identify three appropriate interview behaviors.
   B. Identify three inappropriate interview behaviors.

17. Describe why it is important to be clear and concise when inquiring about job requirements and responsibilities during an initial contact with an employer.

18. Explain the importance of good eye contact and clear speech during an interview.

* 19. Describe how you would dress for interviews for the following jobs:
   A. construction worker
   B. secretary

* 20. List four types of information that are usually exchanged during an interview.

21. What are two appropriate methods of following up after an interview.

P T D   P T D   P T D

The Devereux Foundation   The Center for Head Trauma 37

Figure 7-7.   (continued)

COMMUNITY SKILLS

1. Draw a map of frequently traveled community areas.
   A. Indicate road signs.
   B. Indicate landmarks.

2. Obtain the following information about public
   transportation to your residence:
   A. What public transportation is available?
   B. At what times does this public transportation operate?
   C. How do you purchase tickets if required?

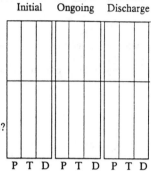

Figure 7-8.   White Level of Community Skills from GROWS.

2. *Folding memos so they could be placed in envelopes.* Adaptive equipment was utilized to aid with the folding of envelopes. This piece of equipment consisted of an 8″ × 10″ piece of sturdy cardboard with a ledge at the bottom and a strip of cardboard at the center of approximately 3½″ in width.

3. *Placing memos in appropriate envelopes (three sizes).* Miss Smith used the following rules: if there were five or less memos, then she would use the small envelope; if there were between six and ten memos, she would use the medium envelope, and for eleven memos or more, she would use the large envelope.

4. *Placing mailing labels on envelopes.* Labels were placed in folders according to the color code utilized on the mailboxes. (These folders corresponded exactly to the mailboxes.)

Step-by-step checklists were developed to execute tasks 5 and 6.

After the various compensatory strategies and adaptive equipment were in place, training on the job commenced. A job coach as well as video taping were utilized for training. The job coach was with Miss Smith for the entire work session during the first two weeks, and for one-hour sessions each day during the next week. During the fourth week, the job coach assisted Miss Smith for two sessions of one hour each. At this juncture, job coaching was eliminated and video taping implemented. The philosophy underlying video taping was to aid Miss Smith in problem-solving skills. For example, what should she do when the envelope gets stuck in the postage machine or she forgets which label she is to place on the envelope.

Currently, Miss Smith is employed in this competitive job placement. She is independently carrying out all job duties successfully. It is anticipated she will continue in this line of work for the duration of her stay at CHT, possibly increasing the number of hours per week and/or her job responsibilities.

Innovative Work Programs for Adults with Neurophysiologic Problems

BRAINTREE HOSPITAL'S
COMPREHENSIVE DRIVER EDUCATION PROGRAM

It is estimated that 1,500,000 employable disabled persons are unemployed because of lack of transportation. Braintree Hospital's Comprehensive Driver Education Program for the physically disabled is based on the premise that restriction of mobility is a serious problem that limits an individual's vocational, educational, social, and recreational opportunities and ultimately an independent lifestyle.

Extensive research and investigation, particularly of accident reports, have revealed that most disabled persons can be licensed as safe, competent drivers. However, the lack of essential medical input in commercial driving schools has kept many from succeeding.

Braintree Hospital's program, which is an extension of the rehabilitation process, provides clinical evaluation of the disabled client's driving potential. When indicated, on-the-road training in specially modified vehicles is also part of the program. Clients may refer themselves or be referred by a physician, rehabilitation counselor, or other health care professional. Referrals are most timely when the client has completed any active therapy programs and has attained his or her maximum functional potential.

At the time of the referral medical history, seizure history, a list of current medications, and discharge summaries from completed therapy programs are requested. This information is used to determine the client's appropriateness for the predriving evaluation and assists in answering questions such as, Is the program timely with respect to the client's disability and rehabilitation progress? and, Is driving a realistic goal for this client?

To date, clients with the following disabilities have participated in the program:

Cerebral vascular accidents
Traumatic brain injuries
Traumatic spinal cord injuries
Progressive neuromuscular disorders such as multiple sclerosis and
    muscular dystrophy
Amputations
Congenital defects such as spina bifida and cerebral palsy
Developmental disabilities such as mental retardation and minimal
    brain dysfunction

Program components include (1) a predriving evaluation completed by an occupational therapist, (2) an on-the-road evaluation, and (3) a physical medicine evaluation and medical certification letter to the Massachusetts Registry of Motor Vehicles.

Clinical Predriving Evaluation

The predriving evaluation has been designed to determine the client's driving potential through the assessment of his or her (1) physical skills, that is, range of motion, muscle strength, coordination, mobility, transfer skills, reaction time, and endurance; (2) perception; (3) cognition; (4) vision; (5) language skills; and (6) need for adaptive driving equipment and vehicle modification. The evaluating therapist also determines if additional therapy is needed before the client begins to drive.

When driving is contraindicated by the evaluation results, the following options are available:

Therapeutic intervention for remediation of residual deficits, for example, muscle strengthening or cognitive retraining
Recommendation for reevaluation of current medications, for example, for spasticity
Recommendations for equipment needed to transport the client safely as a passenger

When the evaluation results demonstrate that the client has the potential to drive, further recommendations may include a 30-hour classroom drivers' education program or an on-the-road training program in a specially modified vehicle. The amount of on-the-road training that the client will require depends on the complexity of the adaptive driving equipment and the client's prior driving experience, endurance, and ability to integrate new learning. The following indicates the average amount of drivers' training recommended for clients with various disabilities:

Disability	Amount of Training (hours)
Spinal cord injury	20–30
Lower-extremity amputations	10
Cerebral vascular accidents	10
Traumatic head injuries	15–20
Congenital defects	20

Besides classroom and on-the-job training, continued therapy for transfer training, wheelchair management, and muscle strengthening; specialized adaptive driving equipment that compensates for physical deficits (e.g., left foot accelerator, steering knob) (Fig. 7-9); or handicapped plates may be recommended. These plates, obtained from the Registry of Motor Vehicles, enable the client to use designated handicapped parking spaces.

On-the-Road Evaluation

The two-hour on-the-road evaluation is completed only when the client's performance during the predriving evaluation demonstrates borderline deficits in cognitive, perceptual, or visual skills. Before the evaluation, the predriving evaluator and the driver trainer plan functional tasks or situations that can be simulated in the vehicle to evaluate further the client's cognitive processing, attention span, impulsivity, reaction time, visual scanning, and depth perception.

The on-the-road evaluation is not a driving lesson but rather an assessment used to supplement clinical findings and determine if the client can return to driving.

Physical Medicine Evaluation and Medical Certification Letter

When all the evaluation components have been completed, a physician reviews them with the therapist and writes a letter explaining the results of the evaluation to the Registry of Motor Vehicles and recommends either a return to driving or suspension of the client's operator's license. In addition adaptive equipment needed for driving is summarized, and license restrictions are recommended. This letter is sent to the medical affairs branch of the Registry. The final step for obtaining a valid operator's license—completion of the road competency test—is the client's responsibility.

Results

Braintree Hospital's Comprehensive Driver Education Program has been in existence since 1977. During this time it has seen much success and an increased need for its services. The program's combination of

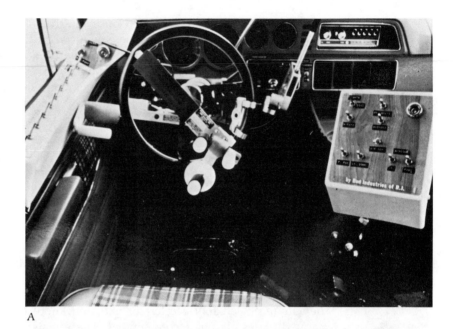

A

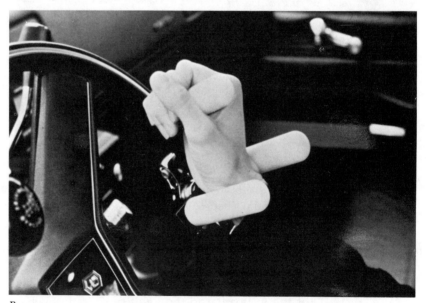

B

Figure 7-9.   A. Adaptive driving equipment and vehicle modification for a van. B. Close-up of adaptive hand device. (Courtesy of Braintree Hospital.)

thorough clinical evaluation and individualized driver's training has enabled 100 percent of the clients who complete the training to obtain a valid license. A license enables the disabled client to utilize fully the skills acquired through the rehabilitation process. This hospital-based driving program helps strengthen the link between rehabilitation and independent living.

Following are two case studies from the Braintree Hospital program:

Case Study 1*

D. M., a 23-year-old woman, was involved in a motor vehicle accident that put her in a coma for four weeks and resulted in head injury, left eye blindness, and multiple fractures. Acute hospitalization lasted 2½ months and included status post tracheostomy and gastrostomy. When medically stable, D. M. was transferred to a brain injury unit for rehabilitation. After 4½ months, she was discharged and went home to her family for 24-hour supervision. As an outpatient D. M. received occupational, physical, and speech therapy for an additional six months. Current medications include phenytoin sodium (Dilantin), 200 mg per day, for seizure prevention. D. M.'s neurologist provided an on-medication agreement stating that she had been seizure-free since the time of the accident. Massachusetts law requires that an 18-month seizure-free period be established before one can return to driving.

On completion of therapy D. M. worked as a secretary in a supervised job that had been arranged by her state vocational rehabilitation counselor in preparation for returning to competitive employment.

Before her motor vehicle accident, D. M. had had five years of driving experience. She also reported having successfully completed the classroom driver education safety course.

A predriving evaluation was completed 24 hours after injury. Physical, visual, perceptual, and cognitive skills were evaluated with regard to D. M.'s ability to drive. Physically, D. M.'s upper extremities demonstrated a functionally adequate active range of motion and generally fair muscle strength. The right upper arm demonstrated normal muscle tone with below-average coordination. However, her left upper arm demonstrated minimal hypertonicity, with associated reactions. Her left-upper-extremity tremors increased when she was frustrated, anxious, or angry, although overall coordination was minimally impaired. Therefore, her left arm was considered to be nonfunctional for driving. As a result, she would need to steer using her right hand with the aid of a steering knob and power steering.

D. M.'s right lower leg demonstrated a functional active range of motion and muscle tone, fair muscle strength, and slower-than-average reaction times. The left lower leg demonstrated increased hypertonicity with associated reactions and clonus and therefore was considered nonfunctional for driving. Because of these deficits, D. M. would be restricted to operating a car equipped with power brakes and an automatic transmission.

D. M. could walk independently without assistive devices. She entered and exited a car independently.

D. M.'s visual acuity was corrected to within Registry of Motor Vehicles requirements. The speed and accuracy with which she was able to scan her environment was impaired but within normal limits. D. M. suffered traumatic blindness in her left eye. The registry ruling on one-eyed vision states that the field of vision must be at least 135. D. M.'s visual field met Registry standards at 155. Depth perception was minimally impaired. Night vision and glare recovery were severely impaired. As a result, D. M. would be restricted to daytime driving. Color vision and traffic color recognition were within normal limits.

---

*This case study was provided by Holly T. Ehle, OTR, Braintree Hospital, Braintree, Massachusetts.

Perceptually, D. M. demonstrated below-average spatial relation skills; however, figure-ground discrimination and auditory memory were functional. Visual memory was minimally below passing standard. Her speed of visual processing was one-third slower than average. However, her accuracy was functional when she was asked to alternate between two stimuli. Her behavior during the clinical evaluation included periods of impulsivity and low frustration tolerance.

The clinical predriving evaluation with the head-injured client is limited; identified deficit areas must be further assessed on the road. D. M.'s performance on the road demonstrated perceptual and behavioral impairments that interfered with her ability to drive safely. The most serious deficit was her slowed mental processing—impaired ability to solve problems demanding quick, accurate responses. She was unable to control her frustration, anxiety, and impulsivity, as was clearly demonstrated when she uncontrollably withdrew her hands from the steering wheel. D. M. acknowledged her behaviors but was unable to realize their implications with regard to safe driving.

On the basis of the clinical predriving evaluation and the on-the-road assessment, it was recommended that D. M. remain a passenger and not drive. It was also recommended that her license be suspended and not renewed. Various alternative activities were suggested to assist D. M. in developing the necessary predriving skills. D. M., her family, and her vocational counselor were informed that D. M. would be eligible for reevaluation if major progress could be demonstrated.

Case Study 2*

At age 15 B. J. sustained a C6 spinal cord injury in a driving accident. A spinal fusion, C5 through C7, was surgically performed for neck stabilization. He received rehabilitation at a regional spinal cord injury unit. During rehabilitation spasticity in his legs resulted in a right hip dislocation. He had surgical correction of his right hip and tendon releases for spastic abductors. After six months of rehabilitation he was discharged to his home, where he functions from an electric wheelchair and receives assistance from his family. The home was modified for electric wheelchair accessibility, including ramping and bathroom modifications.

B. J. returned to high school and hopes to attend college after graduation. He plans to study computers with the goal of full-time employment in business. The state vocational rehabilitation commission referred B. J. for an evaluation of driving potential and adaptive equipment needs.

B. J. did not have driving experience before his spinal cord injury. He completed classroom drivers' education at high school. B. J. depends on private wheelchair van companies for all transportation.

A predriving evaluation was completed 18 months after injury. Physical, cognitive, perceptual, and visual skills were evaluated in terms of B. J.'s potential to drive safely and of his adaptive driving equipment needs. B. J.'s arms had the physical strength, active range of motion, sensation, coordination, and reaction times necessary for learning effective driving of a van with full hand controls. With his right arm, B. J. demonstrated the abilities necessary to steer with reduced-effort power steering and a tri-pin steering device. With his left arm, B. J. demonstrated the abilities necessary to accelerate and brake with a right-angle–type hand control mounted on the left side of the steering column. A left wrist splint was needed for driving, to provide a secure interface with hand control and to maximize left arm strength. All driving functions had to be modified for activation with either right or left arm.

B. J.'s legs were nonfunctional for driving tasks because of the lack of voluntary movement. Full seat belting including shoulder, chest, lap, and leg belting was recommended. B. J.'s legs had to be secured away from conventional floor gas and brake pedals because of his spasticity. Since B. J. required

*This case study was provided by Karen Haggerty-Weake, OTR, Braintree Hospital, Braintree, Massachusetts.

assistance for all transfers, he had to drive from his electric wheelchair with a wheelchair tie-down system. His dependence on an electric wheelchair for mobility necessitated a specially modified van with an automatic wheelchair lift.

All cognitive and perceptual skills evaluated were within functional limits for learning to operate a van. Drivers' training was recommended to maximize these skills and to prepare for the registry road test.

All visual skills were evaluated with prescription lenses, and the results were within registry requirements.

The following actions were taken by the evaluating therapist:

1. A medical certification letter was mailed to the medical affairs branch of the registry, providing clearance for B. J. to begin drivers' training in a specially modified van.
2. Twenty-five hours of drivers' training was recommended for B. J. to learn safe use of adaptive driving equipment and to prepare for the registry road test.
3. On successful completion of the road test, B. J. would receive a restricted driver's license.
4. Because of B. J.'s permanent physical disability, handicapped plates were recommended for his specially modified van.

The following restrictions would appear on B. J.'s driver's license:

Automatic transmission
Power steering
Power brakes
Steering device
Full hand controls
Hand-operated parking brake
Hand-operated dimmer switch

The state vocational rehabilitation commission assisted with payment for drivers' training and adaptive equipment. After 25 hours of training in his modified van, B. J. successfully completed the registry road test and has become a licensed driver.

LIBERTY MUTUAL MEDICAL SERVICE CENTER*

Liberty Mutual Insurance Company, the country's largest underwriter of Workers' Compensation, has been a forerunner in the field of providing rehabilitation for the industrially injured patient. Its outpatient facility, the Liberty Mutual Medical Service Center, provides three types of rehabilitative services: an acute care clinic, general rehabilitation, and a functional restoration program.

The Center was founded in 1943 to provide comprehensive rehabilitation for Workers' Compensation policyholders, both locally and nationally. The fulltime intensive program addresses physical function limitations for a wide variety of orthopedic injuries such as cumulative trauma disorders, traumatic amputations, lumbar and cervical injures, fractures, burns, and all types of hand injures.

The Liberty Mutual Back Education and Rehabilitation (LIMBER) pro-

*This section was written by Valerie Shaw Jones, OTR/L, Patricia Gagnon-Stryke, OTR/L, Sherlyn L. Fenton, OTR/L, and Patricia A. McGauley, OTR/L.

gram addresses chronic low back injuries. The intensive four-week functional restoration program has a multidisciplinary approach incorporating occupational therapy, physical therapy, general fitness, cardiovascular fitness, psychology, nursing, vocational counseling, and physician supervision. Upon completion of LIMBER, the participants will have established a physical demand level appropriate to return to work or further vocational counseling. Participants are provided with an individualized home program to maintain their level of fitness, which is monitored during periodic evaluations.

Evaluation

Occupational therapy is inherent to the three rehabilitative services provided at Liberty Mutual Medical Service Center. On admission to the Center the client participates in a comprehensive occupational therapy (OT) evaluation. A broad overview of the primary components included in various OT evaluations are shown in Table 7-1.

The type of evaluation corresponds to the nature of the client's illness or injury and may require a single session or many sessions to establish treatment plans addressing short-term and longterm goals. The following is a brief example of the results of an evaluation of a client with a below-elbow amputation of the dominant hand:

1. Short-term goals:
   Increase range of motion shoulder and elbow
   Decrease hypersensitivity
   Improve skin/stump condition
   Increase functional use of affected upper extremity
   Increase bilateral strength of upper extremities
2. Long-term goals
   Develop effective use of prosthetic device
   Maximize independence in activities of daily living
   Return to work or vocational counseling
3. Treatment
   Upper extremity exercise with and without resistance, using the Occupational Therapy Resistance Apparatus
   Issuance of and instruction in necessary adaptive equipment
   Functional activities to facilitate use of affected upper extremity
   Prosthetic training
   Job simulation/work hardening

Innovative Treatment Modalities

The LIMBER program provides clients with a unique yet realistic therapeutic experience. At the multiwork station, which resembles a section of a two-story house under construction (Fig. 7-10), clients can test their ability to return to strenuous work. It enables them to develop their capacity to handle some of the more physically demanding tasks associated with their jobs such as climbing ladders, staging, lifting, working overhead, using heavy wrenches, pipe cutting and threading, electrical wiring, tiling, siding, and painting.

Table 7-1. Primary Components of Occupational Therapy Rehabilitation Evaluations

	Category	*Examples*
Physical capacity	Range of motion	Standard upper extremity and cervical active/passive range of motion
	Strength, endurance	Standard upper extremity and methods time measurement (MTM), Jamar dynomometer measurements, maximum capacity evaluation
	Sensation	Semmes/Weinstein monofilaments
	Edema	Volumeter
	Pain	Body pain chart filled out by patient
Functional capacity	Sit, stand, walk, climb, stoop, etc.	Subjective report from patient
	Activities of Daily Living (ADLs)	Assessment Checklist for personal, home and recreational management
	Adaptive needs	Equipment, muscle reeducation, energy conservation techniques
Work capacity	Physical demand level	Maximum weight/frequency to lift, carry, push, pull; work hardening; job simulation
	Impairment	Pre-injury physical demand level per job description versus current physical demand level
	Body mechanics	Educational video
	Job history	Ergonomics, job site visit
General intake information	History of present illness Past medical history Medication/allergies Education Psychosocial information	

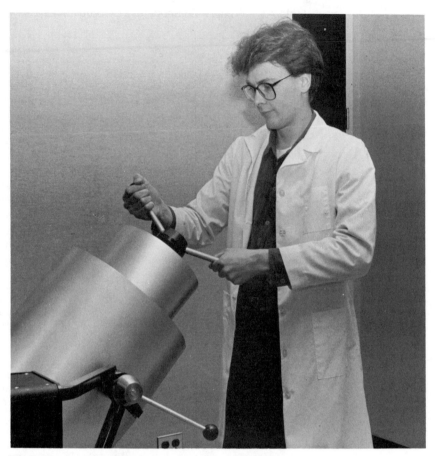

Figure 7-10.   Therapist demonstrating use of OTRA, a computerized work simulator. (Photograph by Liberty Mutual.)

When the client has an upper extremity injury, the Occupational Therapy Resistance Apparatus (OTRA) may be used. The OTRA (Figs. 7-10 and 7-11) is a versatile exercise machine designed to simulate work tasks. The device accomodates a wide range of resistances. Adapted tools such as a steering wheel or lathe handle are coupled to the shaft of the head console to simulate work activities. Data on angular position, force, torque, speed, and acceleration are collected for evaluation of each client's progress, feedback to the client for motivational purposes, and research statistics to help develop new exercise protocols.

For those clients returning to a position involving material handling, occupational therapy provides job specific tasks, including use of two-wheel trucks, loading docks, sand pits, brick laying platforms, and other items that will increase patients' work capacity (Fig. 7-12).

A cross-section of a truck cab is used to simulate the job of the truck driver (Fig. 7-13). The cab has been modified to offer adjustable resistance to the steering wheel, clutch, and stick shift. An audiotape or videotape is used in conjunction with the above to simulate the auditory and visual dimensions of actual driving situations.

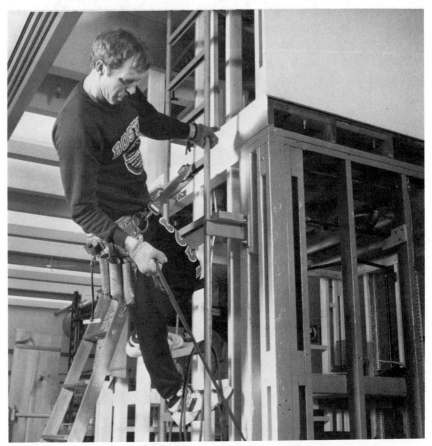

Figure 7-11.   Multiwork station with client practicing skills to return to work as a lineman. (Photograph by Liberty Mutual.)

Case Study 1

B. S. is a 59-year-old man who worked as a senior air conditioning mechanic. While repairing a carding machine, B. S. caught his right dominant arm in the machine. B. S. reported pulling his arm out fast in order to prevent the whole arm and body from being pulled in but a traumatic below-elbow amputation occurred. After 14 days' hospitalization, B. S. was discharged. B. S. was motivated to return to work and did so, using left non-dominant hand and right stump once it became less sensitive.

Five months after the injury B. S. was admitted to Liberty Mutual Medical Service Center for fulltime therapy. This included occupational therapy two times per day initially, physical therapy two times per day, and general fitness once a day, as well as prosthetic fitting, psychological support, and ongoing medical supervision.

A full history was taken including previous injury, prior medical conditions, medication, allergies, education, psychosocial situation, and work history. A physical evaluation was then performed for bilateral upper extremity range of motion, manual muscle strength, endurance, gross motor coordination, fine motor coordination, grasp, prehension, and sensation. Activities of daily living skills were reviewed and B. S. was given a rocker knife with tines, long handled sponge, and fingernail suction cup brush. Plans were made for B. S. to make his own suction cup nail clipper for one arm use. B. S. was found not to be

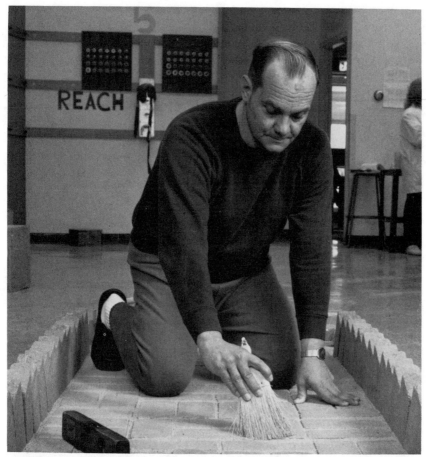

Figure 7-12.   Occupational therapy provides clients with an opportunity to restore their professional skills. (Photograph by Liberty Mutual.)

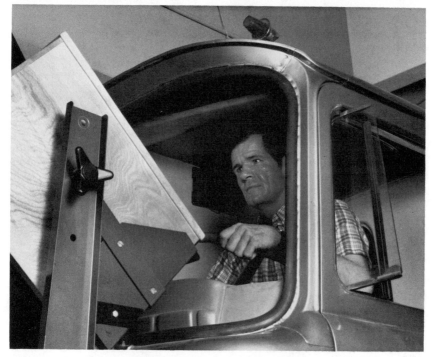

Figure 7-13.   Simulating actual job tasks builds physical tolerance and self-confidence. (Photograph by Liberty Mutual.)

responsible for home management activities and capable of driving his automatic vehicle with no difficulty.

B. S.'s deficit areas were as follows:

Decreased residual right upper extremity strength
Decreased bilateral upper extremity endurance
Slight increased sensitivity in right forearm stump
Decreased sensation over right forearm skin graft
Inadequate knowledge of prosthesis and ability to use it
Lack of knowledge of job capabilities with prosthesis

These deficits lead to the following short-term goals:

Increase right upper extremity strength
Increase bilateral upper extremity endurance
Decrease sensitivity in stump
Review safty awareness techniques
Increase knowledge about and functional use of prosthesis
Determine and increase job capabilities with prosthesis

Long-term goals were also developed, as follows:

To physically and emotionally prepare B. S. for prosthetic fitting
To enable B. S. to tolerate a full day of wearing his prosthesis

Safety techniques were reviewed first to avoid any further injury to stump. Desensitization techniques were then started, using graded tapping, pillow pounding, therapy putty, and buckets of beans, rice and corn. Strength and endurance exercises were carried out with manual resistance from therapist as well as graded theraband exercises to both upper extremities. He continued to have a small sensitive area, but this spot was not aggravated by the prosthesis.

B. S. received his conventional prosthesis after six weeks. He was then discharged from PT and continued with fitness and began prosthetic use. B. S. was scheduled for short sessions in OT multiple times throughout the day. B. S. was able to master donning and doffing as well as opening and closing his voluntary opening dorrance hook starting with two rubber bands around the hook and then three. B. S. was successful with grasp and release of small objects in all planes. Fine motor tasks as well as gross motor tasks were performed and practiced with prosthesis alone and bilateral arms. Functional use of prosthesis was also practiced for feeding, hygiene, dressing, and writing.

Once B. S. mastered the use of his prosthesis job simulation was started. Bilateral coordination became very important for hand tool use as well as holding and carrying small, medium, and large items. B. S. demonstrated very good problem solving and spatial relations, which assisted tremendously with prosthetic use. It became increasingly harder to simulate the actual job, and three days after receiving his prosthesis B. S. was discharged from the Center. He would require more practice for total confidence; however, this would take place in familiar surroundings. B. S.'s employer was understanding and agreed to give him any required assistance. He returned to work on December 18, with gradual increase of duties.

Case Study 2

M. G. is a 36-year-old male who was admitted to the LIMBER program four months after he sustained a low-back injury while moving boxes weighing approximately 50 lbs. He was sitting and twisting when lifting these boxes while at his job as a senior technical writer. M. G. was a tall, well-developed male in no acute distress, demonstrating normal gait without evidence of a limp. A diagnosis of low back strain syndrome with possible left leg radiculitis was made.

The ADL evaluation revealed moderate dysfunction in self-care tasks involving sustained standing positions (shaving, showering) and dressing (putting on pants, socks, shoes). M. G. had difficulty with daily activities that involved carrying (laundry, groceries), reaching and forward bending (bed making and changing, cleaning the bathroom, sweeping, and vacuuming), and he reported a severe increase in low-back pain when driving time was longer than 15 minutes.

M. G. reported the majority of his pain in the low back, with occasional pain in the buttocks and left leg that increased when sitting longer than 30 minutes. When rating his pain on scale of 0 to 10 (0 being no pain and 10 being emergency), patient rated his present pain level at a 4, 2 when his best and 7 when at worst. With repositioning and weight shifting, he could tolerate sitting for 30 minutes, standing for 15 minutes, and walking for 30 minutes.

A functional capacity evaluation indicated that M. G. should have the capacity to push/pull, lift, carry 50 lbs. occasionally (up to 32 times in an eight-hour day) and 10 lbs. constantly (more than 200 times in an eight-hour day).

M. G.'s pre-injury physical demand level was determined from his job description. He was admitted to the LIMBER program as his functional capacity was less than needed for his job. Also, he demonstrated physical deconditioning, minimal knowledge and use of body mechanics, and a great fear of re-injury.

M. G. participated in the intensive, highly structured four-week LIMBER program.

OT addressed increasing ease and independence with ADL and ability to return to his job. This was accomplished through lecture, demonstration, and instruction in the use of body mechanics, and through participation in ten 10-minute task stations that emphasized strength, endurance and flexibility, as well as specific job components. M. G.'s job primarily involved intermittent sitting (4–6 hours/day), as well as bending, reaching, twisting and stair climbing. These components were integrated into the program. At the end of the program, M. G. was re-evaluated. Now he had minimal pain increase with ADL tasks. His driving time had increased by 30 minutes. His pain level at discharge was 1, with a range of 1–5. He was able to lift 82.5 lbs. occasionally, 41 lbs. frequently, and 16 lbs. constantly.

The patient reported feeling much more confident regarding his physical capabilities. His overall strength, endurance, and flexibility had dramatically improved, as had his automatic use of proper body mechanics.

The employer approved the substitution of a more ergonomically designed chair, as recommended by the physician. M. G. returned to his job three days after the completion of LIMBER and will return to the Center for a three-month and one-year follow-up, which involves a complete evaluation by the entire LIMBER team.

ALFREDA REHABILITATION UNIT

The Alfreda Rehabilitation Unit is another example of a short-term, outpatient care facility providing treatment for the client with acute and chronic physical problems such as peripheral nerve lesions, fractures, back disorders, strokes, and sports, hand, and head injuries. The unit is state financed and affiliated with the Queen Elizabeth Hospital located in Royal Park, Australia.

The unit's objective is to enable clients to achieve the optimal level of work performance and life-style in a relatively short period of time. The rehabilitation program aims at providing comprehensive education in health maintenance and preventive health care—diet, recreation, stress management, exercise [1, 2].

Occupational therapists are integral staff members in this multidisciplinary approach to rehabilitation that involves physicians, physical and speech therapists, social workers, and physical education and trade skill instructors. Although the role of occupational therapy is diverse, it entails assessment and treatment of each client as an individual. Dean, Cox, and Auricht [3], occupational therapists at the unit, have described their role as having major emphasis: (1) direct client contact, (2) community health promotion, (3) occupational therapy administration, and (4) education and research.

Direct Client Contact

Client *assessment* at the unit takes two forms: initial assessment to determine the goals of therapy within the rehabilitation program (Figs. 7-14 and 7-15), and ongoing assessment to monitor progress.

The following *specific therapy* is provided:

1. Prescribed activities to improve function in specific areas
2. Back care: individual back care education (given to clients with back injuries and also as a preventive measure to those "at risk"), using visual aids, models, and supervision of workshop activities to reinforce postural awareness and good working habits; graded lifting program to reinforce correct lifting techniques and increase endurance and confidence; group back care sessions, conducted as a health promotion project, using visual aids and models
3. Joint preservation techniques for arthritis clients, using visual aids, demonstrations, and suggestions of aids and adaptations
4. Upper limb assessment and retraining, using standardized tests, remedial equipment, and activities
5. Sensory assessment and retraining
6. Assessment and retraining of higher cortical function (including perception and cognitive functions)
7. Splinting
8. Assessment or review of activities of daily living; when appropriate, instruction on methods of increasing independence and on use of aids

The work-related activities of the occupational therapy program include the following:

In *work assessment* general assessment of the worker's abilities and an assessment of the worker's abilities on specific tasks are carried out.

In *work simulation* activities that simulate the client's work situation are given when possible.

Counseling on suitable alternative employment areas and *training* in job application skills and interviewing skills are provided.

In *work simplification and application of ergonomics* individualized education is given, using visual aids, handouts, and, when necessary,

DISABILITY: ONSET:

OCCUPATION:

HISTORY:

SOCIAL SITUATION:

HOME CONDITIONS:

TRANSPORT:

FUNCTIONAL ABILITY:

Mobility:
   Posture   Squatting
   Lie to sit   Kneeling
   Sitting tolerance   Rolling
   Sit to stand   Walking
   Standing tolerance   Lifting

Trunk:
   Forward flexion   Side flexion
   Extension   Twisting

Results of Lower Back Function Questionnaire:

UPPER LIMB FUNCTION: (use upper limb assessment for more detail)

LOWER LIMB FUNCTION:

                                       Left   *Right*
Hip
Knee
Ankle
Strength
Sensation

ACTIVITIES OF DAILY LIVING:

Personal:
Domestic:

LEISURE ACTIVITIES, HOBBIES:

COMMUNICATION:

PERSONALITY, MENTAL STATE, ATTITUDES:

Figure 7-14.   Form used in initial client assessment at the Alfreda Rehabilitation Unit.

EDUCATION:

WORK HISTORY:

PRESENT WORK SITUATION:

Name of Employer:

Contact Person:

Length of Employment:

Job Description:

GOALS: OT PROGRAMME:

Figure 7-14.   (continued)

demonstration or supervision. Ergonomic principles are applied to make the work situation as safe and efficient as possible.

To foster *communication with the employer* the therapists communicate with the client's employer (1) to minimize misunderstandings that may arise between employer and employee, (2) to promote an understanding of the rehabilitation process, (3) to negotiate suitable return to work conditions (this may be graded on a part-time basis to allow redevelopment of confidence, endurance, and skills), and (4) to discuss matters arising from work site visits. Ideally, the therapist communicates with the client's immediate boss, because a higher-level manager may have limited contact with the client.

Visits to the client's work site are arranged by the occupational therapist; other members of the rehabilitation team may also participate. The purposes of such visits are (1) to assess the client's work (Table 7-2); (2) to advise on possible modifications to work; (3) to advise on suitable alternative duties; (4) to develop an understanding of the rehabilitation concept among the employers, supervisors, and co-workers; (5) when necessary, to supervise the return-to-work process; and (6) when appropriate, to make follow-up contact to review the employee's progress.

The *client is introduced to skills* such as typing or welding to assess his or her potential in specific skills and, when further training is required, to guide the client into relevant community facilities.

General life-style programming, in the Alfreda Unit, emphasizes the development of general fitness through the use of an individualized graded activity program. Stress management—including relaxation training, techniques in time management, and coping and self-awareness exercises—is also taught. The client is encouraged to attain or to maintain a positive attitude toward the future. Therapists provide counseling on options for work and leisure and experience in selected activities to promote the development of skills. Adaptation to residual disability is encouraged. The occupational therapist may also communicate with family and significant others to foster an understanding of the client's situation and to encourage the family to assist in the client's rehabilitation. Supporting the client and family in adapting to role

Lower Back Function Questionnaire

Date: _____

Name: _____   Age: _____

How long have you had back pain? _____ years _____ months _____ weeks

How long have you had leg pain?   _____ years _____ months _____ weeks

PLEASE READ BEFORE COMPLETING THE QUESTIONNAIRE:

This questionnaire has been designed to give information as to how you function in everyday life with your back condition. Please answer every section, and mark in each section only the *ONE* box which applies to you. We realise you may consider that two of the statements in any one section relate to you, but please *just mark the box which most closely describes your* condition.

Section 1—Personal Care (washing, dressing, etc.)
- ☐ I can look after myself normally.
- ☐ I can look after myself but I am slow and careful.
- ☐ I need some help but manage most of my personal care.
- ☐ I need help every day in most of my personal care.

Section 2—Lifting (Think in terms of everyday things such as a 2-kg bag of sugar, etc.)
- ☐ I can lift heavy weights, for example _____
- ☐ I cannot lift heavy weights off the floor, but can manage if they are conveniently positioned, e.g., on a table.
- ☐ I can lift light to medium weights, for example _____
- ☐ I can lift light to medium weights if they are conveniently positioned.
- ☐ I can lift very light weights, for example _____

Section 3—Walking
- ☐ I can walk any distance.
- ☐ I can walk for about 1 hour.
- ☐ I can walk for about 30 minutes.
- ☐ I can walk for about 15 minutes.
- ☐ I can walk for about 5 minutes or less.

Section 4—Sitting
- ☐ I can sit in any chair as long as I like.
- ☐ I can sit in certain chairs as long as I like.
- ☐ I can sit for about 1 hour.
- ☐ I can sit for about 30 minutes.
- ☐ I can sit for about 15 minutes.
- ☐ I can sit for about 5 minutes or less.

Section 5—Standing
- ☐ I can stand for as long as I want.
- ☐ I can stand for about 1 hour.
- ☐ I can stand for about 30 minutes.
- ☐ I can stand for about 15 minutes.
- ☐ I can stand for about 5 minutes or less.

Figure 7-15. Lower back function questionnaire used at the Alfreda Rehabilitation Unit.

Section 6—Sleeping
☐ I sleep the same as before I had my back condition.
☐ My sleep is sometimes disturbed by my back condition.
☐ My sleep is often disturbed by my back condition.
☐ My sleep is always disturbed by my back condition.

Section 7—Sex Life
☐ My sex life is not affected.
☐ My sex life is slightly restricted.
☐ My sex life is moderately restricted.
☐ My sex life is severely restricted.
☐ My sex life is absent.

Section 8—Social Life
☐ My social life is the same as it was before I had my back condition.
☐ My back condition has no significant effect on my social life apart from limiting my more energetic interests, e.g., dancing.
☐ My social life is restricted and I do not go out as often.
☐ My social life is restricted to my home.

Section 9—Travelling (by your usual means of transport, i.e., car, bus, motorbike, bicycle)
☐ I can manage journeys anywhere.
☐ I can manage journeys of about 2 hours.
☐ I can manage journeys of about 1 hour.
☐ I can manage journeys of about 30 minutes.
☐ I can manage journeys of about 15 minutes or less.

Section 10—Pain Management
☐ I can cope with the pain I have without having to use painkillers.
☐ Even when the pain is bad I manage without taking painkillers.
☐ Painkillers give complete relief.
☐ Painkillers give some relief.
☐ Painkillers give very little relief.
☐ Painkillers give no relief.

Section 11—Pain Intensity
Put a cross on the line to indicate your level of pain when

I am at my best. |———————————————|
                        No pain   Pain so
                                                   severe I
                                                   would con-
                                                   sider suicide

I am at my worst. |———————————————|

How I feel at this moment. |———————————————|

Figure 7-15.   (continued)

Table 7-2.   Topics Covered in Work Site Visit

Physical environment
  Lighting
  Noise level
  Dust, fumes
  Housekeeping, e.g., obstacles on floor, adequate storage areas
  Type of building, e.g., under cover, open to weather
  Architectural barriers, e.g., steps, ladders
  Flooring or ground surface
    Slippery
    Uneven
    Duckboards available
  Temperature
    Cold
    Hot
    Air conditioners
    Heaters
  Situation of toilets, lunchrooms
  Access
Safety
  Signs
    Large
    Appropriate
    Different languages
  Fire extinguishers
  Safety officer
  Educational sessions, e.g., on lifting techniques
  Surfaces on floor, benches
  Guards on machinery
  Lifting devices
  Availability of earplugs, safety shoes, spectacles
  Protective clothing
  State of repair of equipment
Psychological and social work environment
  Attitude of employers
  Attitude of workers
  Stress
    Bonus systems
    Other workers relying on client
  Isolated (working alone)
  Able to hold conversations with others
  Music
  Concentration required
  Responsibility
  Initiative
  Situation of lunchrooms; tea and lunch breaks
  Peer group
  Opportunity for change
  "Rehabilitation corner" (generally detrimental to separate handicapped
  worker from usual work environment; better to modify usual work)

Table 7-2. (continued)

Actual job demands
  Range of movement, mobility
  Tolerance, endurance
  Weights lifted, moved
  Repetition
  Work positions
  Variety of work
  Frequency of breaks
  Time limits
Shift work
  Communication
  Relying on others or vice versa
Considerations
  Will employer accept part-time return to work?
  Does client need to be "passed fit" by the industry's medical officer?
  Negotiate part-time return to work initially if possible and if rehab staff feel
  this would be most beneficial to client
  Is job able to be modified?
  Will employer modify job if necessary?
  Are appropriate alternative duties (rather than "lighter" work) available?
  Will modified work affect rates of pay?
  Will other workers accept injured worker on modified duties?
  Attitude of unions?
  Confidentiality: Rehab staff are acting on behalf of the client; it is generally
  prudent to say little or be as positive as possible about the client's program
  Previous work history, attendance record
  Promotions?
  Time off
  Client's attitude regarding return to work

From P. Dean, R. Cox, and R. Auricht [3].

changes and other alterations to life-style is another function of the therapist. The therapist may also explore and teach the planning and organization of leisure time. When appropriate, clients are encouraged to participate in voluntary work or community groups. Therapists also report relevant information about the client to the treatment team and participate in case conferences. Finally, discharge or separation and follow-up review are planned with treatment team.

Community Health Promotion

When unit resources are available, the occupational therapist and the physical therapist present a back care seminar in one community.

Occupational Therapy Administration

Occupational therapists at the Alfreda Unit perform the following administrative duties:

1. Communication with other staff members, such as the trades instructor and the assistant trades instructor
2. Ensuring an adequate range of activities to achieve objectives (e.g., communicating with instructors regarding design and adaptations to equipment and choice and supply of materials)
3. Communication with regional administrative staff regarding

workshop staff coverage, the purchase of equipment and materials, and participation in staff meetings and supervisors' meetings

4. Public relations, that is, disseminating information about the unit to visiting individuals and groups
5. Arranging for specialist community speakers to address unit clients
6. Providing statistics on occupational therapy services to regional administration and committees

Education and Research

The occupational therapy department provides in-service training and ongoing education and occupational therapy student affiliates to the unit. When funding is available, the therapists also conduct research into the importance of occupational therapy at the unit [3].

INSTITUTE OF REHABILITATION MEDICINE*

The Institute of Rehabilitation Medicine (IRM), New York University Medical Center, is a 150-bed comprehensive rehabilitation center for severely disabled adults and children. Its occupational therapy department comprises many specialized units, one of which is the prevocational evaluation area. The therapist's case load in this area includes both inpatients and outpatients; the most common disabilities are spinal cord injuries, cerebral vascular accidents (CVAs), and traumatic brain injuries.

Staff vocational counselors refer clients to the prevocational area for evaluation. Concurrently, occupational therapists provide functional information on the client. Specific criteria for client referral have been developed for the major disabilities (Table 7-3).

The client's program varies according to individual needs and interests. Work samples and tests are included in the following areas:

1. Clerical evaluations including bookkeeping, accounting, and business school work samples and TOWER tests; computer operator evaluation
2. Computer programming evaluation: aptitude testing (IBM test) and BASIC language instruction
3. Electronics evaluation (Heathkit assembly)
4. Drafting evaluation (TOWER series and mechanical drawing texts); computer graphics introduction
5. Mechanics evaluation: engine model assembly, carburetor assembly
6. Sheltered workshop and factory assembly: variety of standardized manual dexterity tests such as Purdue Pegboard, Pennsylvania Bimanual Work Sample, Minnesota Rate of Manipulation Test, TOWER workshop assembly tasks

*This section was developed from information provided by Dorothy Milner, OTR.

Table 7-3.   Criteria for Patient Referral for Prevocational Evaluation

Patient Group	Goals	Criteria
Quadriplegics High-level	To return to school or work	Cervical traction has been removed and sitting posture is upright Assistive devices such as balanced forearm orthoses have been used in OT Use of a mouthstick for typing, painting, and turning pages has been started in OT Patient has expressed the wish to develop skills related to school or work
Low-level	To return to school or work	Sitting posture is upright Patient has expressed the wish to develop skills related to school or work
Hemiplegics	To return to work or the evaluation of existing skills for a new vocation	Cognitive and perceptual deficits are minimal; learning potential and carry-over are fair Deficits in attention span and concentration are minimal; potential for improvement is evident from response to activities in OT clinics Dominance retraining has been initiated in OT; handwriting is fairly legible Functional Communication Profile scores with input from speech therapists regarding reading, writing, and arithmetic ability Evidence of patient's denial, which may interfere with testing, may be present Prevocational screening test is completed; submit test results with referral
Patients with traumatic brain injury	To return to competitive or noncompetitive employment	Visual and spatial orientation is present Attention and concentration abilities are fair Manual dexterity with one or both hands is fair When higher-level skills are present, include criteria for hemiplegics

The Functional Communication Profile (FCP) was devised in 1969 by Martha Taylor Sarno, M.S., Director of Speech Therapy at the New York Institute of Rehabilitation Medicine. The Profile is a speech therapy test based on studies of premorbid functioning. The therapist obtains a percentile score of functional language (100% being the highest score). Depending on the results of the evaluation, a prevocational therapeutic referral may be appropriate.

A microcomputer has been used in the prevocational area since 1980. It has been useful as an evaluation and training tool for most clients. Specifically, a client's potential to enter the programming field can be assessed by instructing the client in BASIC and subsequently having him or her write and run original programs. Academic software is used to evaluate the potential for high school and college training. Many CVA hemiplegics have computer experience from their former jobs. Thus microcomputers using standard business software are viable assessment tools for them. Occupational therapists at IRM are researching computer interfaces for high-level quadriplegics and other individuals with severe disabilities who may not be able to use the conventional keyboard. (Fig. 7-16).

Quadriplegic clients are referred to the prevocational area to develop communication skills and independence in performing desk-top work such as typing; writing; and using equipment including a tape recorder, telephone, calculator, and computer. In addition, the therapist constructs out of any low-temperature plastic material finger loop writing devices and typing fingers for C5 or C6 and lower-level quadriplegics to facilitate increased independence in page turning and using a telephone, typewriter, and other push-button equipment (Fig. 7-17).

Paraplegics with normal hand function are referred to prevocational evaluation for a general skills assessment in their interest areas, such as electronics, drafting, and mechanics.

The occupational therapist and the home-planning consultant collaborate to plan home and office modifications for the spinal-cord-injured patient and others who may need a special setup.

CVA clients and brain-damaged clients are given the prevocational screening test before referral for a full OT evaluation. (Fig. 7-18). This test was developed to determine a baseline work competency level. These clients are then evaluated to determine their ability to return to their former jobs or to less demanding vocations.

Clients from the pediatric service are referred to the prevocational area by the vocational counselor to assist with high school curriculum planning. Disabilities in patients from this service include spinal cord injuries, spina bifida, cerebral palsy, and other congenital and acquired disabilities. The assessment tools are geared to the teenaged population and include academic testing.

---

*Case Study 1**
Mr. C., a 30-year-old C5 quadriplegic, attended the prevocational area one hour a day from June 20 to October 8, 1984. Injured in a truck accident last winter, Mr. C. is realistic about his vocational future. He can no longer be a truck driver and hopes, instead, to open a small sporting goods business, which would be popular in his hometown in upstate New York.

Initially, Mr. C. was dependent on bilateral balanced forearm orthoses for activity. As endurance and strength improved, he could type and write without them, using dorsal wrist extension splints and vertical holders.

Equipment needs and basic store planning became the responsibility of the

*This case study was prepared by Dorothy Milner, OTR, Institute of Rehabilitation Medicine, New York, New York.

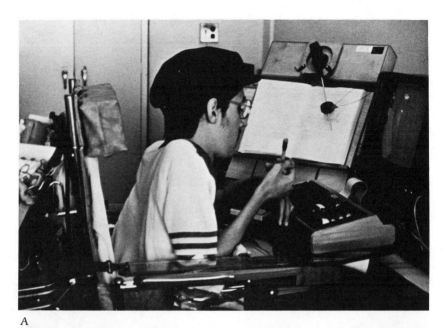

A

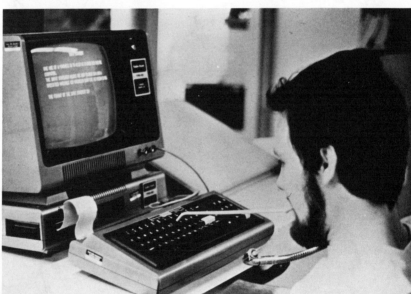

B

Figure 7-16.   A. Muscular dystrophy quadriplegic using chin mouth-stick in his fingers with the computer and an electronic page turner. B. C3 quadriplegic using microcomputer with mouthstick.

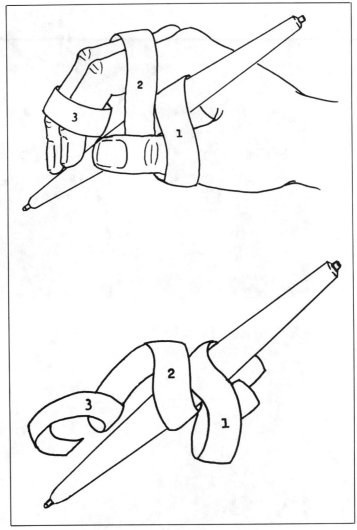

A

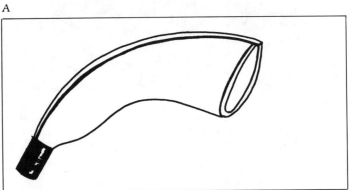

B

Figure 7-17.   Devices developed for quadriplegics by Dorothy Milner, OTR. A: Finger loop writing device, made out of any low-temperature plastic material. B. Typing finger, made from any low-temperature plastic material.

1. 74   35 $10.00
   +83   +78   −   8.57   8 × 17 =   5 × 11 =   24 ÷ 12 =   150 ÷ 15 =

2. A store purchased 450 balloons for $67.50 and sold them for 20¢ each. What was their profit?

3. Number the names in alphabetical order: Matthew Gold
                                              Susan Goodman
                                              Jennifer Jacobs
                                              Mary Jones
                                              Louise Dunn

4. If you bought a hamburger for 89¢, how much change would you receive from $1.00?

5. Write the telephone extension listed for Dr. Rusk using the Medical Center Directory.

Some of the items below are circled, some are underlined, some have boxes around them, and others have checkmarks or initials behind them. You are to find each item that is underlined or has initials after it. Put an X through these items with your pen.

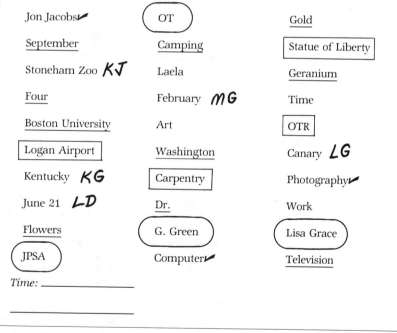

Time: _____

_____

Figure 7-18.   Prevocational screening test used at the Institute of Rehabilitation Medicine. (Used with permission.) (continued)

If the two dollar amounts are the same, circle the S (for same). If they are different, circle the D (for different).

1. $43.99	$43.99	S	D
2. $27.02	$27.02	S	D
3. $83.62	$93.62	S	D
4. $4875.73	$4885.73	S	D
5. $43.70	$43.70	S	D
6. $5297.09	$5927.09	S	D
7. $379.58	$36.68	S	D
8. $23.29	$23.39	S	D
9. $906.06	$906.06	S	D
10. $90.20	$70.02	S	D
11. $6395.58	$6396.58	S	D
12. $73.82	$37.82	S	D
13. $57.03	$57.03	S	D
14. $573.29	$572.29	S	D
15. $9206.72	$9206.72	S	D
16. $345892.01	$345892.01	S	D
17. $6540095.00	$6540095.00	S	D
18. $6910103.	$6910103.	S	D
19. $6430325.99	$6403325.99	S	D
20. $97934.78	$97934.78	S	D

Time: _____

Figure 7-18.   (continued)

prevocational and home-planning services. Table heights, accessible display cases, and convenient placement of all necessary equipment were taken into consideration. The evaluation of a suitable cash register (cash box) and printing calculator as well as other necessary equipment needs was accomplished. Prices were submitted to the insurance company.

Mr. C. was conscientious and well motivated throughout the evaluation, often finding solutions to problems on his own, given the basic equipment.

Case Study 2*
Mr. J. a 49-year-old right hemiplegic with severe receptive-expressive aphasia, initially attended the prevocational area on May 8, 1984. Having suffered a CVA three years ago, he came to the institute primarily for vocational services. Attendance is regular, three days a week for one-hour sessions. As a former plumber's assistant, he has followed a program in the following areas: (1) recognition of word similarities, matching; (2) simple arithmetic skills such as making change; and (3) evaluation of one-handed skills, including assembly tasks, carpentry, electronic wiring, and use of hand tools.

Mr. J.'s right upper extremity is nonfunctional. He walks with a cane and is

*This case study was provided by Dorothy Milner, OTR, Institute of Rehabilitation Medicine, New York, New York.

Please complete the application form at the bottom of the page using the information in the following letter:

25 Johnson Drive
Northborough, MA 01867
January 1, 1985

McDonald's
111 Needham Street
Newton, MA

Dear Sir:

I am interested in applying for a position as a cashier at your store. I am 18 years old, single, and a high school graduate. I worked as a cashier at a summer camp for two months during the summer of 1984, and enjoyed the work very much.

I would appreciate your sending me an application form.

Sincerely,

Erica Osborn

Erica Osborn

APPLICATION
Name of applicant _____

Address _____
         (street number)   (street)   (city)   (state)

Telephone _____

Age _____ Height _____ Weight _____

Marital status _____

Date of application _____

Previous experience _____

_____

Time: _____

Figure 7-18.   (continued)

Answer the following questions using the sample check and stub below:

1. What day was the check written? _____

2. What is the amount of the check? _____

3. To whom is the money being paid? _____

4. Whose account will the money come from? _____

5. Where is the bank located? _____

6. What is the number of the account? _____

7. What is the number of this check? _____

8. What is the balance in this account after the check is paid? _____

Figure 7-18. (continued)

independent in self-care activities. He can follow only demonstrated instructions and imitates models for copying.

Mr. J.'s aphasia has affected his calculation ability. He can add two digits; however, his speed is nonfunctional, and his answers are not consistently correct. Subtraction, multiplication, and division are impossible for him. He cannot make monetary change.

Mr. J. can match names, a functional skill for a job in mail sorting. His speed is slow but should improve with continued practice.

One-handed hand skills are good. He has excellent dexterity with his non-dominant left hand. Specific hand skill testing results are as follows:

1. Hand tool dexterity test (use of pliers, wrench, screwdriver): slow speed but demonstrates good use of tools
2. Doorlock (TOWER): average speed with one hand; no errors
3. Plug jack assembly (TOWER): use of putty as a stabilizer; average speed with one hand; no errors
4. Washers and pins (TOWER): some difficulty noted closing pin with ten washers on it
5. Nuts and bolts: Theraplast as stabilizer; fair speed with one hand
6. Electronic wiring: good dexterity noted; has difficulty reading schematics for color of wire needed; learning ability good after repetition
7. Small carpentry assembly: unable to use hammer and nails without maximum assistance

Mr. J.'s drafting skills are limited to copying simple forms and shapes. He measures accurately and draws neatly; however, his aphasia affecting reading and arithmetic preclude further training in this area.

Compare the two checks to each other. They should be identical. Circle any differences you find on the bottom check:

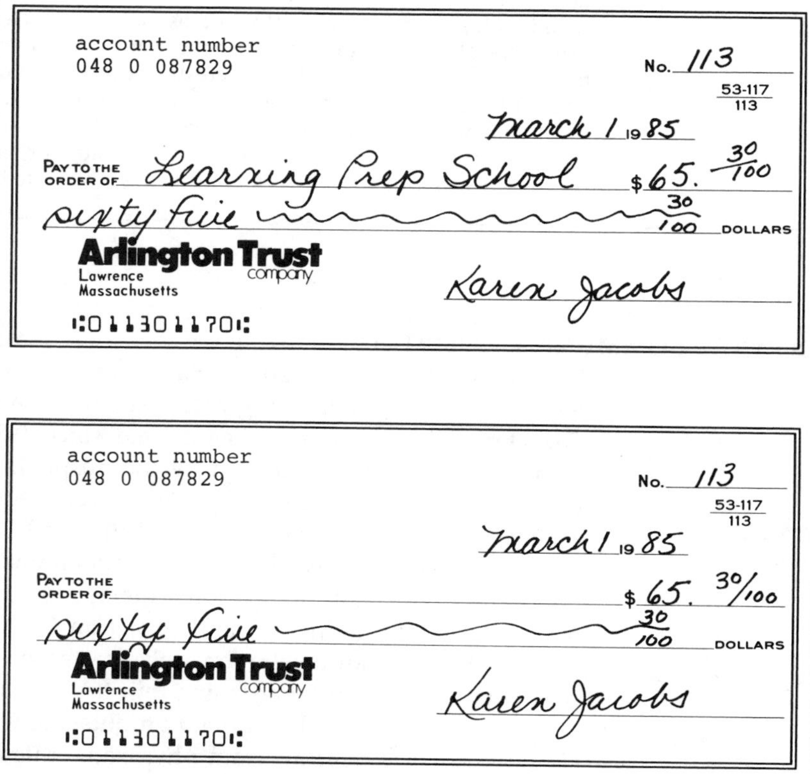
account number
048 0 087829
No. 113
53-117
113
March 1 19 85
PAY TO THE ORDER OF Learning Prep School $ 65. 30/100
sixty five 30/100 DOLLARS
Arlington Trust company
Lawrence Massachusetts
Karen Jacobs
⑆0113011170⑆

account number
048 0 087829
No. 113
53-117
113
March 1 19 85
PAY TO THE ORDER OF $ 65. 30/100
sixty five 30/100 DOLLARS
Arlington Trust company
Lawrence Massachusetts
Karen Jacobs
⑆0113011170⑆

Figure 7-18. (continued)

In summary, Mr. J. displays good hand skills and a potential for learning new and unfamiliar tasks. Speed improves with repetition and increased familiarity with the required job. He cannot read or write, but he can follow demonstrated one-step-at-a-time instructions.

*Case Study 3**

Mr. D., a 50-year-old right-dominant right hemiplegic, was evaluated in the prevocational area from January 23 to April 2, 1984. After his CVA in December 1983, he contracted meningitis, which left him deaf bilaterally. Before his illness Mr. D. had worked as an electronics maintenance engineer with a major broadcasting company. He is considered an expert in the field of cathode-ray oscilloscopes, and his employers offered their assistance with the evaluation, eager to have him return after his rehabilitation program.

Mr. D.'s primary concern initially was dominance retraining, that is, left-handed writing. He learned the basic techniques easily and practices on his own. He exhibited exceptional coordination with his left hand during various assembly tasks and learned one-handed stabilization techniques without difficulty.

*This case study was provided by Dorothy Milner, OTR, Institute of Rehabilitation Medicine, New York, New York.

Mr. D. was evaluated in basic electronics, building a small Heathkit radio. He proved that he can solder safely with one hand and managed the small parts and wiring involved with amazing facility. He had no problems in reading both written and schematic instructions. Final tuning of the radio was impossible for him because of his hearing loss.

At this stage of the evaluation, his employers were asked to assist us. They delivered malfunctioning oscilloscopes for Mr. D. to repair. Mr. D. proceeded with this task eagerly and performed as well as expected.

Because of Mr. D.'s loss of hearing, certain communication problems relating to his job were anticipated, as were the functional limitations caused by his CVA. Mr. D. will never be able to walk; he must use a wheelchair. He is independent performing his job tasks, except for reaching and lifting heavy objects. His employers agreed to a three-month probationary period of employment, with final decision as to his being rehired to be made after that time.

DOWNEY COMMUNITY HOSPITAL*

Downey Community Hospital is a 171-bed non-profit hospital located near major industry in the greater metropolitan area of Los Angeles. The Downey Hand Center has existed since 1974 and is part of the rehabilitation services provided by the hospital. In 1979 it was found that a gap existed between the optimal level of function a patient could achieve in the hand clinic setting and the level of function required to return successfully to work. Using a model found successful at Rancho Los Amigos Hospital, occupational therapists Kay Golgi and Lois Barber, Dr. Leonard Matheson, and physician Dr. Garry Brody, together with the hospital administration, collaborated on the planning and implementation of a work hardening unit to fill this void in rehabilitation services. The program has gained an outstanding reputation and consistently receives referrals from physicians, therapists, insurance companies, and vocational counselors. While upper-extremity rehabilitation is a specialty, the work hardening center has expanded to serve a wide variety of diagnostic groups including back-injured and head trauma clients.

The Downey Community Hospital Work Hardening Center provides a program of maximal reconditioning before return to work or to optimal occupational role. Rather than exercise, graded work samples such as shoveling gravel or assembling nut and bolt units are used in three-to-six hour treatment sessions (Fig. 7-19). The therapists can simulate a specific task or job and evaluate a client's specific activity tolerance (Fig. 7-20). The information regarding a client's work tolerance can then be shared with the physician, the client, the vocational counselor, and the employer.

The principal goal of work hardening is to return a person who has experienced a decrease in function to his or her previous occupation or to an optimal occupation if the residual level of dysfunction precludes return to usual and customary work. In support of this global goal are several subgoals:

*Most of this section was written by Karen S. Schultz, M. S., OTR.

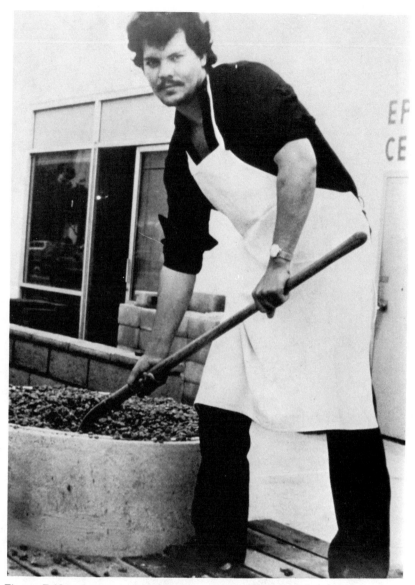

Figure 7-19.   An example of work hardening. Client who will be using shovel in usual and customary work as a mold maker builds tolerance for this task by shoveling gravel. (Photograph courtesy of Karen S. Schultz, M.S., OTR.)

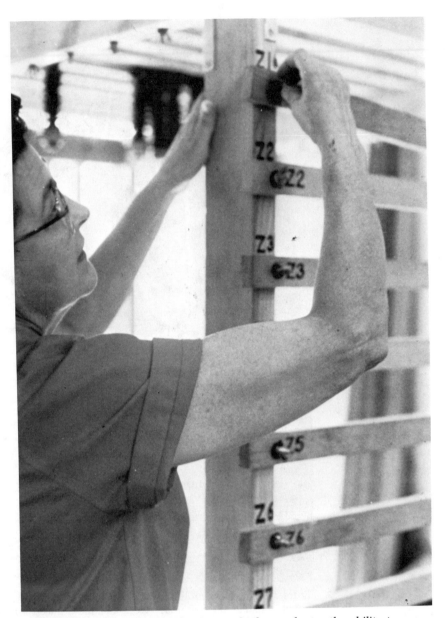

Figure 7-20.   Client performs work sample that evaluates the ability to manipulate objects at various planes of the body. (Photograph courtesy of Karen S. Schultz, M.S., OTR.)

1. To provide optimal physical reconditioning for work (maximize range of motion, strength, stability, endurance)
2. To increase the client's confidence in his or her ability to return to work or to productive activity
3. To identify problems that may require adaptation of a goal occupation or may alter the choice of goal occupation
4. To maintain or reintroduce the worker role to the client
5. To provide optimal psychosocial and cognitive reconditioning before return to productive activity

Clients who require a program with the above-stated goals are appropriate candidates for work hardening. On admission to the program each client receives a thorough intake evaluation, including a physical status evaluation (range of motion, strength, sensibility), a functional tolerance evaluation, and a review of future job or activity demands at either the usual and customary work or at a new vocation (Fig. 7-21). The program is geared to bring a client from his or her current level of function to a level that will permit gainful employment or purposeful activity. When a client reaches this level of function, discharge is recommended and a report is provided to the client and to his or her physician. A client may be discharged if he or she is unable to use the facility appropriately. A client is also recommended for discharge when a plateau is reached and no further gains are made in a one- to two-week period.

Bridging the gap between medical rehabilitation and vocational rehabilitation, the occupational therapist makes a unique contribution. He or she can evaluate the client for specific parameters of physical functioning and can perform an activity analysis of the client's goal task or job. With this information, the therapist can design a graded work hardening program of work simulation to increase the client's ability to perform critical tasks. The ability to identify specific skills and then translate these skills into functionally relevant—and therefore vocationally relevant—information is key to returning an injured person to his or her optimal occupational role.

Case Study*

George, a 23-year-old right-dominant man, was employed as a telephone cable splicer at the time of his injury. On May 25, 1983, he fell 28 feet from a ladder and sustained a fracture-dislocation of his right elbow and multiple fractures of his right wrist as well as other orthopedic injuries to his lower extremities. He underwent open reduction and internal fixation (ORIF) of his right elbow and right wrist.

George began a hand therapy program 4½ months after his injury, after prolonged immobilization in various casts. At six months after injury he was evaluated for the work hardening program. At this time his grip strength had plateaued at 40 pounds, and his maximum active and passive wrist extension was 20 degrees. George was unable to grip forcefully with his fingers and simultaneously maintain wrist extension; his wrist collapsed into flexion. A program of work samples including woodworking, block wall assembly, pipe

*This case study was provided by Karen S. Schultz, M. S. OTR, Downey Community Hospital, Downey, California.

WORK HARDENING
WORK CAPACITY EVALUATION
UPPER EXTREMITY

| DOMINANCE   L   R | | EVALUATOR |
| INVOLVED   L   R | | DATE |

RANGE OF MOTION

| Joint exam attached |
| Significant limitations present |
| L R Limitations: Scapula |
| L R Limitations: Shoulder/Arm |
| L R Limitations: Elbow/Forearm |
| L R Limitations: Wrist |
| L R Limitations: Fingers |
| L R Limitations: Thumb |

FINGER PADS FROM PALMAR CREASE: if touch use +

| L | I___cm M___cm R___cm L___cm |
| R | I___cm M___cm R___cm L___cm |

FINGER TOUCH PALM: if touch, use+, if not use

| L | I___cm M___cm R___cm L___cm |
| R | I___cm M___cm R___cm L___cm |

DISTANCE THUMB TIP FROM FINGER PADS:

| L | I___cm M___cm R___cm L___cm |
| R | I___cm M___cm R___cm L___cm |

DISTANCE THUMB TIP FROM HEAD OF 5th MC

L___cm   R___cm

STRENGTH/ENDURANCE

| Muscle exam attached |
| L R Limitations: Muscle Strength |
| L R Limitations: Endurance |
| L R Cocontraction |

GRIP (JAMAR), (lb)	LEFT	RIGHT
I = Narrowest Comments:	I	
	II	
	III	
	IV	
	V	
PALMAR PINCH (lb)		
LATERAL PINCH (lb)		
C/A Circumference		
Hand Volume		

SENSIBILITY

L   R

AMPUTATED ■   IMPAIRED ▒   ABSENT ▨

| Detailed exam attached |
| L R Limitations: Functional Sensibility |
| L R Limitations: Protective Sensibility |
| L R Paresthesias (Describe): |
| L R Limitations: Stereognosis |
| L R Limitations: Proprioception |

OBJECTIVE SENSIBILITY

| L R Limitations: Color |
| L R Limitations: Turgor |
| L R Limitations: Rugal Folds |
| L R Limitations: Skin Temperature |
| L R Limitations: Sweat |

SUBJECTIVE SENSIBILITY

| L R Limitations: Sharp/Dull |
| L R Limitations: Light Touch |
| L R Limitations: Texture |
| L R Limitations: Temperature |

PATIENT

Figure 7-21.   Forms used in upper-extremity work capacity evaluation at Downey Community Hospital. (MP = metacarpophalangeal; PIP = finger proximal interphalangeal; DIP = finger interphalangeal; IP = interphalangeal.)

UPPER EXTREMITY EVALUATION   INITIAL_____ FINAL_____

TESTER_____

CLIENTS NAME _____   DATE _____

INVOLVED R   L   ACTIVE RANGE OF MOTION   DOMINANT R   L

SHOULDER	INVOLVED	NORMAL
FLEXION		0-180
ABDUCTION		0-180
INT.ROT.		0-80
EXTERN.ROT.		0-60

ELBOW	INVOLVED	NORMAL
FLEXION		0-150
EXTENSION		150-0
PRONATION		0-80
SUPINATION		0-80

WRIST	INVOLVED	NORMAL
FLEXION		0-70
EXTENSION		0-60
ULNAR DEV.		0-30
RADIAL DEV.		0-20

LEFT SIDE

RIGHT SIDE

SHOULDER	INVOLVED	NORMAL
FLEXION		0-180
ABDUCTION		0-180
INT.ROT.		0-80
EXTERN.ROT.		0-60

ELBOW	INVOLVED	NORMAL
FLEXION		0-150
EXTENSION		150-0
PRONATION		0-80
SUPINATION		0-80

WRIST	INVOLVED	NORMAL
FLEXION		0-70
EXTENSION		0-60
ULNAR DEV.		0-30
RADIAL DEV.		0-20

FINGER	MP	PIP	DIP
NORMAL	0-90	0-100	0-70
INDEX			
MIDDLE			
RING			
LITTLE			

THUMB			
MP			
IP			
CM ABD.			
CM ADD.			

FINGER	MP	PIP	DIP
NORMAL	0-90	0-100	0-70
INDEX			
MIDDLE			
RING			
LITTLE			

THUMB			
MP			
IP			
CM ABD.			
CM ADD.			

MANUAL MUSCLE TEST

MANUAL MUSCLE TEST

Figure 7-21.   (continued)

tree assembly, and a simulated cable-splicing activity was initiated in conjunction with progressive wrist splinting and aggressive resistive exercise of the entire upper extremity, with emphasis on the wrist extensors. It was noted that the wrist extensors were caught in scar at the ORIF site at the wrist and thus could not achieve their optimal excursion. A program of vibration and vigorous massage of the scar was added.

George was discharged to return to work as a cable splicer on January 25, 1984, after two months of work hardening. His grip strength was 58 pounds; his active wrist extension, 45 degrees. He was able to demonstrate good hand balance when forcefully gripping and could maintain wrist extension with strong finger flexion. The client was confident of his ability to return to his usual and customary work. In his program he had lifted and carried objects similar in size and weight to those used in his previous job. He had also used tools that required the same types of grip and pinch required in his usual and customary work.

HAND THERAPY AND REHABILITATION ASSOCIATES*

Hand Therapy and Rehabilitation Associates was founded in 1976 in Los Gatos, California, by Thelma Wellerson Hook. It comprises two divisions: the hand service (the original practice) and a vocational division, the work evaluation unit.

The hand service is a private, medically oriented hand therapy and rehabilitation practice that serves private, industrial, and hospital-based physicians in northern California. Its offices are located in an urban area in Santa Clara County, a location central to hand surgeons, orthopedic surgeons, plastic surgeons, rheumatologists, and other practicing physicians in northern California.

The sole purpose of this medically prescribed treatment program is to treat industrial and private patients with traumatic hand injuries and hand dysfunctions. The program is designed to assess the special needs of each patient. An individualized therapeutic program is prescribed by the referring physician. Each member of the staff is committed to returning the patient to his occupation and accustomed lifestyle as soon as medically feasible.

The hand service program includes continuous intensive hand evaluations and tests. Some examples of the specialized therapeutic programs are (1) reduction of edema, (2) scar care, (3) therapeutic exercises, (4) custom fabrication of dynamic or static splints, (5) prosthetic evaluation and training programs for upper-extremity amputees, (6) joint protection techniques, (7) activities of daily living, and (8) physical evaluation abilities or on-the-job assessment. All of these programs assist the physician in restoring the injured hand to functional capacity and in determining the patient's readiness to return to work.

Work Evaluation Unit

As an adjunct to the highly successful hand therapy division, a separate vocational division was established in November 1982. This work evaluation unit is a private practice, non-medically-oriented office. It serves industrial, government, and private rehabilitation counselors, consul-

*This section was written by Thelma Wellerson Hook, M.A., OTR.

tants, claims adjustors, nurses, self-insured company administrators, casualty adjustors, applicants' attorneys, benefits managers, and corporate industry in northern California.

The work evaluation unit is located near the hand therapy division in an urban area adjacent to the high-technology industry of the Santa Clara Valley.

The primary purpose of the work evaluation unit is to assess traumatic hand injuries and hand dysfunctions of industrial and private clients, whose injuries may or may not be classified as permanent and stationary. The program is designed to provide information to the referring agent, and to the client, on the client's physical ability to meet specific job requirements and occupational goals. A comprehensive written report with specific recommendations is given to the referring agent. The work evaluation unit increases the client's motivation to work and assists in his or her rapid return to employment, which results in reduced corporate costs.

Staffed by therapists with training in occupational therapy, guidance, and personnel work as well as in hand therapy and vocational rehabilitation, the work evaluation unit offers the following programs and services: work tolerance screening, work capacity evaluation, work hardening, job analysis, on-the-job assessment, job site modification, and corporate consultation.

Work tolerance screening takes from two to four hours, and the ratio of supervision is one to one. The screening assesses the client's hand and extremity physical abilities by measuring range of motion, muscle strength, grip strength, pinch strength, edema, tolerance to hot and cold, and sensation limitations. In addition there is a limited appraisal of the client's physical ability to use the injured hand and upper extremity on a minimum number of nonspecific job samples and tests. These require fine and gross manipulation of tools and equipment and hand and arm range of motion under load.

Work capacity evaluation is an individualized program lasting one to seven six-hour days. The ratio of supervision to clients is one to four. The evaluation assesses the client's hand and upper extremity physical abilities, with the additional goal of an in-depth appraisal of the client's ability to use the injured hand and upper extremity at work. Numerous systems are used to make this assessment. These include standardized evaluations such as (1) the Wide Range Achievement Test, (2) the Raven Progress Matrices, (3) the Gates-McKillop-Horowitz Reading Diagnostic Test, (4) Work Evaluation Systems Technology (WEST), (5) the Purdue Pegboard, and (6) the Minnesota Rate of Manipulation Test; standardized work samples such as the TOWER system or work samples especially developed to simulate jobs indigenous to the Santa Clara Valley industrial area; and situational assessment, exemplified by observation of the client's performance on the job for a limited time. The goal is to observe the client using the injured hand and arm in a realistic work situation. The job situation is chosen on the basis of a client's real, or perceived, occupational goal.

Work hardening is an individualized physical conditioning and training program in half-day sessions lasting for a period of two weeks. The ratio of supervision to clients is one to six. The purpose of work hardening is to build up the physical ability to meet the demands of the work day. The work tasks, amount of work time, and resistance are graded throughout the duration of the program.

Job analysis is a systematic description of the work performed by the client before or after injury. The goal of this assessment is to aid the referring agent in understanding the job skills that are required of the client. This analysis is provided on an hourly basis.

On-the-job assessment evaluates a client's work endurance, stamina, tolerance to pain, and physical performance on a given job. The objective of this service is to observe the client at work, analyze the actions required of the client's injured hand or arm, and analyze the client's physical ability to perform those actions within the context of industrial performance and standards. The assessment, provided on an hourly basis, includes recommendations for placement in a specific job and consideration of physical limitations in job placement.

Job site modificatioin analyzes the job, the client, and the place of work. The objective of this service, which is also provided on an hourly basis, is to determine what changes in the job, client, and work place will enable the worker to perform the job satisfactorily. The analysis includes recommendations for either client or job site modification. Such recommendations may include use of ergonomic principles, fabrication of adaptive equipment designed especially for the client, instruction for the client in compensatory body mechanics, and modification of job skills and equipment that will enable the client to meet industrial standards.

Corporate consultation is a service available to industry to aid in the prevention of on-the-job injuries to employees' hands and upper extremities. Through evaluation of jobs and recommendations for changes, corporate costs can be reduced.

Case Study 1*
Diagnosis 1. Primary diagnosis is not available from medical histories
2. Frozen shoulder, right
3. Flexion contracture, right elbow
4. Causalgia, right upper extremity
Surgery 1. Manipulation of right shoulder and elbow
2. Stellate blocks (medical history available reports three)

Occupation: Machine operator, pill packaging

Objectives of Referral
The client was referred for a half-day work tolerance screening with the following objectives:

1. To determine physical ability of right arm and hand
2. To determine physical ability of right arm and hand in performance of former job
3. To determine physical ability of right arm and hand in clerical work

*This case study was provided by Thelma Wellerson Hook, M.A., OTR, Hand Therapy and Rehabilitation Associates, Los Gatos, California.

Evaluation

Pain
The client reported pain in right middle, ring, and little fingers and numbness in all three digits. She stated that the numbness was constant. She also complained of pain and burning from the right neck area through the right shoulder blade and down the right arm. This occurred when the neck is flexed approximately 10 degrees after working for approximately 50 minutes.

Sensation
Two-point discrimination testing showed normal sensibility in all digits (Fig. 7-22). An EMG report was not available to evaluator.

Edema
The water displacement test for measurement of swelling in the right hand had the following results: right, 345 ml of water displacement; left, 310 ml.

Range of Motion
Dominant right hand; injury on right. There was loss of range of motion in the right shoulder (Fig. 7-23) as compared to the left:

Abduction (away from the body to the right)	–10 degrees
Flexion (away from the body forward)	–40 degrees
Extension (away from the body behind)	–10 degrees
Internal rotation (hand to middle back)	–11 degrees
External rotation (hand behind neck)	–55 degrees

There was loss of range of motion in the right elbow extension as compared to the left:

Extension (straighten elbow all the way)	–30 degrees
Flexion (hand to shoulder)	Normal

There was loss of range of motion in the right wrist as compared to the left:

Dorsiflexion (raise cocked fist)	–10 degrees
Plantar flexion (drop hand down)	Normal
Radial deviation (move hand to the left)	–05 degrees
Ulnar deviation (move hand to the right)	–10 degrees

All digit range of motion is within normal limits.

Grip Strength
The norm group for the client is women aged 45 to 49 years. The client was well below the tenth percentile for grip strength on the right for women of her age group, and at the tenth percentile on the left for women of her age group (Fig. 7-24).

Pinch Strength
Palmar pinch (fingertip to thumb tip) was at the tenth percentile on the right and at the ninetieth percentile on the left. Three-point pinch (as in holding a pencil) was at the fiftieth percentile on the right and above the ninetieth percentile on the left. Lateral pinch (as in turning a key) was at the seventy-fifth percentile on the right and above the ninetieth percentile on the left.

Filing Test
A TOWER filing test was given to test the ability to alphabetize names with 4″ × 6″ index cards and a file box. The task was explained orally with an interpreter and a demonstration was given.

Results
1. No difficulty in alphabetizing; average speed and accuracy.
2. Complaints of numbness in right middle, ring, and little finger after 1

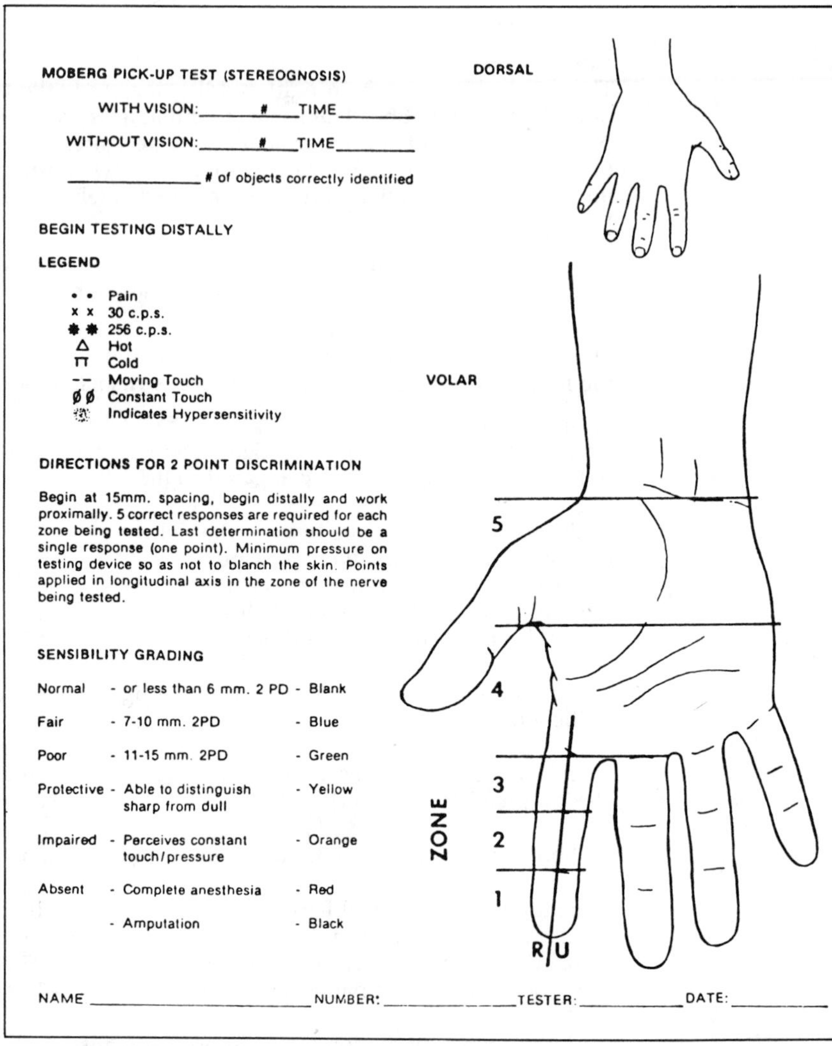

MOBERG PICK-UP TEST (STEREOGNOSIS)

DORSAL

WITH VISION:_____ # ____TIME_____

WITHOUT VISION:_____ # ____TIME_____

_____ # of objects correctly identified

BEGIN TESTING DISTALLY

LEGEND

- • • Pain
- x x 30 c.p.s.
- ✱ ✱ 256 c.p.s.
- △ Hot
- ᴛᴛ Cold
- − − Moving Touch
- ∅ ∅ Constant Touch
- ⊠ Indicates Hypersensitivity

VOLAR

DIRECTIONS FOR 2 POINT DISCRIMINATION

Begin at 15mm. spacing, begin distally and work
proximally. 5 correct responses are required for each
zone being tested. Last determination should be a
single response (one point). Minimum pressure on
testing device so as not to blanch the skin. Points
applied in longitudinal axis in the zone of the nerve
being tested.

SENSIBILITY GRADING

Normal	- or less than 6 mm. 2 PD	- Blank
Fair	- 7-10 mm. 2PD	- Blue
Poor	- 11-15 mm. 2PD	- Green
Protective	- Able to distinguish sharp from dull	- Yellow
Impaired	- Perceives constant touch/pressure	- Orange
Absent	- Complete anesthesia	- Red
	- Amputation	- Black

ZONE

5

4

3

2

1

R | U

NAME _____ NUMBER: _____ TESTER:_____ DATE:_____

Figure 7-22.   Peripheral nerve sensibility evaluation (cps = cycles per second; 2PD = two-point discrimination.)

NAME _____ No._____ (Right Major)

Circ. (inches) Biceps_____ / _____ Wrist _____ / _____
 Forearm _____ / _____ Hand _____ / _____

MOTIONS: Report as a fraction (injured/uninjured) in degrees of Active Motion

Shoulder: Abd.____70/90____ / _____   Forearm Pron. _____ / _____
 Flex._0-140/0-180__ / _____   Sup. _____ / _____
 I R.____34/45____ / _____
 E R.____35/90____ / _____   Wrist   D F ___65___ / ___75___
 Ext.____50/60____ / _____   P F ___73___ / ___73___
 Add._____ / _____   R D ___25___ / ___30___
 U D ___30___ / ___40___

Elbow: Ext.____140/180____ / _____
 Flex.____60/60____ / _____

Thumb: (ABD.___50___ / ___56___ (degrees)

 (ADD. Tip misses head of 5th MC._____ / _____ inch

	Proximal	Middle	Distal	Report as a fraction inj./uninj.

Thumb	(Ext ((Flex		XXXXXXX XXXXXXX		Finger tips miss palm: inches
Thumb (Flex)	40/40	XXXXXXX	85/76	
Index (Ext) (. (Flex)	80/80	103/102	63/70	T
Middle (Ext) ((Flex)	80/80	173/180 105/105	64/78	T
Ring (Ext) ((Flex)	80/83	176/180 110/112	60/65	T
Little (Ext) ((Flex)	83/85	113/112	64/71	T

Grip   (dynamometer readings)   8444

Right Inj.   Uninj. Left   Pinch   Right   Inj.   Uninj. Left
07/12/08/11/12/ 35/53/35/31/ 24   Thumb-Index   8.5   16
_____ / _____   Lateral   13   18
_____ / _____   Jaw Chuck   5.5   19
In case of bilateral disability state estimated normal as ABD. 140/160 (EN 180).

MEASUREMENTS NOT SHOWN ARE CONSIDERED NORMAL
All measurements should be made in accordance with the standard method as described in the book "Evaluation of Industrial Disability."

Figure 7-23.   Range of motion, grip strength, and pinch strength measurements of client with frozen right shoulder, flexion contracture of right elbow, and causalgia of right upper extremity.

hour 26 minutes seated at standard desk chair (18 inches floor to seat) and desk (height 28 inches). Chair height was changed to 14 inches from floor to seat. The client asked to continue the task.

3. After working 15 minutes at a new chair height, the client complained of her right neck, shoulder, and arm hurting and burning. The client asked to continue the task.

4. Chair height was changed to 19 inches. The client complained of "bent neck" making arm go to sleep. Chair height was changed to 17 inches. There were no further complaints at this height. The client asked to continue the task.

5. Total working time was 2 hours 25 minutes with one break.

Attitude

The evaluator discussed with the client and her rehabilitation counselor the possibility of obtaining another opinion from a member of the American Society of Hand Surgeons concerning the alleviation of pain and the possibility of increased range of motion in the client's right arm and hand. The client stated that she no longer wants to participate in a medical program. She said she wants to return to her former job or to some form of work within her present physical limitation.

NAME _____ No._____ (Right Major)
Circ. (inches) Biceps _____ / _____ Wrist _____ / _____
                Forearm _____ / _____ Hand _____ / _____

MOTIONS: Report as a fraction (injured/uninjured) in degrees of Active Motion

Shoulder: Abd. _____ / _____   Forearm Pron. _____ / _____
            Flex. _____ / _____   Sup. _____ / _____
            I R. _____ / _____
            E R. _____ / _____   Wrist   D F   45 / 55
            Ext. _____ / _____   P F   45 / 50
            Add. _____ / _____   R D   05 / 30
                                                                U D   30 / 45
Elbow: Ext. _____ / _____
            Flex. _____ / _____

Thumb: (ABD.   52 / 60 (degrees)
            (ADD. Tip misses head of 5th MC. ___ T / T ___ inch
                  Proximal   Middle   Distal
                  Report as a fraction inj./uninj.

		Proximal	Middle	Distal	Finger tips miss palm: inches	
Thumb	(Ext		XXXXXXXX			
	(Flex	60/59	XXXXXXXX	60/60		
Index	(Ext					
	(Flex	90/90	91/90	64/67	T	
Middle	(Ext			145/180 *		
	(Flex	95/96	85/90	74/70	T	
Ring	(Ext					
	(Flex	90/90	93/91	62/62	T	
Little	(Ext			163/180		
	(Flex	90/90	92/86	53/60	T	

Grip   (dynamometer readings)   8444   *Swan Neck Childhood Injury

Right Inj.   Uninj. Left   Pinch   Right Inj.   Uninj. Left

15/32/26/31/27/ 45/65/60/51/49   Thumb-Index   12   19
_____ / _____   Lateral   20.5   25
_____ / _____   Jaw Chuck   16   20

In case of bilateral disability state estimated normal as ABD. 140/160 (EN 180).

MEASUREMENTS NOT SHOWN ARE CONSIDERED NORMAL
All measurements should be made in accordance with the standard method as described in the book "Evaluation of Industrial Disability."

Figure 7-24.   Range of motion, grip strength, and pinch strength measurements of client with bilateral Colles' fractures.

Assessment Summary

1. The client complains of pain, numbness, and a burning sensation in the right upper extremity and hand that interfere with her functional capacity to work at a clerical table.
2. The client has loss of range of motion in the right shoulder in abduction and flexion that contributes to her right shoulder pain and to her discomfort when she is working at a standard desk. The loss of range of motion in elbow extension and wrist does not prohibit functional use of the elbow and hand at desk tasks.
3. The grip strength is at the tenth percentile but does not prohibit functional ability in clerical tasks.
4. The pinch strength ranges from the tenth percentile to the seventy-fifth percentile and is sufficient for functional use of pinch in clerical tasks.
5. The client was able to work for 2 hours 25 minutes with one authorized break. However, there were numerous complaints of pain, numbness, and burning.
6. The evaluator feels that because the client has not worked for three years she would benefit from a work hardening program of three weeks or a work capacity evaluation of five days before proceeding with a vocational evaluation.

7. The evaluator was unable to address the physical ability of the client's right arm and hand as a machine operator in pill packaging, owing to lack of a job description. An evaluation on the job is needed for further determination.

Recommendations
1. Consultation with a member of the American Society of Hand Surgeons for possibility of alleviation of pain and increase in range of motion if the client so desires
2. A work capacity evaluation of five days or a work hardening program of three weeks to increase the client's potential for employment; both of these in clerical skills
3. On-the-job evaluation of the client in machine operation, pill packaging, position

Case Study 2*

Objectives of Referral
The client was referred by her vocational rehabilitation counselor for a five-day work capacity evaluation to assess the following:

1. Physical capacities as they relate to drafting tasks (note problem areas)
2. Physical capacities as they relate to computer aided design (CAD), which is performed largely at a terminal
3. General physical tolerances (to be used in broad vocational exploration)

Physical Evaluation

Pain
The client stated on initial contact that she experienced pain in the knuckle of the right thumb when she used a pencil; numbness day and night in the right middle, ring, and little fingers; and a "hot poker" feeling in the middle of her palm day and night. During the evaluation the client did not complain of the above, but instead of pain in the lower back from "sitting too long" and a "rubber band pulling at the right shoulder and forearm" when the work was flat. She reported that her right wrist and thumb and the base of her left thumb on the radial side hurt.

Range of Motion
There is a slight decrease in right index finger touch to palm and a decrease in range of motion in straightening out the index finger (Fig. 7-25). The minimal loss of range of motion does not interfere with function in either traditional drafting or CAD.

Grip Strength
The grip strength of the client's right hand is below the tenth percentile for women aged 50. That of the left hand is at the fiftieth percentile.

Pinch Strength
Palmar pinch (as in picking up a pin) is below the tenth percentile in the right and left hands. Three-point pinch (as in holding a pencil) is at the tenth percentile in both hands. Lateral pinch (as in turning a key) is at the twenty-fifth percentile in both hands. Muscle strength is within normal limits in all areas.

Sensation
Sensation is normal (two-point discrimination is 4 mm in all fingers).

*This case study was provided by Thelma Wellerson Hook, M.A., OTR, Hand Therapy and Rehabilitation Associates, Los Gatos, California.

Date __5-2-83__

NAME _____ No._____ (__Right__ Major)

Circ. (inches) Biceps _____ / _____ Wrist _____ / _____
                Forearm _____ / _____ Hand _____ / _____

MOTIONS: Report as a fraction (injured/uninjured) in degrees of Active Motion

Shoulder: Abd. __WNL_____ / _____ Forearm Pron. _____ / _____
           Flex. __140/145_____ / _____   Sup. _____ / _____
           I R. __WNL_____ / _____
           E R. __WNL_____ / _____ Wrist   D F __63/62__ / _____
           Ext. __52/40_____ / _____   P F __63/67__ / _____
           Add. _____ / _____   R D __25/20__ / _____
                                                                  U D __40/30__ / _____

Elbow: Ext. ___180/180_____ / _____
           Flex. ____30/30_____ / _____

Thumb: (ABD. __65/69__ / _____(degrees)

           (ADD. Tip misses head of 5th MC. __T____ / __T____ inch

           Proximal   Middle   Distal
                  Report as a fraction inj./uninj.

Thumb	(Ext		XXXXXXXX		Finger tips miss palm: inches	
	(Flex	70/74	XXXXXXXX	60/60	Right	
Index	(Ext	160/180		167/180		
	(Flex	74/84	102/100	66/70	-1/2	T
Middle	(Ext	160/180	175/175			
	(Flex	77/95	107/100	71/75	-1/4	T
Ring	(Ext					
	(Flex	85/95	100/95	65/65	T	T
Little	(Ext					
	(Flex	91/85	94/85	65/70	T	T

Grip (dynamometer readings)   Injured

__Right__ Inj. __Left__ Uninj. _____   Pinch   Right   Left
10/30/19/18/17 _____ / 19/17/17/17/11
_____ / _____   Thumb-Index   2.5   5
_____ / _____   Lateral   10   8.5
                                               Jaw Chuck   7   6

In case of bilateral disability state estimated normal as ABD. 140/160 (EN 180).

MEASUREMENTS NOT SHOWN ARE CONSIDERED NORMAL
All measurements should be made in accordance with the standard method as described in the book "Evaluation of Industrial Disability."

Figure 7-25. Range of motion, grip strength, and pinch strength of client with arthritis. (WNL = within normal limits.)

Edema
Measurements increased during the course of five working days: right hand, from 395+ to 405+; left hand, from 360+ to 390.

Work Evaluation

Session 1
Equipment and Tools
Manual pencil sharpener, sandpaper, two pencils with carbon lead, T square, triangle, roll of drafting paper, scissors, drafting board with top tilted 7 degrees, table height 29½ inches, chair height 25 inches with back support.

Work Sample
The client was requested to produce 12 geometric figures from TOWER drafting test 5. The scale was 1 inch to 4 inches. The client completed the task 15 minutes before lunch break. After break she completed five figures in 13 minutes.

Results
The client reported at the end of the day that her left hand and wrist were beginning to hurt and that her back bothered her. She was told to try the option that had been offered her of working while seated, and it was found that sitting alleviated the back pain.

Session 2
Equipment and Tools
Electric eraser (1¼ lbs.), erasing shield, dust brush, drafting board (top tilted at 10 degrees, table height 29½ inches, chair height 22 to 25 inches with no back support, masking tape, square scissors (1″ × 1″) 36 minutes, hexagon scale (1″ × 1″) 36 minutes.

Work Sample
The client was asked to repeat TOWER test. Standard time is 2 hours 7 minutes. The client completed the test in 59 minutes, in superior time range.

   The client used the electric eraser with her right hand and the erasing shield with the left. She lifted masking tape with the thumb and index finger of right hand. She held the scissors in her right hand and pushed forward to cut against the static edge of the scissors. She used the dust brush with her right hand.

Results
The client complained that the 25 inch chair height bothered her lower back. The chair was lowered to 23 inches.

Session 3
Equipment and Tools
Drafting table with top at 65 degrees, 24-inch perch stool with back support, manual pencil sharpener, two pencils with carbon lead.

Work Sample
TOWER test 5, repeat of geometric forms, 1 hour 27 minutes. Circles and half-circles, 59 minutes. Floor plan office space 1, 1 hour 27 minutes.

Results
The client complained of a "tired back last night." She was given "back" booklet.

   The client alternated standing and sitting at standard drafting table 29¾ inches high and 42″ × 29½″. The table tilts from 25 to 65 degrees. The chair height was at 22 inches. The client stated that if the board was "too flat" her back was affected, but if the table was tilted too high her right arm had to be raised and she felt a "rubber band pull" at the outside of her shoulder and along the top of her forearm. A good position appears to be a chair height of 2 feet with the table tilted 30 degrees.

Session 4
Client and therapist went to the Mission College campus where the client tried out CAD

Equipment
Computer table height 29 inches
Keyboard 31½ × 15″ × 10″
Screen height 47 inches to center of monitor
Total screen height 50 inches
Monitor 18″ × 7½″
Eye to screen 21½ inches
Digitizer 28 inches to the right of the client
Pad 17″ × 14″

Work Description
The stylus is positioned with the right hand. It is necessary periodically to press a button on the stylus with the right index finger. Very light pressure is required.

The client looks forward at screen while using the cursor with the right hand. The full arm is stretched 36 inches forward and to the right approximately 45 degrees.

The client uses two hands, one on the digitizer and one on the Hipad with the cursor. Her head is to the right momentarily then returns straight ahead to monitor screen.

Results
The client did not complain of pain, fatigue, or discomfort during the evaluation period.

Session 5
The client continued using a traditional drafting board, model 3042-ST, alternately standing and sitting on perch chair at 22 inches. She continued working on Office Floor Plan 2 for two hours. Her complaints remained the same.

Session 6
Equipment
Drafting table model 3042-ST, Vemco drafting machine elbow; 0.5-mm Pentel P205 lead pencil; electric eraser (1¼ lbs); erasing shield; lead sharpener; masking tape; drafting paper; templates—circles, architecture, and electric; perch chair.

Mixed Drawing and Printing
Work Sample. The client alternated standing and sitting with the table at full 65-degree tilt and chair at 2 feet. The left hand constantly pulls up the elbow, which weighs 2 pounds, from 1 to 1 ¼ inches. This motion positions the verticle and horizontal 18- and 12-inch scale. While the left hand controls the elbow, the right hand draws the required line. The thumb and first finger are in constant pinch position. In addition to constant pinch, the drafter must twirl the pencil continually so that the lead will not flatten. These motions are necessary for all drafting requirements, including lettering. The client stated that product bill of parts on the job is 12 pages long with a minimum of two pages of printing lines ½ inch apart.

Results
The client worked 90 minutes without complaints of discomfort. At the end of that time, she complained of pain in her right thumb and left wrist. She rested and then worked for another 30 minutes before she stopped and changed jobs.

The therapist tried a larger-diameter pencil to relieve constant pinch. This was ungainly and unacceptable to the client. The client worked on lettering with the chair at 2 feet and the table at a 25-degree tilt for approximately one hour. She complained of discomfort as described, both left and right hand.

Attitude and History
The client was cooperative and knowledgeable in all areas of her job. The client first noticed arthritis in her hands about 20 years ago. She presently sees her physician every three weeks. She has received therapy twice weekly for two months. Therapy was discontinued seven months ago.

The client developed right carpal tunnel syndrome in 1967, with surgery in

June 1980, and a left carpal tunnel syndrome in 1970, with surgery in August 1980.

The client stated she has had scoliosis since 14 years of age. This causes tension across her back. She was in a body cast for two years but had no surgery.

The client stated that her right eye is normal but since five years ago she has been unable to read with the left with correction.

The client has arthritis in C5 and C6.

The client started drafting in junior high school. She has had two years of college. She started drafting with Bell in 1948. In 1951 she worked as a cartographer for Rand McNally for three months and then started drafting with EIMAC. She continued with EIMAC when Varian bought out EIMAC.

The client stated that her interest is computers in addition to various hobbies that she pursues when her hands permit.

The client has looked into a Masters School course in CAD and took a minicourse in 1977 for six weeks. She learned how to do tape-ups. She has taken two Saturday courses at Radio Shack on computers.

The client said she would like to take a 20-week CAD course offered by the Masters School. The school requires a 20-week computer-aided manufacture (CAM) course as a prerequisite. She states that she already knows the CAM material and does not want to take this course, but Masters will not allow her to take the CAD course without first taking the prerequisite.

Assessment Summary

1. The client has pain in left wrist, right palm, base of right and left thumb, and lower back. She is able to control the pain while working on traditional drafting by changing positions and tasks.
2. Range of motion loss in right hand is minimal and does not interfere with traditional drafting or CAD.
3. Grip strength loss below the tenth percentile on the right and at the fiftieth percentile on the left does not interfere with traditional drafting or CAD.
4. Pinch strength loss does not interefere with traditional drafting or CAD.
5. Muscle strength in both extremities is within normal limits.
6. Sensation is normal in both hands.
7. Swelling in both hands, which increased during the course of the five-day evaluation, does not interfere with traditional drafting or CAD.
8. Traditional drafting causes constant discomfort to the client. The client suffers the least discomfort in the hands and lower back when the drafting table has a 30-degree tilt, her chair with back support is in the 22-to 24-inch range, and she alternates standing and sitting and changes tasks frequently. Traditional drafting will continue to cause the client discomfort and pain in both hands.
9. CAD is best performed by the client in a support chair at the 22-to 24-inch range from seat to floor. If the Hipad with cursor position becomes a problem to the client, the pad should be moved from the right to the left of the computer keyboard. CAD is not as physically demanding to the client and does not appear to cause constant discomfort and pain.
10. The client's attitude is excellent, and she is motivated to learn CAD.

Recommendations

1. If the client is to pursue traditional drafting, the best position for the drafting table is a 30-degree tilt with a 29¾ inches table height. The chair should have a support back and the seat should be between 22 and 24 inches from the floor. The client should be able to change positions and tasks frequently.
2. If the client is to pursue CAD, the best chair height is 22 to 24 inches, and the chair should have a back support.
3. A short course of training in CAD and placement are recommended.

*Case Study 3**

A 26-year-old right-dominant Guyanese man was referred for an upper-extremity work tolerance screening (WTS). He had been employed as a wrapping machine operator at the time of his injury. He sustained two injuries to his hands while operating this machine. In 1981 the right middle and ring fingers were amputated through the distal interphalangeal joints. He returned to his usual and customary work 2½ months after that injury. Eight months after his return to work, he sustained a left index finger distal phalanx crush with an open fracture. When he recovered from the second injury, his treating physician questioned whether or not the client had adequate coordination to perform his work on such a machine.

Although assessment of upper-extremity coordination and dexterity was the stated purpose of the WTS, another problem surfaced as a major reason for the client's decreased ability to perform his work safely. During the sensory evaluation of the hand, it was found that the tips of the right middle and ring finger stumps were hypersensitive. The client jerked his hand away when the stumps were stimulated. In a further interview the client stated that he had not been able to perform his work in the usual manner since his first injury because of his need to protect the hypersensitive fingertips of his right hand. On a standardized test such as the Crawford Small Parts Dexterity Test (Fig. 7-26) and a standardized apparatus such as the WEST 2, the client demonstrated excellent hand coordination, dexterity, and attentiveness to detail as long as the right amputation stumps were not involved or inadvertently touched. Right hand skill deteriorated in the presence of stimulation of the right stumps. This information was summarized and presented to the referring counselor. The occupational therapist recommended a program of desensitization.

SCHOOL FOR THE DEVELOPMENTALLY DELAYED

The Walter E. Fernald State School, founded in 1848, was the first publicly supported residential training facility for the mentally retarded. Historically, occupational therapy has played an important role in client care at Fernald, particularly with respect to work-related programming. In the early 1970s occupational therapists were actively involved in the development of Fernald's vocational training workshops. The introduction of vocational rehabilitation services to the school provided the catalyst for the occupational therapy department to redirect some of its resources from vocational training workshops to prevocational skills and behavior training.

Prevocational skills and behavior training are viewed as a fundamental part of a total habilitative plan to teach work skills, behaviors, and attitudes. As formulated by Carolyn Austin and John Basile [4], "An idealized long-term goal of prevocational training is competitive employment. However, a more realistic goal is the development of the client's work-related skills to their fullest potential with an increased sense of self-identity and accomplishment achieved through purposeful and meaningful activity." The prevocational programming is conceptualized on a continuum of increasing difficulty and includes prevocational training, a comprehensive training center, sheltered workshops, and on-the-job training. The transition from lower to higher levels of

*This case study was provided by Karen S. Schultz, M.S., OTR, Hand Rehabilitation Specialists, Santa Monida, California.

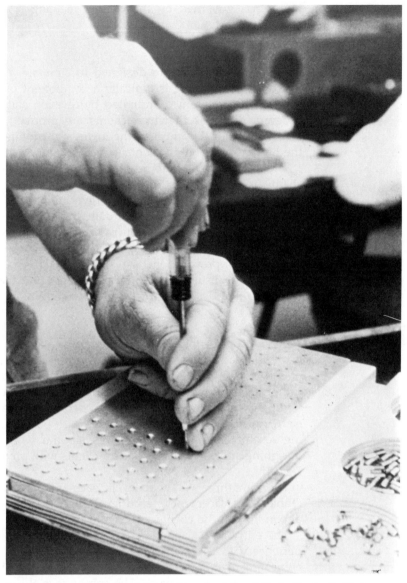

Figure 7-26.   Client performing Crawford Small Parts Dexterity Test, which assesses fine manipulation, small tool use, and endurance. (Photograph courtesy of Hand Rehabilitation Specialists.)

training is governed by the client's meeting specific predetermined admissions criteria.

Prevocational Training

Presented in a classroom designed to simulate a work environment, prevocational training is typically a component of the comprehensive day activity program coordinated by division staff. There are six day program divisions in which clients are grouped homogeneously by ability. Division 1 comprises the lowest-functioning clients; division 6, the highest-functioning clients.

The occupational therapist may work on a one-to-one basis with clients or in a group setting using treatment modalities such as sensory stimulation, motor development, prevocational skills development, fine motor training, and activities of daily living (ADL) training. The therapist also provides consultation to the division staff and clinical supervision of direct staff. The *comprehensive training center* specializes in the acquisition of prevocational skills by means of simulated and real work in a more realistic worklike environment. The therapist plays a role similar to that described for prevocational training.

Sheltered Workshops

The philosophy inherent in the sheltered workshop program at Fernald is to assist each client to maximize his or her abilities and acquire feelings of self-worth. This is accomplished by focusing on the client's *ability* rather than disability and by providing realistic work experiences. The occupational therapist is available on a consulting basis to the workshop staff, providing evaluations of clients with perceptual difficulties, making recommendations on task analysis and work simplification, and designing and constructing jigs for clients with physical handicaps (Fig. 7-27) [5].

There are three workshop levels, each with its own admissions criteria (Table 7-4). Placement in each level may be a long-term or short-term, depending on the client's needs and progress.

The entry-level workshops are the first stage in a continuum of experience with contract work (when available) in a real full-time work environment. For many clients these workshops represent their first experience in fulltime work. The emphasis in this level is on the further development of basic work skills.

In the *intermediate-level workshop* clients have had some work experience that has increased their familiarity with the expectations of a fulltime work adjustment program. Emphasis here is placed on the development of more advanced work behaviors and attitudes such as production levels, cooperation, and independence.

The *transitional program* is the final stage of the sheltered workshop continuum. These clients have had work experience and have successfully mastered a variety of work situations and tasks. The goal of complete work-related independence is consistently reinforced, and worker production and peer socialization are emphasized. At this level clients have evolved a fundamental understanding of work attitudes and behavior.

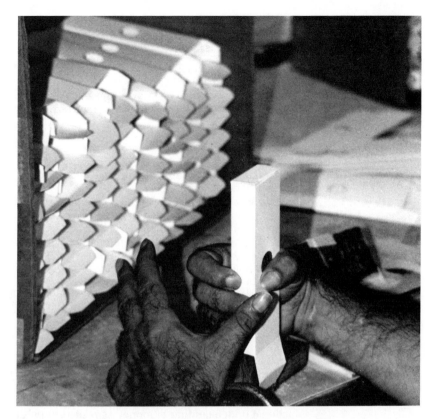

A

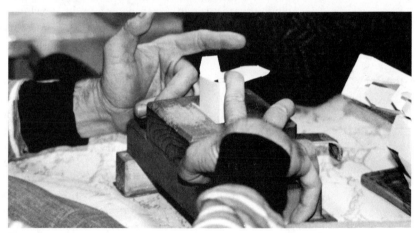

B

Figure 7-27. Jigs developed by therapists at Fernald State School to assist clients in performing sheltered workshop subcontract tasks of (A) assembling box and (B) stuffing and closing box. (Photos courtesy of Matthew Gold.)

Table 7-4.   Workshop Entry Criteria

Entry-level workshops
    Able to attend work daily
    Independence in basic ADL* skills
    Ability to make basic needs known through signs, gestures, or words
    Ability to understand three-step tasks either verbally, visually, manually, or
    in combination
    Sitting tolerance of 50 minutes
    Ability to work independently for approximately five minutes
    Ability to work at least two hours per day five days per week
    Ability to participate in small, structured social groups
Intermediate workshops
    Ability to work in cooperative group setting
    Reinforced by money or verbal praise
    Ability to produce at approximately 10–12% NPA* on most tasks
    Ability to work for approximately 15 minutes with minimal supervision
    Demonstrated ability to acquire additional work skills
    Functionally understands such concepts as larger, smaller, front of, behind,
    between, before, after
    Ability to attend to task for 30–50 minutes with supervision and prompts
    Ability to accept changes in routine
Transitional programs
    Ability to work six hours per day, five days per week with appropriate
    breaks
    Production 20–30% NPA on most tasks
    Ability to use leisure time such as breaks appropriately
    Functional understanding of the supervisor-worker relationship
    Functional understanding of quality control as related to work
    Functional understanding of money as related to production
    Ability to work consistently for approximately 2 ½ hours with supervision
    Ability to participate in a realistic way in the development of vocational
    goals and objectives

---

* ADL = activities of daily living; NPA = normal production average.

On-the-Job Training

Concurrent with the sheltered workshop program is on-the-job training (OJT). The OJT program offers the client the opportunity to learn a wide variety of meaningful activities and tasks in a normalized setting. Many OJT tasks offer an alternative for clients unable to tolerate assembly line tasks, such as those offered in the sheltered workshops. Approximately 45 clients from divisions 2 through 6 participate in OJT. This program, like the sheltered workshops, has specific entry criteria (Table 7-5). A client may simultaneously participate in a sheltered workshop.

Both the sheltered workshop and OJT are certified under the Massachusetts Department of Labor and the Central Office of the Department of Mental Health. These agencies guarantee that clients are paid for their productivity.

On-the-job training areas include a greenhouse, the North Café, the manual porter crew, the Polaroid porter crew, the clerical pool, the marketable crafts program, and individualized placements. The *greenhouse program,* in operation since 1975, uses horticultural therapy to provide prevocational and vocational skills training and leisure activity development. Clients work at the greenhouse approximately 4½ hours

Table 7-5.   Entry Criteria for On-the-Job Training

Skill Area	Criteria
Attending to task	Ability to attend to a learned task for up to ten minutes
Cooperation	Ability to follow directions for secondary and delayed reinforcement such as weekly pay; response to money as a secondary reinforcer
Work tolerance	Ability to stay in work environment up to two hours; experience with day activity programming preferred
Communication skills	Ability to communicate basic needs and follow up to four-step instructions
Cognitive skills	Ability to discriminate by size and shape and to match items if sorted by color; one-to-one correspondence skills
Motor skills	Ability to perform jobs in program (types of work are dependent on training site)

per day five days per week. Throughout the year these clients participate in seasonal horticultural activities. In the spring, for example, clients learn to replant seedlings, plant seed flats, and maintain the greenhouse; in the summer the focus shifts to vegetable and flower gardening, basic landscaping, and replenishing house plants for the greenhouse.

The sale of greenhouse products to the public facilitates a businesslike atmosphere and affords the clients the opportunity to interact with the community in a positive milieu of an exchange of labor for product. The community garden program provides clients with an additional opportunity to interact with the community. Garden plots on Fernald's ground are available to community members, as well as staff and clients. The success of this project with respect to positive public relations with the community has been expressed in the following way: "This project provides a positive setting for the community to become involved with Fernald and to learn more about mental retardation through a positive experience. Since the community gardens began many citizens have expressed positive feelings about Fernald and increased concern for its residents" [4].

The *North Café* is a structured restaurant training program in which clients, under staff supervision, provide a variety of daily luncheon specials for staff and clients. Through restaurant-style experiences clients learn about hygiene, service skills, table setting, and clean-up procedures. The restaurant is also used to help other clients learn how to order a meal, wait appropriately for the meal to be served, and pay for items.

The clients in the *manual porter crew program* are trained in custodial work to maintain three buildings on the school grounds. Clients work four hours per day five days per week on tasks that typically allow them to channel their energy into physical activity. Team cooperation is greatly emphasized throughout the program.

The emphasis of the *Polaroid porter crew program*, which is carried on at the nearby Polaroid plant, is on social adaptation in a community work setting and on developing and evaluating independent work skills. The program provides janitorial training; the work involves cleaning 18 bathrooms daily. Tasks include emptying trash, replenishing supplies, sweeping, mopping, and cleaning toilets, sinks, and shelves. This offers a work experience in a normal environment with normal work expectations. The skills that the clients acquire are assumed to be marketable.

The *clerical pool* consists of five clients who perform various clerical tasks (stapling, folding) for departments at the school.

The *marketable crafts program* provides the client with a creative outlet in the production of salable handcrafted items such as patchwork pillows, draft stoppers, and Christmas wreaths, while reinforcing general work skills and behaviors. At present clients sell their items to local shops, to craft fairs (the Little People's School annual arts and crafts fair—see Chap. 5) and to the Fernald staff. For those clients who are able to perform work duties independently, jobs are available through *individual placement* with the school's boiler house, farm, and grounds department.

Conceptual Framework of Prevocational Program

Austin and Basile have classified work-related skills into a four-category developmental framework: (1) basic work behavior skills, (2) work performance skills, (3) refined work behavior skills, and (4) refined work concepts.

Basic work behavior skills make up the foundation of task-related skill development and refined work behaviors. Such basic skills include attending to the task, sitting tolerance, work tolerance, independent working, compliance, and cooperation. The acquisition of these skills is a prerequisite for the development of more advanced prevocational skills such as performance, refined work behaviors, and work concepts.

Work performance skills are the physical, cognitive, sensory, sensorimotor, and communication skills necessary to perform tasks.

Skills	Examples
Physical	Strength, endurance, range of motion, dexterity
Sensory	Body schema, position in space
Sensorimotor	Coordination of sensory and physical skills
Cognitive	Concept of task completion; concept of "one"; discrimination by shape, size, color, weight; sequencing ability
Communication	Receptive language (ability to follow two- or three-step directions), expressive language (ability to express basic and work-related needs)

Refined work behavior skills are the advanced prevocational skills derived from well-developed basic work behavior skills. Examples of refined skills are work attendance, punctuality, initiative (working independently), frustration tolerance, adaptability to change, cooperation, appearance and hygiene, organizational ability, and appropriate communication.

Refined work concepts include such aspects of successful employment as liking one's job and understanding the relationship between productivity, employment, and success.

Austin and Basile have also identified a continuum of work behaviors from basic to refined (Fig. 7-28).

Case Study*

Jane is a 24-year-old visually handicapped yet functionally sighted resident of Fernald. Primary care and service delivery within the institution have been augmented by federal funding for the past six years.

Jane was admitted to the institution at age 4 with the diagnosis of Down's syndrome. Her functional abilities are limited owing to both her organic disorder and subsequent developmental retardation resulting from extended institutionalization. During the first 14 years of Jane's residency in the institution, anomalies developed in her behavior partially because of her syndrome and partially because of extremely limited service delivery other than custodial care before ancillary funding made available by the federal government.

Jane has been receiving daily structured educational services in her residential building for the past four years. The emphasis has been on the development of self-care, communication, refined motor, cognitive, and work-related skills. Consistent behavioral interventions have been in effect for the last six years.

The residence interdisciplinary treatment team noted that Jane had made considerable progress in all skill areas. The incidence of inappropriate behavior was minimal and almost nonexistent in a structured setting. She was able to communicate basic needs and was receptive to elementary forms of expressive communication. She demonstrated a potential for independence in self-care and a marked ability to learn work-related tasks and to maintain appropriate behavior in a work-related setting.

Prompted by Jane's noted progress, the treatment team recommended her admission to First Step, a comprehensive out-of-building day activity program designed to address all need areas with an emphasis on teaching clients to generalize learned skills and incorporate them throughout their day.

Skill evaluations were conducted by the First Step treatment team, who agreed with the residence treatment team that Jane met the admission criteria to the program and that service delivery from the program would most appropriately meet her needs at that time.

Two years after her admission to First Step, Jane was nearly independent in self-care skills such as dressing, toileting, washing, and grooming, although she did require limited assistance in most of these areas. Her motor planning, strength, and range of motion were within normal limits. Her communication skills had improved enough to greatly facilitate skill development in other areas; the incidence of inappropriate behavior continued to be minimal; and her cognitive, physical, and perceptual abilities had enabled her to learn new work-related tasks, some of which were fairly complex, quickly. Jane appeared to enjoy work and to understand the value of reward for work well done. Staff noted her ability to tolerate sitting and working for extended periods; to tolerate supervision and change in routine; and to work continuously, consistently, and cooperatively in a simulated work setting.

Jane's progress and skills were recognized by the residence and program treatment teams, whose combined efforts had given Jane a continuous opportunity to learn.

Jane's admission to Advance was recommended. Advance is a comprehensive training center that specializes in the development and refinement of basic work behavior skills and work performance skills by means of a wide variety of prevocational tasks including multiple-step assembly and packaging, sorting, cooperative work, and housekeeping. Self-care, communication, and behavior continue to be addressed with an increased emphasis on the development of

---

*This case study was provided by John Basile, Walter E. Fernald State School, Belmont, Massachusetts.

Flow Chart of Work Behaviors

Work Behavior Categories:	Basic		Intermediate		Refined		
Work tolerance	Ability to discriminate between home and work environment as measured by going to and from work.	Ability to remain in the work environment for up to one hour a day.	Ability to remain in work environment for up to two hours a day.	Ability to remain in work environment for 2–4 consecutive hours.	Ability to remain at work for up to 6 consecutive hrs.	Ability to remain at work for up to 8 hours daily.	Ability to utilize vacation and sick time appropriately.
Staying on the job Sitting tolerance	Ability to sit in designated seat for immediate effective reinforcer.	Ability to sit in designated seat up to 45 minutes with intermittent effective reinforcer.	Ability to stay in designated seat up to 45 minutes for social reinforcement and edible contingency up to 45 minutes.	Ability to stay in designated seat for 45-min. period over 4-hr. day. Social praise, workcard, money.	Ability to stay in designated work space with minimal prompts.	Ability to stay and leave and return to workspace independently.	Ability to work independent of supervisor. Report to supervisor when necessary.

Figure 7-28.   Continuum of work-related behaviors.

Attending to task / Task completion / Quality	Ability to perform one subunit of a task for immediate effective reinforcer.	Ability to complete one simple task for immediate effective reinforcer.	Ability to complete a quota of simple tasks for immediate effective reinforcer.	Ability to complete quota of simple tasks for ✓ on workcard; social praise—delayed reinforcer.	Ability to complete task independent of quota for delayed reinforcer.	Ability to complete tasks accurately and fast for social praise and weekly pay.	Ability to complete work for self-esteem and weekly pay.
Following instructions	Ability to respond to one-step instructions: Sit down. Time to work.	Ability to respond to additional one- and two-step simple-task, specific instructions.	Ability to follow 3–4 task-specific instructions.	Ability to follow complex 4–10 task-specific instructions.	Ability to follow general work rules; ability to quality, control work.	Ability to receive corrective feedback and change accurately.	Ability to problem-solve complex tasks and work issues.
Flexibility	Inapplicable	Inapplicable	Ability to tolerate the same tasks weekly if contract determines this.	Ability to accept change of task.	Ability to accept change of task.	Ability to work cooperatively with co-workers and supervisors.	Ability to discuss changes with supervisors and co-workers.

(continued)

Flow Chart of Work Behaviors

Work Behavior Categories:	*Basic*		*Intermediate*		*Refined*		
Responsibility							
Attendance	Staff dependent	Staff dependent	Staff dependent	Ability to attend work daily for reinforcement and with staff prompts.	Ability to attend work daily and arrive on time with prompts.	Ability to attend work daily and arrive on time with minimal prompts.	Ability to accumulate and use sick time and vacation time appropriately.
Appearance	Must be dressed for work.	Ability to remain appropriately dressed with staff supervision.	Ability to dress for work appropriately with minimal supervision.	Ability to dress for work appropriately, independently.	Ability to wear work-related clothing, aprons, uniforms, protective glasses.	Same	Same
Initiative	Inapplicable	Inapplicable	Ability to get more work with prompts.	Ability to get more work with minimal prompts.	Ability to seek help from supervisor with minimal prompts.	Ability to recognize route to success.	Ability to seek promotion and gain peer acceptance.

Figure 7-28.   (continued)

Work Behavior Categories:	Basic		Intermediate		Refined		
Physical Strength Endurance Dexterity	Ability to reach for and grab large table-top objects with either hand.	Ability to manipulate large tabletop objects: Ring on ring stack; ability to repeat fine motor skills necessary to perform simple tabletop activities for up to 45 minutes.	Ability to manipulate smaller tabletop objects; ability to perform more refined finger movements, for example: 3 jaw chuck grasp.	Ability to manipulate one part of tabletop object with one hand while steadying matching part with other hand, e.g., large jar large hand dominance, unilateral coordination.	Ability to use both hands together to manipulate objects of smaller size, e.g., some types of nuts and bolts. Bilateral coordination, ability to sustain 2–4 hrs of assembly work.	Ability to use tools to manipulate objects, e.g., screwdriver, scissors, hammer, holepunch; ability to sustain 4–6 hrs. of object manipulation.	Ability to use machines; e.g., heat-sealer, drills, riveter, factory jigs; ability to do piecework for 8 hrs.
Cognitive Discrimination Matching 1:1 correspondence Task completion	Ability to recognize a change in environment; ability to discriminate between two functional tabletop objects, e.g., cup and plate.	Ability to discriminate between basic 3-dimensional shapes □ and ○ then □△ Ability to complete a subunit of a task, e.g., put all the way down on stack.	Ability to discriminate between additional 3-dimensional shapes; ability to put one subunit in a container, ability to complete up to a 6 subunit of tasks, e.g., one peg in each pouch of egg carton.	Ability to discriminate objects by size, shape, color; ability to object-count up to 5; ability to complete 2–3-step tasks using concept of 1; e.g., putting 1 nut, 1 bolt, 1 washer together.	Ability to discriminate and match objects by length, weight, width, size, color, shape; ability to object-count to 10; ability to complete 3–6-step tasks; e.g., packaging print-coaters.	Ability to discriminate and match letters, codes, numbers, symbols; ability to object-count to 100; ability to sequence multistep tasks.	Ability to quality-control using discriminative and counting skills; problem solving, using simple addition and subtraction.

(continued)

Flow Chart of Work Behaviors

Work Behavior Categories:	Basic		Intermediate		Refined		
Sensory and Perceptual Body schema	Ability to recognize and relocate environmental stimuli.	Ability to locate and recognize environmental stimuli.	Ability to locate and recognize environmental stimuli in relation to self.	Ability to locate position and relationship of objects between self and between objects.	Ability to recognize qualities of objects; e.g., size, shape, color, in relation to each other.	Ability to recognize and reconstruct complex contructions.	Ability to recognize and construct complex constructions.
Sensory-Motor	Ability to manipulate meaningful stimuli, e.g., sit on chair, open door, step over plank.	Ability to manipulate objects in relation to self; in front of, behind self; throw ball.	Ability to manipulate objects in relation to objects; put block on top of door.	Ability to manipulate objects correct distance from self in relation to each other.	Ability to manipulate and match objects using discrimination skills.	Ability to build block patterns; put screw, nut, and bolt together.	Ability to assemble complex constructions and follow directions.

Figure 7-28.   (continued)

monetary skills, frustration tolerance, and other more complex prerequisites for vocational placement.

Jane met Advance admission criteria, and the treatment team agreed that placement in the program would meet her needs.

During the 18 months after her admission to Advance, staff continued to note her consistent progress in communication, behavior, self-care, and other skill areas relevant to work. Her independent travel from residence to program site was monitored by staff. The residence treatment team continued to receive positive reports from the Advance program staff concerning Jane's responsiveness, cooperation, flexibility, and ability to learn in a work setting. After recommendation from Advance staff, the treatment team agreed to screen Jane for placement in an entry-level workshop. Observations and evaluations by workshop staff were completed; eight months after Jane was placed on a waiting list, she was admitted to Work Place, an entry-level workshop program providing services to fifteen clients, four of whom live in the same residential building as Jane. The workshop appeared to be the most appropriate environment to facilitate Jane's advancement toward ultimate normalization and independence.

Using both simulated and contract work (when available), Work Place focuses on increased tolerance to work-related frustrations produced by such features as a supervisor-employee, as opposed to a teacher-student, relationship. Work Place emphasizes the development of more advanced work behaviors, skills, and attitudes leading towards increased work-related independence. The objectives include regular attendance, punctuality, cooperation, appropriate appearance, appropriate communication, and increased tolerance to change, or lack of change, in routine.

Work Place has offered Jane her first experience in a full-time work adjustment situation. Her placement in the workshop may be long-term or short-term, depending on her needs. In this setting, Jane is assisted in developing more advanced work-related skills and an increased sense of self-worth and accomplishment achieved through purposeful and meaningful activity. Now, as at any level in the continuum of prevocational training, Jane has the opportunity, if appropriate for her, to advance to any one of the higher levels of prevocational or vocational training or vocational placement. The options available to Jane include placement in another sheltered workshop (intermediate or transitional level), an on-the-job training program, or both, depending on her needs. Ultimately, if Jane is able to perform work duties independently, certain full-time employment positions within the institution can be made available to her. Moreover, concurrent with the potential for residential placement in the community, a wide variety of enriching employment experiences are available to Jane outside the institution.

DAY HABILITATION PROGRAM*

The United Cerebral Palsy Association of MetroBoston has a community day program, which uses a fine motor/work skills development component (Fig. 7-29) as part of therapeutic programming for adults with developmental disabilities. This program provides clients with the opportunity to develop and apply those work habits, behaviors, and skills that are considered basic to successful participation in the work world. A variety of individual reinforcer programs are utilized to motivate the clients toward their optimum work performance. This aspect of the program serves as the foundation experience for clients who aspire toward less restrictive referral and placement in settings such as sheltered workshops and supported work environments within the community.

*This section was written by C. Shana Krell, OTR/L.

NAME_____

KEY - DEMONSTRATES/-PERFORMS BEHAVIOR OR SKILL:
    A = Always Demonstrated; 4/4 trials
    F = Frequently Demonstrated; 3/4 trials
    S = Sometimes Demonstrated; 2/4 trials
    R = Rarely Demonstrated; 1/4 trials
    N = Never Demonstrated; 0/4 trials
    AJ = Adaptive Jig; to compensate for physical limitations.
    SJ = Structural Jig; to facilitate performance by visual
         cues.

		INIT	YR.	YR.	YR.
A. WORK BEHAVIOR	DATE				
1. Type of reinforcer used					
a. Primary (food, drink)					
b. Social (verbal praise,attention)					
c. Activity (appropriate & pleasurable)					
d. Token-specify in documentation					
e. Combination of above-specify in documentation					
f. No reinforcer found successful at this time					
g. No reinforcer necessary					
2. Schedule of reinforcer					
a. Continuous (after each piece of work)					
b. Fixed ratio (after specific no. of pieces)					
c. Variable ratio (after unspecific no. of pieces)					
d. Fixed interval (after specific time period; specify in documentation, ex, end of work period, 2x daily, end of week)					
e. Variable interval (document variability of reinforcer)					
3. Remains of work station					
a. 21-30 minutes					
b. 31-45 minutes					
c. 45 minutes - 1 hr.					
d. 1 hr. - 1 1/2 hrs.					
4. Attendance - leaves job inappropriately during work period					
a. 0X					
b. 1-4X					
c. 5-8X					
d. 9-15X					

Figure 7-29.   Evaluation of work skill acquisition. (Courtesy Shana Krell, OTR.)

	DATE	INIT	YR.	YR.	YR.

5. Task focus - maintains sustained work effort

a. 0-5 minutes				
b. 6-10 minutes				
c. 11-15 minutes				
d. 16-20 minutes				
e. 21-30 minutes				
f. half hour or more				

6. Work Tolerance

a. Appropriately indicates need for assist when encounters difficulty				
b. Waits patiently if work is delayed or stopped				
c. Continues work after unsuccessful attempts				
d. Continues to work through peer outbursts				
e. Acts out when encounters job difficulty				

7. Adaptability

a. Accepts & adjusts to new tasks				
b. Accepts more difficult tasks				
c. Changes tasks successfully within work period				
d. Adapts to changes in routines (doesn't over-react or lose control)				
e. Performs task following change in instruction				
f. Responds appropriately after correction cues				
g. Works without complaints				
h. Continues to work while being observed				

Figure 7-29.   (continued)

List behavioral factors which impede work performance: <u>Date</u>

_____

_____
_____
_____

_____

	DATE	INIT	YR.	YR.	YR.
B. WORK HABITS					
1. Punctuality					
a. Arrives at worksite ready for work					
b. Begins work task promptly after instruction					
c. Leaves work area at proper times for bathroom use.					
d. Takes appropriate amount of time for bathroom break					
e. Proceeds punctually to break or lunch					
f. Responds positively to productivity cues					
2. Neatness - keeps work station neat:					
a. Picks up materials that have fallen					
b. Arranges disorganized work materials					
c. Maintains task in work space					
d. Places items in indicated places					
3. Task acquisition-generally learns new tasks best by:					
a. Written instruction					
b. Visual indicators					
c. Verbal directives					
d. Gestural cues					
e. Physical prompts					
f. Hand-over-hand guidance					

Figure 7-29.   (continued)

	DATE	INIT	YR.	YR.	YR.
4. Task performance: generally utilizes what type of structure to perform a task:					
a. Written					
b. Visual (pictures)					
c. Verbal					
d. Location of materials					
5. Responds to an instruction that requires compliance after how many verbal prompts					
a. 1					
b. 2					
c. 3					
d. 4					
e. 5+					
6. Responds to instructional cue					
a. Immediately					
b. Within 1-2 minutes					
c. Within 2-3 minutes					
d. Within 3-4 minutes					
e. Within 4-5 minutes					
f. After more than 5 minutes					
7. Memory - general ability to remember and follow how many specific task steps					
a. 7-9					
b. 5-6					
c. 2-4					
8. Adaptability - ability to learn, generalize and perform same number of like steps of a task in a different job					
a. From week to week					
b. From day to day					
c. Within 1 work period					
9. Production Rate - maintains rate of productivity of a learned work task					
a. From week to week					
b. From day to day					
c. Within one work period					

Figure 7-29.   (continued)

	DATE	INIT	YR.	YR.	YR.
10. Performance Quality - generally maintains assembly type work with what amount of accuracy					
a. 10+ steps		%	%	%	%
b. 7-9 steps		%	%	%	%
c. 5-6 steps		%	%	%	%
d. 2-4 steps		%	%	%	%
11. After verbal cues, is generally able to use judgement and correct work mistakes					
a. 100% of the time					
b. 76-100% of the time					
c. 51-75% of the time					
d. less than 50% of the time					
12. Work style -					
a. Indicates when finished					
b. Indicates when in need of materials					
c. Self-corrects work before indicating finished					
d. Works tentatively; lacks initiative to begin when appropriate					
e. Works impulsively; requires cues to wait for supervision					

C.   JOB SKILLS

1. Disassembles item and sorts how many unlike parts				
a. 10+				
b. 7-9				
c. 5-6				
d. 2-4				
2. Assembles product of how many unlike parts				
a. 10+				
b. 7-9				
c. 5-6				
d. 2-4				

Figure 7-29.   (continued)

	INIT	YR.	YR.	YR.
DATE				
3. Sorts objects by (indicate in documentation)				
a. 1 variable (ex., size, shape, color, texture, number, letter)				
b. 2 variables (ex., size & shape, shape & color, size & texture)				
c. 3 variables (ex., color, shape & size, size, color, & texture, etc.)				
4. Packages – into container				
a. 3-7 like items				
b. 8-10 like items				
c. 11-14 like items				
d. 15-20 like items				
e. 3-7 unlike items				
f. 8-10 unlike items				
g. 11-14 unlike items				
h. 15-20 unlike items				
5. Seals				
a. Box top – insert into box				
b. Snap top container				
c. Screw top container				
d. Plastic bag by folding and clipping				
e. Ziptop bag				
f. Tucking envelope flap				
g. Clasping envelope flap				
h. Taping box closed				
6. Envelope skills				
a. Unstuffs envelopes				
b. Inserts 3x5 card				
c. Inserts 4x9 paper				
d. Inserts already collated papers				
e. Places insert with address in window				
f. Seals and stamps envelope				
7. Paper assembly/placement				
a. Folds 8 1/2" x 11" paper in half				
b. Folds 8 1/2" x 11" paper into thirds				
c. Folds paper in thirds and inserts into envelope				

Figure 7-29.   (continued)

	INIT	YR.	YR.	YR.
DATE				
8. Collates and stacks				
a. 2 pieces of paper				
b. 3-5 pieces of paper				
c. 6+ pieces of paper				
d. 6+ pieces, stacks crisscrossed				
9. Collates and places in envelope				
a. 2 items				
b. 3-5 items				
c. 6+ items				
10. Securely fastens/manipulates				
a. Rubber bands				
b. Twist ties				
c. 1" paper clips				
d. 2" paper clips				
e. Squeeze clip				
f. Staples paper				
g. Staples paper at indicated spot (ex., upper left hand corner)				
h. Staple remover				
i. Single hole punch				
j. 3 hole punch				
k. Tape in dispenser				
l. Electric pencil sharpener				
m. Manual pencil sharpener				
n. Stamp and ink pad				
11. Labeling and clerical				
a. Removes self-sticking label from backing				
b. Removes, centers and places label as indicated				
c. Marks envelope with inked stamp as indicated				
d. Inserts punched paper into binder correctly				
e. Alphabetizes by letter into folders				
f. Alphabetizes by letter into file box (8" x 10" or 3" x 5")				

Figure 7-29.   (continued)

REFERENCES

1. Community Service Department of the Queen Elizabeth Hospital. 1202 Old Port Road, Royal Park, Australia 5014. *Alfreda Rehabilitation Unit Fitness for Work and Living* (brochure).
2. Community Service Department of the Queen Elizabeth Hospital. 1202 Old Port Road, Royal Park, Australia 5014. Western Domiciliary Care and Rehabilitation Service The Alfreda Unit (in-house handout).
3. Dean, P., Cox, R., and Aurich, R. *The Role of Occupational Therapist in the Alfreda Rehabilitation Unit* (in-house handout). 1982.
4. Jones, P. D. *Walter E. Fernald State School. A Photo Essay.* Belmont, Massachusetts: Office of Communications, Walter E. Fernald State School (P.O. Box 158, Belmont, Massachusetts 02158), 1983.
5. Jageman, L. W. *Adaptive Fixtures for Handicapped Workers.* Menomonie, Wisc.: Materials Development Center, Stout Vocational Rehabilitation Institute, University of Wisconsin—Stout, 1984.

The Older Worker*

Retailers and other service companies are turning more to retired workers to fill front-line jobs dealing with customers. Most companies are delighted with the results and are planning to recruit more older workers. Some benefits cited:

Older workers anticipate customer needs better than younger workers do.
They provide positive role models for younger workers.
They bring expertise to the job [4].

In the United States there are more than 24 million persons over age 65 (11 percent of the total population); by the year 2030, 18 percent of the population will be 65 or over. As a nation, we can ill afford to support the growing older population with tax dollars. Returning older persons to the work force or assisting them in staying in it appears to be a viable solution.

With the expanding aging population, a new role for occupational therapists exists. As the supply of young workers decreases, older workers will be courted by employers. Occupational therapists can act as liaisons between employers and older workers, as well as advocates for aging workers.

TRENDS IN AGING

Statistics illustrate an unprecedented growth of the "old" population, generally considered to be age 65 to death, and the age group 75+, often known as the "old-old." For by the year 2050, the 65+ age group will represent about 25 percent of the United States population, and the 75+ age group will have grown to the size the 65+ age group is today. The 85+ age group will account for 5 percent of the total United States population [1]. The number of women in all these groups is expected to double by the year 2025 [1].

Because of their implications for future health care and work options, it is important to note the following:

People are living longer, but not necessarily better.
The incidence of chronic mental illness is increasing.
The need for assistance in activities of daily living increases with age.
The need for longterm care will increase over the next four decades.
Over 85 percent of Americans of all ages are uninsured or underinsured against catastrophic and longterm care costs.

*This chapter was written by Nancy MacRae, M.S., OTR.

More people are receiving extended periods of formal care in their own homes and communities.

The prevalence of chronic conditions with high associated disability, such as arthritis and heart conditions, is rising, while death rates for most major causes of death continue to fall [1].

The incidence of part-time work increases with age [1].

The number of older men (ages 55–64) in the labor force is declining, as the number of older working women rises [11].

Almost two million non-working Americans aged 50–64 are ready and able to work [5].

These growth patterns have had and will continue to have a profound effect on health care delivery and the kinds of work and workers that support our society.

A *cohort* is a group of individuals born over a short time span, usually 5 to 10 years [3]. Each new cohort has specific and different expectations of what is entailed in the aging process and working. The expectations of today's 65+ age group are different than they will be for the 65+ cohort ten years from now. Factors that affect each cohort are improved health care and a higher level of education. It is likely that future cohorts will not only expect but demand innovative occupational options that offer more intrinsic satisfaction, as well as health delivery choices that will allow them to cope better with chronic conditions.

Coincidental with improved longevity are the fairly new (historically speaking) concepts of middle and old age and retirement, during which personal growth, career changes, and a variety of leisure pursuits can be pursued.

RETIREMENT

In the 1880s, Bismark designated 65 as the age when a German worker could "retire" from working. The United States adopted Bismark's scheme in 1935 in the Social Security Act. Retirement is now seen by many Americans as a reward for the work they have accomplished during their lifetimes [9], as well as a "symbolic boundary and a rite of passage between middle years and old age" [11]. Technically retirement is considered to be anything less than full-time work [12].

Demographics illustrate that the "graying of America" will present problems for our current system where the young, a diminishing segment of our population, support the old. If the percentage of women who may not have reaped Social Security benefits and the extended life expectancy, particularly of those over 75, who consume 30 percent of health care dollars [1], are factored in, the problem becomes more complicated.

Retirement requires a reallocation of time. People of retirement age move in and out of the work force and seek working arrangements that provide an optimal mix of work and leisure and necessary financial support. Encouragement to plan for retirement options is gaining momentum, with more businesses offering this as a service to their employees.

THE AGING PROCESS AND ITS IMPACT ON THE WORKER

Aging is a normal process, which begins at conception and progresses until death. Although there are changes that go along with aging, such as deteriorating audition and vision, aging is not in and of itself responsible for poor health. Most people over 65 are able to function independently (Figure 8-1). Only 5 percent of the aging population is institutionalized, but a dramatic increase occurs after age 75 [1]. Although medical technology has allowed people to live longer, medicine does not consistently cure.

Chronological age is less important as a predictor of health and ability than is "functional age," the ability to perform tasks, particularly activities of daily living. "Age differences manifest themselves in a slowing of reaction time and speed of performance, but older employees score as well or better than younger employees on creativity, flexibility, facility of information processing, absenteeism, accident rates, and turnover" [10, p. 519].

Only recently has research begun in earnest on "successful agers"—those who remain healthy and active [13]. Such research plus the increasing visibility of aging individuals who remain active participants in society, have begun to dispel the myth that aging equals illness. A balance of play, work, and rest is essential for the physical and mental health and well-being of any individual [8]. Involvement in occupational tasks serves a survival function, enables an individual to realize and demonstrate his or her potential, and enhances social standing and self-esteem via contributions made to society [12]. Such involvement "arises out of innate, spontaneous tendency . . . to explore and master the environment" [7].

Purposeful and meaningful activities that fit into the work–play continuum are the basis of occupational therapy [8]. Work begins as "child's play," a rehearsal for learning about adult roles, extends into adolescence where further practice and exploration of specific work options are pursued, and continues into adulthood, when work provides social status and remuneration. At each of these developmental stages, the proportion of work to leisure—"unobligated discretionary time" [11]—is different. "The concept of the life cycle itself rests in part upon the predominance of work or leisure in various life stages" [11]. Occupation's importance does not diminish as aging occurs, nor does it stop at retirement. With many familial and social responsibilities already met, aging adults may have their first opportunity to make "real" and less-pressured choices about work and leisure.

THE ROLE OF OCCUPATIONAL THERAPY WITH THE OLDER WORKER

The health of our aging population is of prime significance to the practice of occupational therapy. Many occupational therapists are already involved with the delivery of health care to geriatric patients with acute diseases and chronic disabilities. A primary concern of occupational therapy has been helping older clients to maintain and/or improve their ability to perform activities of daily living (ADLs) and thus maintain their independence and quality of life (Fig. 8-2). As the population

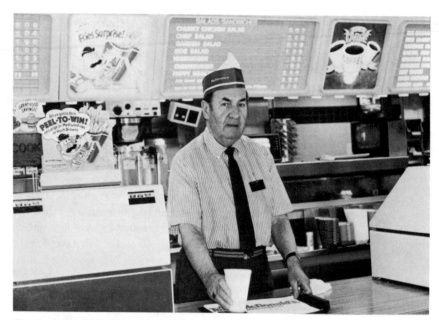

Figure 8-1.   Older workers are becoming one of the prime markets for recruitment in the service companies, such as fast-food restaurants. (Photographer Karen Jacobs.)

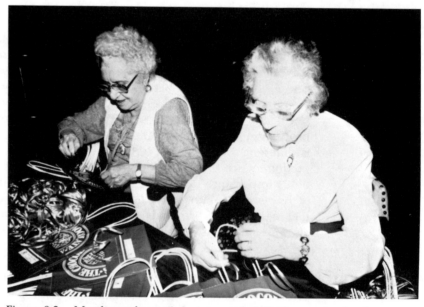

Figure 8-2.   Members of a workshop in a rehabilitation center for the aged completing subcontract work. (Photographer Karen Jacobs.)

continues to age, the variety of available occupational activities will become more diverse. It also enhances an expanding role for occupational therapists in health promotion and functional assessments of aging people who are capable of and eager for work. The recent trend to call this area of occupational therapy practice "gerontics" [6] (of or pertaining to the old) parallels the growing recognition that the majority of the aging population are relatively healthy.

Because of their belief in the crucial importance of meaningful, productive activity, occupational therapists are uniquely qualified to help others find challenge and meaning through activities. Through their functional assessment of the whole person, their knowledge of physiology, psychology, and sociology, and their practical approaches to providing meaningful tasks to assist in gaining or maintaining independence, occupational therapists provide a crucial link to productivity, both intrinsically and extrinsically.

The basic occupational therapy process need not change to work with an older population, but a number of factors need to be considered, including chronic diseases, acute conditions, mental illness, cultural background, gender differences, and social and familial supports. As an example, in order to retain an older worker with low vision, special adaptations will need to be made in the work environment. An occupational therapist can determine what adaptations, such as improved, non-glare lighting, utilization of figure-ground techniques, and judicious selection of color to enhance important elements, are necessary to ensure continued successful employment.

Occupational therapists can use a four-step process called tactical activity planning [2] as part of preretirement planning. The TAP relies on an activity analysis of the use of time and an assessment of the skills developed during a lifetime. It involves the prospective retiree in realistically setting goals and helps promote understanding of the relationship between work and leisure time.

Creativity will be necessary to increase and/or improve the occupational opportunities for aging individuals, particularly those who are institutionalized or homebound. Occupational therapists will need to advocate for more flexibility in work schedules, to help older individuals to work during times when they are most productive, and to accommodate seasonal moves to ensure consistent health status. That work or occupation does not necessarily mean monetary compensation bears repeating. Non-paid activities, such as volunteerism, can be valid in and of themselves and make significant contributions to society.

CONCLUSION

Seniors will demand more opportunities to remain involved in society, both to fulfill their own needs to be productive and to share their wisdom with younger people. Intergenerational dialogue can produce a greater awareness of each group's needs and strengths and how inexorably they are linked. Such acknowledgment can help society gain a wider perspective of future options and help them shape the health care delivery and work options of the future.

Occupational therapists will continue to be an integral part of an interdisciplinary team that provides functional treatment to this aging portion of our population. One of occupational therapy's most important contributions to the future may be advocacy—promoting the well-being of an aging society via wellness concepts, developing adaptive and compensatory techniques, and ensuring the right and the means to pursue work activities throughout life. Enhancing this sense of productivity and contribution will help aging people to maintain a sense of integrity, dignity, and worth.

REFERENCES

1. An Aging Society: Implications for Health Care Needs Impacts on Allied Health Practice and Education, A Report of the National Task Force on Gerontology and Geriatric Care Education in Allied Health *J. Allied Health,* 16(4):301–363, 1987.
2. Bachner, S. C. Retirement Activity Planning. *ROTE,* American Occupational Therapy Association, pp. 179–188, 1986.
3. Bengsten, V., Cutler, N., Mangen, D., and Marshall, V. Generations, Cohorts, and Relations Between Age Groups. In Binstock and Shanas (Eds.). *Handbook of Aging and the Social Sciences,* Second Edition. New York: Van Nostrand Reinhold Co., 1985, pp. 304–338.
4. *Business Review,* 4:4, 1990.
5. Health News. *OT Week,* 4(6):8, 1990.
6. Hopkins, H. L., and Smith, H. D. *Willard and Spackman's Occupational Therapy,* 7th Edition, Philadelphia: J.B. Lippincott, 1988, pp. 272–307, 742–755.
7. Kielhofner, G., and Burke, J. P. A Model of Human Occupation, Part 1: Conceptual Framework and Content. *Am. J. Occup. Ther.* 34(9):572–581, 1980.
8. Lewis, S. C. *Elder Care in Occupational Therapy.* Thorofare, NJ: Slack, 1989, pp. 14–17, 233–237.
9. Morrison, M. H. Work and Retirement in the Aging Society. *Daedulus,* 115(1):269–294, 1986.
10. Palmore, E., Burchett, V., Fillerbaum, G., George, L., and Wallman, L. *Retirement: Causes and Consequences.* New York: Springer Publishing Co., 1985, pp. 81–103.
11. Robinson, Coberly, and Paul. Work and Retirement. In Binstock and Shanas (Eds.). *Handbook of Aging and the Social Sciences,* Second Edition. New York: Van Nostrand Reinhold Co., 1985, pp. 502–527.
12. Rogers, J. C. Why Study Occupation, *Am. J. Occup. Ther.* 38(1):47–49, 1984.
13. Rowe, J. W., and Kahn, R. L. (1987). Human Aging: Usual and Successful. *Science* 237:143–149, 1987.

Prevention of Work-Related Injuries*

Injury is epidemic in America and most other industrialized nations and is, without a doubt, one of America's greatest health problems. The word "epidemic" is a key concept here. Whereas injuries as "problems" must be "managed" and "solved," only when injuries are seen in the context of an epidemic does it become obvious that preventive measures are imperative if we are to halt the spread of this killer and crippler. Physical trauma is of such magnitude that its costs to society overshadow AIDS, all forms of cancer, and cardiovascular disease combined. While cancer and cardiovascular diseases combined were estimated to be responsible for 3.8 million years of life lost in 1980 [6], injuries accounted for 4.1 million years of life lost in the same period. It is the most common cause of death in persons under age 45. The impact of this epidemic has been masked for years by the hundreds of different diagnoses assigned to its victims. Each year hundreds of billions of dollars are spent trying to deal with this problem. Few of us realize that injuries are the major cause of lost years of life under age 65.

A particularly problematic subset of the broad category of injury is accidents related to the work place. Other injury subgroupings such as vehicular trauma and accidents in the home are beyond the scope of this chapter.

Occupational therapy is strategically placed to assume a leadership role in work place injury prevention. The case to be made here for occupational therapists playing a major role in the prevention of work-related injuries is based on almost five years of experience of the Industrial Accident/Injury Prevention Laboratory at the University of Texas Health Science Center at San Antonio. The model of prevention services and some of the specific examples of successful prevention programs are based on the author's experiences with both public and private sector employers who collectively employ more than 30,000 workers, more than one-third of whom have been included in the programs and approaches described here.

*This chapter was written by Richard K. Schwartz, M.S., OTR.

RATIONALE FOR INTERVENTION BY OCCUPATIONAL THERAPISTS

There are two primary reasons for occupational therapists to play new roles in accident/injury prevention. First, the unique professional skills, abilities, and knowledge that occupational therapists bring to injury prevention are essential for any comprehensive safety program. Second, the costs of primary care and rehabilitation for injury-related disabilities comprise a staggering portion of escalating health care costs. Prevention services offered by occupational therapists both minimize the incidence and severity of disability, for a far lower cost than occupational health physicians and other primary care providers have traditionally charged.

Medical costs for the treatment of injuries and diseases have been escalating since at least 1980. Corporations now pay approximately 70 percent of the health care dollars spent each year in America. In 1989 under 6 percent of the gross national product was spent on the military. In this same year over 11.5 percent of the gross national product, or 599 billion dollars, was spent on health care [25]. It is no surprise that medical cost containment has become the number one priority of many corporations.

While detailed consideration of the economics of prevention is beyond the scope of this chapter, some basic concepts need recognition. First, true costs of injuries and accidents go far beyond the obvious medical, rehabilitative, and even compensation costs. Each day that an employee is unable to work, productivity is lost. Work schedules are disrupted while others fill in for the injured worker. Documentation costs for the company may eventually include costs of determining liability and other legal services. If the employee cannot return to work, there are the costs of hiring and training a replacement. The final blow to the company comes with the productivity differential in the output or work capacity of the new employee compared with that of the injured person being replaced.

As if these costs weren't bad enough, state, local, and even federal disability benefits are often financed by taxpayers. So there may also be lost tax revenues, such as FICA, state and federal income taxes, and sales tax revenues, all generated by a healthy worker.

It is a sad comment that most health professionals think that the only costs that need containing are those of other medical professions! This leads physiotherapists, work hardening specialists, occupational safety engineers, occupational physicians and nurses, chiropractors, and others into marketing battles designed to exclude competition. The results of this unnecessary conflict is that corporations are often ignorant of the need for a team approach to prevention and cost containment. A further irony of the competitive service delivery arena is that single-discipline approaches often *do* show improvement in comparison to pre-intervention or no-treatment conditions. Thus, corporations often settle for less than optimal gains in accident/injury prevention and management by going with the provider and discipline that is most effective in marketing specialized services. There are, unfortunately, very few studies comparing one form of intervention to another or comparing single-discipline interventions to multiple interventions.

The core educational requirements for certification of occupational therapists include human anatomy, physiology, kinesiology, pathology, activity analysis, psychosocial functioning, evaluation and measurement, and a broad range of physical and psychological treatment approaches. In addition, many curriculums now include courses in ergonomics, work rehabilitation, work evaluation, work hardening, and accident/injury prevention. However, it is not the knowledge base per se that makes occupational therapy special with respect to prevention. What is unique about the occupational therapy *perspective* is that it acknowledges the multifactorial, multidimensional nature of health and illness and expressly seeks to integrate information that other professions choose to segregate. For instance, it is rare to find an industrial safety engineer who understands the etiology and pathologies of back pain, carpal tunnel syndrome, and other common injuries. Likewise, it is rare to find a physician who is devoted to prevention rather than to diagnosis and treatment of existing conditions. Occupational therapists, on the other hand, view performance, competence, and problems as interdependent. Those who are distressed by our profession's apparent eagerness to be "all things to all people" may fail to recognize the value of approaching problems from many angles and acting in many arenas of intervention simultaneously.

A multifactorial concept of inherently complex behaviors is not, in and of itself, enough to qualify occupational therapists as experts in accident/injury prevention. The unwritten, shared heuristic of occupational therapy has always been that a problem can be solved using one or more of four fundamental approaches:

1. Change the skills and abilities of persons to enable them to perform as needed in a particular environment at a particular time. This approach implies an emphasis on education and training (e.g., exercises, training, counseling).
2. Change the methods and/or tools of performance to allow the individual to achieve the stated goal in an atypical or "adapted" manner. The unique element of this approach is reorganization and/or redesign of tasks rather than people.
3. Change the roles and/or the social/productivity expectations of individuals to allow them to contribute to their own independence and the welfare of society in a manner consistent with residual abilities and limitations. The emphasis here is on redefinition of expectations and reassignment of individuals to "niches" in which each is likely to be successful.
4. Educate the person and all those in direct contact with the person in the principles of preventing further complications or loss of function once something does go wrong. The emphasis here is on first aid and primary medical care being viewed as a form of prevention (i.e., secondary prevention).

Although this approach has proven most effective in the rehabilitation of injured and disabled individuals, it has even greater potential for minimizing disability *before damage is done*. Occupational therapists have skills, attitudes, and methodologies that are ideal for preventive intervention related to work place injuries and accidents.

It is difficult, and at times disturbing, to practice a profession in which complete habilitation or rehabilitation is rare and where one has to settle for relative rather than absolutely satisfactory results. As more is learned about the causes and related risk factors for cardiovascular disease, back problems, repetitive motion trauma, and even some cancers, the question to be asked is not what to do about these, but instead what can be done to prevent them from happening in the first place. A shift to a prevention focus is invigorating. It offers the chance to eliminate, avoid, and prevail over conditions that challenge even the best of us once diagnosed. Prevention can decrease the incidence, severity, and frequency of injuries. Prevention turns control over disease back to the individual and society and preempts the traditional medical establishment. The practice of a prevention service role is unlike that of the traditional clinician in many respects. There are seldom personal thanks for preventing something that each person never believed would happen to them personally. Professional relationships with clients/patients are briefer, less costly, and less personal. Yet the opportunities for occupational therapists to make a difference are staggering.

Prevention demands a set of services that physicians and engineers are poorly prepared to offer. That is, services which are education and training intensive. It is increasingly clear that prevention services provided by an occupational therapist will not only be cost-effective compared to the services of physicians and engineers, but also may yield the highest benefit/cost ratio. Because occupational therapists are trained to call upon physicians, engineers, psychologists, and others when problems exceed their personal and professional expertise, they are likely to incorporate such experts' knowledge and advice in problem-solving strategies. Occupational therapists in preventive medicine employ the services of the traditional medical team for only a fraction of the time and expense there would be if these other professionals were to direct prevention programs.

Finally, prevention does not require traditional third-party financing. Subgroups of employees at greatest risk can be identified and targeted intervention conducted as part of a general benefit/cost maximization strategy. Prevention services can be marketed to private firms, to governmental agencies, educational institutions, labor unions, professional associations and special interest groups, insurance carriers, health care provider agencies, and individuals. Payment can be per hour, per day, per employee, on retainer, by contract, or even on a draw plus commission (based on savings attributable to the program). If all of this is not opportunity waiting for the rush of takers, then what is?

A NEW MODEL FOR INDUSTRIAL PREVENTIVE MEDICINE

Having considered reasons *why* occupational therapists should lead the way in industrial accident/injury prevention, the question of *how* this is to be accomplished needs to be answered. The industrial accident/injury prevention research team at the University of Texas Health Science

Center in San Antonio has been testing the effectiveness of a multistage model of industrial injury prevention. To better understand this model, it is useful to compare it to the older and more traditional model of preventive intervention, the "barrier" model. This older approach is best exemplified by vaccination against disease. Typically, a single intervention is staged for an entire population at risk, and while there may be a few individuals who do not achieve immunity, most will. Of those who do not become immune, the few that will actually be diagnosed with the condition being prevented are considered "failures." As long as these have a small enough incidence, they are considered to pose little or no risk. This model of injury prevention is dichotomous; the condition has either been prevented or not. The most serious drawback of this model is that it fails to take into account the degrees of severity and increased risk that can occur with successive injuries. It also does not take advantage of heightened motivation to comply with safety education following initial and subsequent injuries.

The "penetration" model that we use views prevention as a multistage, multiple-intervention process. It goes beyond traditional injury prevention strategies, which include training and environmental safety engineering, and adds *multiple and successive phases* of preventive intervention both prior to and following the occurrence of each injury. Traditional injury prevention models have viewed work injury as a final outcome, and little attention has been focused on the likelihood or prevention of reinjury. It is hypothesized that intervention following *each* injury will yield important health, safety, and economic advantages to the employer, the worker, and society. This penetration model takes the view that global efforts to reach all workers at a given worksite, or all employees of given enterprise by using the same training program for every worker, is an expensive and less than optimal prevention strategy. Interventions may only affect workers whose risk was slight and whose motivation for changing their behaviors was above average. By targeting successively more intensive interventions for those who have either a known occupational risk or history of harm, the goal becomes preventing disability and serious injury rather than attempting to simply lower the incidence of injuries irrespective of severity.

A single type of problem—low back injuries—will be used to illustrate various risk factors and methods of prevention.

UNDERSTANDING WHY INDUSTRIAL ACCIDENTS/INJURIES OCCUR

The key to treatment of disease is diagnosis of pathology. The key to prevention of accidents and injuries is identification of *risk factors*. A knowledge of contributing factors to accidents and injuries is indispensable in the design and implementation of a successful prevention program. These factors can be divided into two major subdivisions—environmental and human factors.

Environmental Factors

These include such diverse risk factors as noise, vibration, excessive heat or cold, chemical and biological toxins, radiation hazards, architectural and other physical barriers, pollutants, pressure, vehicular/ machine hazards, inadequate illumination, and electrical hazards [8]. Using the human back for illustration, vibration contributes directly to low back syndromes through the repetitive loading and unloading of intervertebral discs. This is especially true for those workers who must operate some form of motorized vehicle, be it forklift, truck, automobile, bus, or train. Since low-frequency vibration leads to an amplification of the imparted motion to the back, secondary resonance waves may transfer harmful mechanical stresses onto structures of the back. Knowledge of this risk factor leads to (1) prescribing a seating system with armrests and lumbar supports, (2) teaching the proper way to sit while driving a motor vehicle, and (3) developing protective equipment such as seat cushions to absorb vibratory shock.

Chemical and biological issues in back injury are best exemplified by tobacco as a risk factor [11]. Smoking is one of the preventable risk factors for back problems. Until recently the evidence upon which these recommendations were based was fairly limited. In the past two years, however, there has been a tremendous increase in evidence of the role of smoking in back problems. [3,7] Smoking (and even chewing tobacco) contributes to back problems in two ways. First, tobacco contains nicotine, which has been shown to adversely affect the nutrition of intervertebral discs. Nicotine is a vasoconstrictor, which causes the blood vessels to tighten up and decrease blood flow [11]. Second, smoking is associated with increased coughing. Each time a person coughs it greatly increases pressure on the intervertebral discs. Chronic coughing wears out the discs prematurely whether or not one is a smoker. The more one smokes, the greater the risk of back problems. This is especially true for those under 45 years of age. Any reduction in smoking translates into a decreased risk for back problems. Even if it is not possible to quit smoking, it will help to decrease the amount smoked per day. This strongly supports the movement toward "smoke-free" work places as one way to promote prevention on the job and to decrease medical costs.

Architectural hazards may force a worker to use unsafe body mechanics in lifting. Materials and tools stored either too high or low or placed behind barriers that prevent keeping the object close to the center of gravity may impose increased risk of back sprains, strains, and even disc problems related to excessive forces being transmitted to the spine during lifting.

In many instances the risk of accident and/or injury is increased because of the structure of tasks. Machine operators and assembly line workers who continuously receive material from either the right or left side may have excessive twisting of the spine associated with routine work. Not only does this lead to asymmetric wear and tear on paraspinal musculature, but it also contributes to overstretching of the longitudinal ligaments of the spine, with resultant loss of integrity and decreased spinal stability.

Tools used to perform productive work often contribute to excessive wear and tear on the body. The knives used by most meat cutters and butchers require excessive forceful wrist motion and appear to be one of the major causes of carpal tunnel syndrome among such workers. A lack of armrests for the driver on most motor vehicles makes it difficult to translate vibratory forces into the seat system rather than absorbing them in spinal structures. As a general rule, individuals at risk for particular conditions or injuries should have machines and/or tools to help them perform work that is harmful for the body without mechanical aids.

Human Factors

Even in the safest possible environment, with the best tools, and an ergonomically designed work process, there will still be injuries and accidents! Human error has always been a risk factor in work-related accidents and injuries.

Cognitive Factors

It is only recently that cognitive factors in injury and accident prevention have even been addressed. In this context it is useful to consider that each worker must have three distinct kinds of knowledge concerning the safe performance of work tasks.

1. First and foremost, the employee must know *what* to do to perform a task safely. This kind of information is termed "declarative knowledge" and usually is represented by oral or written statements concerning the task, potential dangers, and how they can be avoided.
2. The employee must have the psychomotor skills, including the physical and perceptual abilities, to carry out the task safely. This kind of knowledge is termed "procedural knowledge" and consists of knowing *how* to do the job safely [2].
3. The individual must know how to employ general rules of body use under specific conditions. This third type of knowledge is termed "conditional knowledge" and has only recently been recognized as a factor in accidents and injuries [12,26].

To illustrate the issues and difficulties of cognitive approaches to prevention, the example of back schools is most informative. A number of intervention programs called "back schools" have evolved to prevent initial episodes and/or reduce the recurrence of back pain through education. Such programs typically consist of classroom training in proper use of the body or "body mechanics." There have been uniformly positive findings that such intervention can reduce the incidence and severity of back pain [21]. Back schools have been shown effective as both primary and reinjury prevention measures. Most primary programs work with small groups of 10–20 workers in one or two sessions lasting one to two hours each. Lectures, demonstrations, films, slides, models, and group practice in exercises and proper body mechanics are employed during the training sessions. Participants are usually trained in a classroom environment, taking notes as they are instructed and referring to manuals provided during the session.

Post-injury prevention programs (often called "re-education" programs) are offered to those already having suffered back impairment of some kind. These differ from primary programs mainly in that they are often conducted either one-on-one or in small groups at a therapy or rehabilitation facility, and they emphasize the precautions related to each participant's particular injuries or condition.

The success of training programs in comparison with no intervention has been documented in most studies of "back schools." Yet there are intrinsic flaws in the rationale and methodology of these programs. For example, it might appear that the primary goal of such educational programs would be to teach proper methods of lifting, carrying, pushing, and pulling (procedural knowledge). This goal is unrealistic, however, because most workers have established habits and patterns for performing work activities. Such habits cannot be easily altered simply by creating a new cognitive structure—describing the steps of safe lifting and material handling. What is essential is to sensitize workers to the dangers and possible loss of function from *not following safe and prudent body mechanics.*

The purpose of training should be primarily to teach how to employ general rules or principles of body use under less than ideal circumstances (conditional knowledge). Workers must learn to make decisions about the *best choices under the circumstances* rather than ideal actions. Learning must be relevant both to the individual worker and to the unique circumstances of each job.

Biomechanical Factors

Kinesiologic and ergonomic aspects of performance have received a great amount of research attention [11, 14]. Research on lifting and carrying has led to the National Institute of Occupational Safety and Health (NIOSH) "action limit" and "maximum permissible lift" formulae. Training in proper body mechanics is a major portion of most "back school" programs for both primary prevention and re-education of those with diagnosed back pain. The emphasis has been on identifying basic principles of safe usage of the body and employing these in skills-training programs. Training programs that address both declarative and procedural knowledge have been developed for back problems [27], for carpal tunnel syndrome [28], and for sprains and strains [23]. There is no information, however, concerning the conditional knowledge required to prevent these conditions.

Affective Factors

While affective state may play a role in many forms of injury, it is a difficult area to research. Emotional states are transient, subjective, and not always fully conscious. The theory that anger may be distracting, that depression may make one less alert and vigilant, that high arousal may make it difficult to focus attention is logical, but there is no direct evidence yet of their role in accidents and injuries. Stress, on the other hand, is emerging as a definite injury factor.

Over the past two decades, an enormous body of literature has evolved on the effects of stressors on health and well-being. In 1967, Holmes and Rahe created interest in the measurement of stress by publishing the results of their studies using the "Social Readjustment Rating Scale" [16], a tool designed to assess the impact of significant life events requiring change. Using this and other scales, a number of studies have shown positive correlations between the magnitude of stressors experienced by individuals and their subsequent health status [15, 20]. Recently, Lazarus and colleagues [18] have engendered interest in less obvious stressors that occur on a daily basis.

Little of the research on stress has examined the relationship between stress and accidents [10]. One retrospective study [22] examined the life stress profile of injured workers before and after their accidents. As anticipated, the injured workers showed significant increases in stress both before and after their accidents. Moreover, the injured workers reported a significantly higher level of stress than the control group. Considerable debate has evolved over both conceptual and methodological issues associated with the measurement of life stress [29, 32]. Maddi, Bartone, and Puccetti [24] have recently provided a compelling argument in support of the validity of such research.

Motivation

Motivation is a behavioral tendency to persevere at a task independent of behavioral reinforcements and should be useful in assessing the proclivity of workers to adhere to injury prevention guidelines. Individual differences in the tendency to persevere have been reflected in various constructs, including achievement, locus of control, and success or failure. Since none of these constructs efficiently predicts behavioral compliance, Dishman and Ickes [9] have argued that a trait-like construct of self-motivation could offer an improved approach to predicting perseverant behavior. This is supported by medical compliance research, which suggest that behavioral tendencies of a patient at the onset of therapy may effectively predict their adherence to therapeutic regimens [13].

Self-Concept/Identity

It has been suggested that some workers lack the motivation to participate fully in safety programs *because they view themselves as invincible.* Unlike affective and motivational factors, which are subject to the daily flux of life events and therefore may change rapidly from one situation to the next, self-concept factors are assumed to be relatively stable. In many respects, self-concept is even more immune from change than cognitive variables such as declarative, procedural, and conditional knowledge, which may be altered through even relatively brief training sessions [30, 31]. To date this is an area that appears to be unexplored in relation to accident/injury prevention.

Almost 100 years ago, William James framed a fundamental issue of personal identity by asserting that the self or "the me" is the sum total of all that one can call one's own. Included in this framework were "the material me," "the social me," and "the spiritual me" [17]. James suggested that the physical self could be considered a construct independent of one's total identity. He further argued, "We all have a blind impulse to watch over our body" [17]. Recognizing that conflict of the "mes" would be inevitable and that integration of material, social, and spiritual selves is necessary, James argued that "a tolerably unanimous opinion ranges the different selves . . . in an hierarchical scale, with the bodily me at the bottom, the spiritual me at the top, and the extracorporeal material selves and the various social selves between" [17].

From this, it is not unreasonable to infer that the industrial worker, faced with the "social me" pressures of co-workers, supervisors, family, and friends, might be inclined to neglect "material me" concerns such as risk of accident/injury. Likewise, an actual injury would command attention and become an organizing principle of behavior, if it in turn threatened social and spiritual selves.

Allport [1] framed the nature of the ego in terms of its function rather than its form(s). He reviewed the literature of the day and concluded that the degree to which there was active ego involvement determines the degree to which there are consistent personality traits. He noted that "employees in industry are not 'economic men' so much as they are 'ego men.' What they want above all else is credit for work done, interesting tasks, appreciation, approval, congenial relations with their employers and fellow workers" [1]. When the ego is highly involved in a task or activity, there is greater consistency in behavior; memory and retention are enhanced; and learning is facilitated.

If Allport's theory is applied to the case of industrial accident/injury prevention, it would be logical to postulate that the worker who considers him- or herself at risk for accidents/injuries (a "vulnerable" worker) will be more ego-involved and therefore better able to learn, remember, and act consistently in relation to safety training and injury prevention education programs than the worker who feels invincible.

Kihlstrom et al. [19] present an information-processing view of the self, suggesting that the "self" is a hierarchical encoding of self-concepts in memory. These self-concepts are considered to be context-specific and to represent the self in a variety of situations. Thus, workers from different backgrounds might have highly dissimilar self-concepts even though they work side by side. The authors also suggest that there is a memory structure for one's "future self" and that the nature of this representation may, at least in part, determine one's motivation in relation to future goals. For example a person who is raised to have fatalistic expectations based on religious and cultural experiences may have less motivation to participate in safety programs and to change behavior as the result of such training. On the other hand, a worker from a background that emphasizes the importance of good works (e.g., the "Protestant ethic"), of responsibility for one's fate, or the nobility of striving to better oneself may be highly motivated.

It is a current limitation of both industrial psychology and occupational medicine that there are no measures of self-concept for predicting which workers will benefit from accident/injury prevention training. The classification of workers along a dimension of *concern for safety* needs to be accomplished psychometrically. The development of these screening tools could greatly increase the efficiency and effectiveness of injury prevention programs in industry.

The ability to identify workers' self-concept in relation to the dimension of vulnerability/invincibility has enormous practical consequences. First and foremost would be the ability to target only those likely to benefit from training for prevention programs. More importantly, there would be a way of identifying workers with the highest risk for injury and then using these subjects to develop training programs targeted to their particular personalities and self-concepts.

DESIGNING EFFECTIVE INTERVENTION PROGRAMS

To effectively offer occupational therapy services to business and industry, it is imperative to understand their goals vis-a-vis prevention of accidents and injuries. First and foremost is medical cost containment. This includes not only direct costs such as workman's compensation insurance, health insurance, and direct medical payments, but also a host of less direct costs including lost time from work, changes in productive output capacity due to personnel loss, employee replacement costs, and costs of on-site medical records/documentation management.

Medical Care Cost Containment: Prevention and Wellness Promotion

The following should be considered whenever the ultimate goal of preventive programs is medical care cost containment.

A common medical cost-containment strategy is to pass along an increasing share or percentage of medical expenses to the employee. Any program that seeks to have workers share an increasing fraction of total costs must also have an educational program to make employees aware of risk factors and healthy behaviors. Since a change in behavior is almost always antecedent to the reduction of the incidence and severity of injuries and accidents, an approach that simply increases the motivation of the employee to work more carefully but does not educate the worker as to *how* this may be done is not likely to be effective.

In addition, passing along costs without educational programs and engineering controls to reduce injuries is likely to decrease employee morale. On the other hand, when employers demonstrate a commitment to institute engineering controls, eliminate environmental hazards, and create a healthy work environment, employees are more likely to comply with work rules and safety measures and thus reduce loss time. A hidden benefit of successful programs is that they help to reduce adversarial relationships between employees and management.

Incentive programs for individual workers and job groups or job classes increase compliance with health and safety programs and thus reduce demands on health care services. If a portion of the savings realized through medical care cost containment measures is returned to the work force, there will be increased motivation to avoid medical problems.

On-the-job wellness and health programs have a benefit above and beyond their direct effect on the particular health problem or need addressed. Studies of the Industrial Accident/Injury Prevention Lab consistently find that programs to reduce back problems actually reduce other medical problems in addition to those targeted by training sessions!

Targeting of populations at risk for particular health problems is superior to all forms of global screening and/or training. Successful health and wellness promotion depend on the identification and minimization of known risk factors for illness and/or accidents. It is now possible to create comprehensive injury databases for a given employer and statistically analyze the nature, extent, and distribution of injuries and lost time throughout the organization. Factor analytic models, analysis of variance procedures, and contingency analysis may be used to assess factors contributing to existing problems and create models of risk factors that are specific to a particular group. Where this is done, management may implement prevention programs that are custom-tailored to a particular work environment and specific employees.

Risk managers, insurance companies, and upper level corporate managers need to be trained how to put together a mixture of human and engineering services that address unique groups of workers in particular settings. Traditionally, engineering has been favored over educational approaches; however, *both are essential to realize full benefit from a prevention and wellness program*. Programs designed to train management teams to design and conduct their own prevention activities (called training-the-trainers programs) are ideal since they free companies from longterm dependence on outside consultants to manage prevention efforts.

Occupational therapists need to be aware of local, state, and federal safety regulations. The best known of these are the guidelines from the federal government's Occupational Safety and Health Administration (OSHA) and nongovernmental standards such as those published by the American National Standards Institute, for which compliance is voluntary.

The occupational therapist may also contribute both directly and indirectly to the management of liability for employee injuries and accidents. A well-designed prevention program that documents the precise nature of training provided to employees is convincing evidence that a company does not take the welfare of its workers lightly. When workers are given every opportunity to follow safe practices, when environmental hazards are minimized, and where workers are trained in safe job performance, claims of negligence become difficult to prove.

Employee Relations

Prevention programs send a clear message to workers that the well-being of each employee is important to the company. Under ideal circumstances, employees from both management and the rank and file should have an opportunity to participate in the design and implementation of prevention and wellness programs. Companies that are genuinely committed to the health and safety of workers and take steps to prevent accidents and injuries benefit not only in economic terms, but also with respect to employee morale. It seems that this is especially true when the company brings in "experts" from outside or takes other extraordinary steps to protect workers.

Educational Considerations

Classroom training has very little relation to most hazardous work activities. While simulation may be of some benefit, *workers should be trained in the actual environments and under the actual work conditions in which they will be expected to use such learning.* That was shown by the recent work of Carlton [5], who failed to find that body mechanics instruction made any difference between two groups, one trained in body mechanics and one untrained, even though the trained group showed greater procedural knowledge on the novel research task.

The specific nature of each criterial task or the particular evaluation methods used to assess learning in large part determines what will be recalled and used in the future [4]. Most prevention programs do not use a formal set of evaluation activities, known in educational psychology as "criterial tasks" [4], which are used to enhance worker attention to newly learned information and to assess the degree of understanding and retention of new learning. In any learning situation there are numerous ways to success. For example, in teaching joint protection to people with arthritis, one can ask the patient to demonstrate what has been learned, set up a practical test of knowledge and see how many actions the arthritic performs using joint protection, give a multiple-choice test concerning these techniques, or simply ask the patient, "Do you feel you understand what we have been going over? If not, ask me about the things you don't understand." (This final example is, unfortunately, a method of assessment used by some occupational therapists.)

Case Studies

The following are brief descriptions of projects that have been undertaken by the UTHSC-SA Industrial Accident/Injury Prevention Lab over the past few years. They are offered as examples of the types of programs (both consultation and research) that fit the model of preventive interventions.

Cognition and Learning in Industrial Accident/Injury Prevention: An Occupational Therapy Perspective

One hundred ten workers and approximately eleven representatives of corporate management were trained. Of this group, all were males except for one female. A majority of the workers were manual material handlers. Spotters (persons who drive "mule" tractors to move trailers around the "yard"), traffic control specialists, fork lift operators, pallet repair workers, and maintenance personnel were also included in this group. All training was done during normal working hours. While participants were required by management to receive training, they were also paid their normal wages for attending the sessions.

Of the management personnel, most were floor supervisors and the remainder were middle-management supervisors. A unique feature of this program was that managers were trained before workers. The managers were then given the responsibility for ongoing assessment of workers based upon the principles outlined by the consultant. No punishments were used as part of the follow-up and reinforcement strategy. Supervisors were told to request workers who were not performing safely to try and show the supervisor a better way to do the job than the one that they had just used. By assuring that the supervisors understood the principles of safe body mechanics, there was always a source of educational support and reinforcement present.

Also, a detailed set of 23 safety recommendations was provided to management to act upon. Most notably, all training took place in small groups of three to six workers at their actual workstations. No classroom, reading, or writing was used, based on the assumption that the most relevant learning would be through conversation and experiential learning. The estimated benefit to the company of this program was approximately $90 per year per employee, or about $9900 saved in the first year. Most important with respect to programmatic goals was an almost 40-percent reduction in lost time *from all causes*. Clearly a program targeted at back problems, but that focuses on principles of safe and efficient movement, appears to have the potential of contributing to the prevention of problems other than those involving the back. One of the long range goals of this program is to refine and develop better methods of worker education in accident and injury prevention.

Prevention of Back Problems in HEB Fleet Drivers
This was a contractual consulting agreement that provided for the training of the entire HEB Fleet including supervisors and safety personnel. Over 240 workers were trained during the summer, and a report detailing comprehensive measures required to reduce accidents and injuries for the fleet was submitted to management. A unique feature of this program was that the occupational therapist spent considerable time riding with drivers and making deliveries prior to designing the training program. The actual training was done in group sessions using a truck cab simulator designed by the consultant. This simulator included the steering column, seat, and all controls from an actual truck. The seat and backrest were then covered with a set of LED-activating pressure sensors, which showed a computer image of how the worker was seated during the training simulations. A more than 50-percent reduction in back-related problems has been maintained during the two years following this program.

Effects of Training and Prophylactic Lumbosacral Bracing on Prevention of Low Back Problems in Asymptomatic Industrial Warehouse Workers
This study was conducted using a group of 90 warehouse workers randomly selected from over 800 employees with the same job classification in the same division of the H.E. Butt Grocery Company in San Antonio, Texas. Those individuals being treated for back pain or back injury were excluded from the study.

All subjects had their abdominal strength assessed with a calibrated cable tensiometer. A special chair was designed to standardize the positioning of the subject and eliminate substitute motions of trunk flexor muscles. All subjects were given a brief (25 question) multiple choice test concerning care of the back and proper body mechanics. Group 1 (control group) had no intervention. Group 2 (experimental) received a one-hour training session in back pain prevention and proper body mechanics on the job. Group 3 (experimental) also received this same training session, and then wore a simple back support (lumbosacral brace) during their working hours for a period of six months.

At the completion of the study period, all subjects had their abdominal strength assessed and again filled out the questionnaire on knowledge of proper lifting, carrying, and care of the back. H.E. Butt Grocery Co. furnished the health records of all subjects to determine if they reported any back pain, back injuries, or lost time from work during the six months of this study and to identify those with a history of prior back pain/back injury for comparison with those without such history.

This study provides preliminary evidence of the relative effectiveness of an accepted method of prevention (educational programs) compared to an unexplored method of education plus prophylactic bracing. Those workers who received no training had no gains in knowledge, decreased productivity, increased frequency of accidents, and an average increase in lost time of .8 days per worker per year. Those receiving training only had increased knowledge, increased productivity, decreased frequency of accidents, and an average decrease in lost time of 1.2 days per worker per year. Those receiving both brace and training had increased knowledge, increased productivity, no change in accident frequency, but an average decrease in lost time of 4.9 days per worker per year! There were no effects of the brace on strength of the workers.

CONCLUSION

Prevention is cost effective. It is a better investment than health insurance or liability insurance. It minimizes loss of human life, function, and productivity. It is also labor intensive and requires a broad range of knowledge including kinesiology, neurosciences, psychology, education, pathology, economics, labor relations, and corporate/industrial management. Of all the weapons available in rehabilitation, it is the most powerful and the most under-utilized. There is soon to be an explosive demand for prevention services. Whether it be under the rubric of "wellness," "risk-management and cost-containment," or some other label, it is going to become an economic and legal imperative for employers to act before the fact to prevent accidents and injuries.

But it is not only occupational therapists who are already involved with work hardening who will have the opportunity to focus on prevention. A pilot project with 111 third-graders in San Antonio demonstrated that even brief experiential training programs can lead to demonstrable changes in understanding and knowledge of back safety. Biomechanical habits are acquired early and difficult to modify later in adulthood. Accident/injury prevention needs to be part of every school curriculum. Injury prevention work is not limited to occupational therapists practicing in physical disabilities or work-related areas. Opportunities abound for pediatric, psychiatric, and geriatric therapists as well. Those in geriatrics already know the role that accidents and injuries play in problems of the elderly. Falls alone account for thousands of hip fractures that result in hospitalization, loss of function, and even death. As the numbers of older people in the work force increase, there will be greater demand for work simplification, safety training, and worksite design, which are all needed to minimize disability in the elderly.

Prevention is the only logical future for occupational therapists engaged in work-related rehabilitation and training programs. Either we will join forces with industrial safety engineers, occupational medicine practitioners, supervisors, and trainers to eliminate the causes of work disabilities, or we will join the myriad of medically based professions that are as much a part of the problem as of the solutions they profess to offer. Professions define themselves by doing the things that a very small number of their members have shown is effective and in demand. It is always the examples of those at the cutting edge of the profession that create the models and opportunities for the entire profession. Occupational therapy will become identified with work injury prevention when occupational therapists shift a major portion of their attention from rehabilitation and remediation to education and safety in the work place.

REFERENCES

1. Allport, G. The ego in contemporary psychology. *Psychol. Rev.* 50:451–478, 1943.
2. Anderson, J. R. *Cognitive Psychology and Its Implications.* San Francisco: W. H. Freeman and Co., 1980.
3. Battie, M. C., Bigos, S. J., et al. A Prospective Study of the Role of Cardiovascular Risk Factors and Fitness in Industrial Back Pain Complaints. *Spine* 14:141–147, 1989.
4. Bransford, J. D. *Human Cognition: Learning, Understanding, and Remembering.* Belmont, CA: Wadsworth, 1979.
5. Carlton, R. S. The effects of body mechanics instruction on work performance. *Am. J. Occup. Ther.* 41:16–20, 1987.
6. Centers for Disease Control. Table V. *Morbid. Mortal. Weekly Rep.* 31:599, 1982.
7. Deyo, R. A., and Bass, J. E. Lifestyle and Low Back Pain: The Influence of Smoking and Obesity. *Spine* 14:501–506, 1989.
8. Diffrient, N., Tilley, A. R., and Harman, D. *Humanscale 4: Human Strength and Safety.* Cambridge, MA: The MIT Press, 1981.
9. Dishman, R. K., and Ickes, W. Self-Motivation and Adherence to Therapeutic Exercise. J. Behav. Med. 4:421–438, 1981.
10. Dohrenwend, B. S., Krasnoff, L., Askenasy, A. R., and Dohrenwend, B. P. Exemplification of a Method for Scaling Life Events: The PERI Life Events Scale. *J. Health Social Behav.* 19:205–229, 1978.
11. Frymoyer, J. W., Pope, M. H., et al. Risk Factors in Low Back Pain. *J. Bone Joint Surg.* 65:213–218, 1983.
12. Hale, A. R. Achieving Safe Behavior. In Gardner, A. W. (Ed.) *Current Approaches to Occupational Health—3* Bristol: Wright, 252–264, 1987.
13. Haynes, R. B., Taylor, D. W., and Sackett, D. L. *Compliance in Health Care.* Baltimore: Johns Hopkins University Press, 1979.
14. Heliovaara, M. Risk Factors for Low Back Pain and Sciatica: Invited Review Article. *Ann. Med.* 21:257–264, 1989.
15. Holmes, T. H., and Masuda, M. Life Change and Illness Susceptibility. In Dohrenwend, B. S. and Dohrenwend, B. P. (Eds). *Stressful Life Events: Their Nature and Effects.* New York: Wiley, pp. 45–72, 1974.
16. Holmes, T. H., and Rahe, R. H. The Social Readjustment Rating Scale. J. Psychosom. Res. 11:213–218, 1967.
17. James, W. Psychology: Briefer Course. In *The Works of William James.* Cambridge, MA: Harvard University Press, 159–190, 1984.
18. Kanner, A. D., Coyne, J. C., Schaefer, C., and Lazarus, R. S. Comparison of Two Models of Stress Measurement: Daily Hassles and Uplifts Versus Major Life Events. J. Behav. Med. 4 (1):1–39, 1981.
19. Kihlstrom, J., Cantor, N., et al. Information Processing and the Study of the Self. In L. Berkowitz (Ed.) *Advances in Experimental Social Psychology.* San Diego, Academic Press, 1988.
20. Kobasa, S. C., Maddi, S. R., and Kahn. Hardiness and Health: A Prospective Study. *J. Personality Social Psychol.,* 42:168–177, 1982.
21. LeBlanc, F. E. Scientific Approach to the Assessment and Management of Activity Related Spinal Disorders: A Monograph for Clinicians. *Spine, Euro. Ed.* 12(7):s1–s59, 1987.
22. Levenson, H., Hirschfeld, M. L., and Hirschfeld, A. H. Industrial Accidents and Recent Life Events. *J. Occup. Med.* 1980.
23. MacLeod, D. *Strains and Sprains: A Worker's Guide to Job Design.* Detroit: International Union UAW, 1982.
24. Maddi, S. R., Bartone, P. T., and Puccetti, M. C. Stressful Events are Indeed a Factor in Physical Illness: Reply to Schroeder and Costa (1984). *J. Personality Social Psychol.,* 52(4):833–843, 1987.
25. New York Times Wireservice. Health Careers Gaining Strength: Increase Gives Experts Some Cause for Fear. *San Antonio Express News,* March 18, 1990.

26. Paris, S. G., Lipson, M. Y., and Wixon, K. K. Becoming a Strategic Reader. *Contemporary Educational Psychology* 8:293–316, 1983.
27. Paris, S. V., and Porter, R. W. *Workbook for Prevention and Reeducation.* Atlanta: The Back School of Atlanta, 1985.
28. Pearce, R. B. *Hand and Wrist Owner's Manual: A Guide to Hand and Wrist Injuries.* Daly City, CA: Krames Communications, 1985.
29. Schroeder, D. H., and Costa, P. T., Jr. Influence of Life Events Stress on Physical Illness: Substantive Effects or Methodological Flaws? *J. Personality Social Psychol.*, 46:853–863, 1984.
30. Schwartz, R. K. Cognition and Learning in Industrial Accident/Injury Prevention: An Occupational Therapy Perspective. *Occup. Ther. Health Care,* 5(2):67–85, 1989.
31. Schwartz, R. K. Occupational Therapy in Industrial Accident and Injury Prevention. *Work Programs Newsletter,* Vol. 3:2–7, 1989.
32. Zimmerman, M. Methodological Issues in the Assessment of Life Events: A Review of Issues and Research. *Clin. Psychol. Rev.* 3:339–370, 1983.

Home-Based Employment*

As long as women have taken in knitting and writers have set up typewriters in their living rooms, people have been working at home for pay. Betsy Ross, for example, stitched the American flag in her own home. Today's rising use of the personal computer and advanced technology, such as modem hookups and facsimile (fax) machines, have greatly expanded the range of occupations that can be completed successfully at home. Along with these expansions has come an increase in the *types* of individuals able to do these jobs. Many physically and mentally challenged individuals who are unable to work outside the house can now do meaningful, productive work, *without* leaving home.

For example, in 1972, Coralee Smith Kern started the "Maid to Order Incorporated Cleaning and Party Service" after she was diagnosed with lupus and ordered to stay in bed. Initially, she ran the business from her bedroom. Currently, Kern works out of a "work apartment," adjacent to the apartment in which she lives. Kern employs 460 workers and works an average of 40 hours per week. As a pioneer of the future workstyle, Kern coined the term "electronic cottage," which means "using computers in some way to produce a good or service out of your home" [7]. In addition to the cleaning service, Kern publishes the *Mind Your Own Business at Home Newsletter* (circulation 35,000) and the *Cottage Connection Newsletter* and founded the Nonprofit National Association for the Cottage Industry. Through her publications, Kern receives correspondence from many job displacement victims, parents of small children, and handicapped people who describe a "home occupation as the best solution" [7].

According to the Manhattan-based Link Resources Research Firm [1], the number of home professionals now totals 9 million. In 1990 approximately 13 million, or 11.4 percent of the United States work force worked out of the home [1].

Possible options for home employment include four major categories:

Computer Utilization	Involves data entry and analysis, software applications, word processing, and programming
Telemarketing	Involves information gathering, direct sales, product marketing, and public relations
Service Functions	Involves clerical responsibilities, small business, and professional assistance

*This chapter was written by Theresa L. Breen, Kim Ann Clark, and Michelle Moran.

Table 10-1.   Companies with Options to Work at Home

A growing number of firms now allow employees to work at home, at least part of the time. Of the companies listed here, some have full-fledged telecommuting divisions; others have pilot programs. Employees work at home anywhere from one to four days a week. In most cases, the programs are open only to current employees.

Bell Communications, Livingston, N.J.
Boston's Beth Israel Hospital, Boston.
Corning Inc., Corning, N.Y.
Detroit Free Press, Detroit.
Gannett, Washington, D.C.
GTE California, Thousand Oaks, Calif.
Hartford Insurance Group, Hartford, Conn.
IBM, Armonk, N.Y.
JCPenney Company, Dallas.
Johnson & Johnson, New Brunswick, N.J.
Merck, Rahway, N.J.
Pacific Bell, San Francisco.
Southern California Assn. of Governments, Los Angeles.
Southern New England Telephone, New Haven, Conn.
State of California Department of General Services, Sacramento, Calif.
The Travelers Corporation, Hartford, Conn.
Time Inc., New York City.
Unum Life Insurance Company, Portland, Me.
US West, Englewood, Colo.

Light Manufacturing   Involves construction of parts of whole units for industry in accordance with the law

"Telecommuter" is a term used to describe home-based employees doing computer utilization and/or telemarketing. Since 1984, the roster of companies offering telecommuting has gone from 200 to 350 [1]. Among these companies are Bell Communications, IBM, JCPenney, Johnson & Johnson, and Time Inc. (Table 10-1) [3].

ADVANTAGES TO HOME-BASED EMPLOYMENT

As with any other type of work, home-based employment is not well suited to everyone. To benefit from working at home, one must be able to work independently, without strict supervision. The home-based worker must be well-disciplined, able to screen out distractions, and have the ability to attend to the job at hand. Most importantly, the individual who works at home must possess goal-setting qualities and strive to attain these goals.

There are many advantages that can be enjoyed by the home-based worker. Working out of the home minimizes the cost of commuting, childcare, lunch, clothes, and dry cleaning. The convenient, flexible hours are another benefit, especially to those with low stamina. By offering the physically and mentally challenged a chance to succeed, home-based employment meaningfully reduces the high level of unemployment for persons with disabilities. Consequently, the opportunity for home-based employment can substantially increase not only the self-esteem, but also the overall quality of life, for individuals unable to work at conventional, on-site jobs.

DISADVANTAGES TO HOME-BASED EMPLOYMENT

There are also disadvantages to home-based employment. The general lack of social interaction and intellectual stimulation can lead to feelings of isolation. Recently, some evidence has suggested that home-based employees have a propensity to gain weight. In addition, due to decreased visibility, telecommuters and other home employees are often passed up for promotions. Also, some companies do not offer their home-based employees many benefits or comprehensive insurance coverage, holidays, or sick pay. However, with the increase in numbers of people working at home, this may soon change.

EMPLOYER BENEFITS FROM HOME-BASED EMPLOYMENT

In several respects, employers benefit from placing their employees in the homesite. It appears that employers enjoy greater productivity from employees who are happier working out of the home. Travelers and Mountain Bell Telephone Company in Denver hail their telecommuters as 35 to 40 percent more productive than their in-office counterparts and state that they develop "independent work habits and learn to set goals" [1]. Home-based employment is cost effective in that it abates the cost of "the rental of office space, related equipment, and maintenance costs" [12]. In addition, employers are able to pay less for benefits and can profit from tax breaks. Companies say that other incentives for home-based employment include the opportunity to "recruit from a wider area and keep employees who need to move" [9]. Although employers have less control over their home-based employees, the advantages of hiring employees for work at home greatly outweigh this drawback.

FINDING HOME-BASED EMPLOYMENT
Video Resumes

One aid for obtaining jobs that is gaining in popularity is the video resume. Now used by conventional job seekers, the video resume has long since been a popular tool of actors, broadcasters, dancers, musicians, and artists. Most video resumes are three to five minutes long and show the applicant from the waist up, talking about himself or herself, his or her job history and experience, and the kind of position he or she is seeking. Throughout the video, the potential employee answers questions posed by a narrator. Although video resumes have received mixed reviews from employers, employees like them because they allow the applicant to speak freely about what he or she feels is important, without feeling pressured to offer information that he or she is reluctant to discuss. Some employers use video resumes as a "screening tool for three basic requirements: appearance, command of the language, and presentation abilities" [6]. Other employers are reluctant to view video resumes for fear of potential discrimination lawsuits if the applicant is rejected [6].

Massachusetts Rehabilitation Commission and Massachusetts Commission for the Blind

The Massachusetts Rehabilitation Commission (MRC) and Massachusetts Commission for the Blind (MCB) are state agencies that provide evaluation, adjustment training, and on-site placement services that benefit the blind and the physically and emotionally challenged. In 1987, MRC and MCB compiled a client talent pool based merely on "word of mouth" interests from the field offices. Their available client work force now numbers nearly 100 capable, employable individuals who operate at various levels of performance. These clients can undertake a full range of entry level, professional employment situations including clerical assistance, data entry, and computer programming. Some clients are new to the work world, while others possess excellent experience. Some of these individuals have been disabled since birth, others for only a short while [12].

MRC's Home-Based Employment (HBE) program is headed by vocational rehabilitation counselors. When a job arises from "Jobsearch" (database) and/or want ads, the counselor scans his/her client pool for a compatible employee. The counselor then contacts the client, verifies his/her qualifications, checks for interest in the job, and sets up an interview. If this process is successful, the vocational rehabilitation counselor will place his/her client.

REGULATIONS FOR HOME-BASED EMPLOYMENT

The complex *Laws Relative to the Control of Industrial Homework* [2], the *Occupational Safety and Health Administration (OSHA) Workplace Regulations* [8], and *the Building Owner Authorization* [8] are some of the legal and regulatory guidelines (Table 10-2) governing the implementation of home-based employment. The *Laws Relative to the Control of Industrial Homework* are designed to protect home workers from exploitation by employers. They require meticulous, specific methods of record keeping for hours worked.

The *OSHA Workplace Regulations* are aimed at keeping the work place free from hazard and consequently maintaining the safety of employees. These regulations require the installation of smoke detectors, fire extinguishers, appropriate furniture, and certified electrical facilities. The *Building Owner Authorization* is required for any electrical or telecommunications cabling.

FUNDING FOR HOME-BASED EMPLOYMENT

Government programs have been established to aid in funding employment programs for the physically and mentally challenged. One such program is the targeted jobs credit [5], which grants employers federal tax credit for each worker hired from one of nine targeted groups. Beginning with the employee's initial day on the job, the employer may

Table 10-2.   Regulations that Concern the Home Worker

Regulation	Purpose	Example
U.S. Dept. of Labor, part 530	Limits what kind of work is legal to perform from the home, and provides guidelines for employer and employee.	Part 530 does not allow the manufacturing of women's apparel, jewelry, gloves, mittens, and belts.
Occupational Safety and Health Administration (OSHA)	Keeps work place free from hazards to maintain safety of employee.	Smoke detectors and fire alarms are types of safety devices found in the work place.
Building owner authorizations	Ensures that the landlord will allow modifications of the worksite.	Landlord may not allow the telephone company to place another cable in for telemarketing work done in the home.

Adapted from Kuhlman, G. A. Follow-Up of a Word Processing Training and Employment Program for Homebound Persons with Disabilities. *J. Rehab.* 54:2, 1988.

claim the credit for two years. The credit itself equals half of the worker's first $6,000 in wages for the first year, with a maximum of $3,000 awarded. In the second year, the credit matches one-fourth of the employee's first $6,000.

One targeted group consists of individuals deemed "economically disadvantaged" by local job services. Persons in this group include:

1. 18- to 24-year-olds who are self-supporting
2. 16- to 19-year-olds in cooperative education programs
3. 16- to 17-year-olds in summer jobs
4. Vietnam veterans
5. Ex-convicts

The remaining groups in the program are recipients of various forms of assistance: state or local general funding, Aid to Families with Dependent Children, and Supplemental Security Income (which benefits the needy, aged, blind, and handicapped). Disabled individuals referred from state rehabilitation or Veteran's Administration programs are also members of a targeted group.

Another source of aid for the disabled employee is the Dole Foundation, which, in 1987 awarded a $500,000 grant for job training of the disabled. For more information on these and other state programs, contact the MRC or local state job service agency directly.

ROLE OF OCCUPATIONAL THERAPY IN HOME-BASED EMPLOYMENT _____

Vocational rehabilitation counselors are currently coordinating the few operating home-based employment programs. However, potential involvement by occupational therapists (OT) in these programs is great. The following is a description of the prospective role of the OT in a home-based employment program.

Once a client had completed a rehabilitation program, the OT would determine whether or not home-based employment was appropriate for the client. This process would include evaluation and analysis of the client's physical and emotional capabilities. Melnik has compiled a useful analysis, the "Home Movement Analysis," which could aid in assessing the physical and emotional readiness of the client to return to home work [10].

If the client appeared ready to return to home work, the OT would then decide whether home-based employment was a viable option. The OT would assess the client for necessary criteria for success in a home-based employment program, including promptness, the ability to manage money, good concentration capabilities, and effective time management skills. Sidler's Occupational Therapy Questionnaire [11] could be adapted for use in evaluating criteria for home-based employees (Figure 10-1).

Once home-based employment was identified as appropriate for the client, the OT would then assess the home for a viable work space. The OT Home Assessment Report [4] could easily be adapted and used as a tool to assess the potential work area within the home (Table 10-3). In the comment column of the assessment, the OT could make recommendations for adaptive equipment needed to ensure that the client established the highest possible level of productivity.

Next, the OT would implement a job readiness program designed to train or retrain the client in skills required to obtain a job. The OT would teach the client interview skills and coach him or her in role-play situations. In addition, the OT would work on problem solving and goal setting with the client. When the client was ready, the OT would search the database for a job to match the client, set up an interview, and, if successful, place the client.

Unlike a vocational rehabilitation counselor, the OT would follow through on the program in the client's first weeks of work. The OT and/or Certified Occupational Therapy Assistant (COTA) would perform job coaching as necessary. This part of the program would consist of teaching effective time management and tactics for screening out distractions. Evaluating the client at the worksite, the OT would focus on training the client in good body mechanics and would also be able to suggest ergonomic approaches to work. Once the client was working independently, the OT would follow up periodically and evaluate any problems that arose.

CONCLUSION _____

Home-based employment is a challenging arena for today's occupational therapist. The fundamental skills occupational therapists possess

Name _____ Date _____
Expected worker status   Part time _____   Full time _____
Expected homemaker status   Part Time _____   Full Time _____
Is client responsible for child care?   Yes _____   No _____
If yes; is it   Part time _____   Full time _____   Children's ages _____

	Good	Fair	Poor	Comments
1. Manage money and/or checks; pay bills on time				
2. Remember to do important things on time				
3. Get along with family members				
4. Get along with roommates or neighbors				
5. Work on a job				
6. Get along with a boss				
7. Get along with co-workers				
8. Support/help family financially				
9. Use public transportation/drive car				
10. Call people on phone				
11. Concentrate on a task				
12. Follow task through to completion				
13. Learn new things readily or with little difficulty				
14. Make decisions; act independently				
15. Interest and motivation to accomplish goals				
16. Express self effectively				
17. Invent and initiate own ideas				
18. Manage time well				

Question	Yes/No	Comment
1. Do you feel you need others to help you manage your time and tasks?		
2. Do you feel you handle changes and new experiences without feeling too nervous?		
3. Do you entertain family and friends in your home? If so, how often and when (day or evening)?		
4. What do your household duties include? How often do you perform these tasks?		

Adapted from Sidler, Marilyn Occupational Therapy Questionnaire [11].

Figure 10-1.   Criteria for home-based employees

Table 10-3.   Occupational Therapy Home Assessment for Home-Based Employment Programs

Work Area	Criteria	Adequate/Inadequate (±) Recommendations
1. Stairs, railing, lights	Number, railing size, height	
2. Doors, doorways	Width, threshold, direction of opening, operation of knobs and locks	
3. Maneuverability	Furniture, carpeting, mobility on surfaces, adequate turning radius, throw rugs	
4. Plugs, switches	Location, height, ease of operation	
5. Furniture	Location, height, transfers	
6. Distance from house traffic	Quiet work area away from distractions	
7. Phone accessibility	Emergency numbers visible, location, type, operation, warning light	
8. Working surfaces	Countertop heights, depth, direction of approach	

Adapted from Hopkins, Helen L. and Helen D. Smith. *Willard and Spackman's Occupational Therapy (6th ed.).* Philadelphia: Lippincott, 1983.

make them highly qualified for creating many additional aspects of a home-based employment program. With their fine-tuned observational and evaluation skills, occupational therapists can develop and refine a home-based employment program best suited for their client. As teachers, occupational therapists are adept at helping clients learn new skills. Through work simulation tasks, occupational therapists teach their clients to adapt and improve job skills and worker habits. In keeping with the ideology of occupational therapy, home-based employment programs would be designed to increase the client's overall quality of life. Thus, OT-created home-based employment programs would be comprehensive and efficient.

Occupational therapists must face the challenge of overcoming the often stereotypical and negative attitudes of employers toward the disabled. Through the creation of employer education programs, occupational therapists can illustrate the value of home-based employment to both the employer and the employee. Hence, the area of home-based employment affords a variety of opportunities for the occupational therapist.

Case Study

Ryan, a 19-year-old respirator-dependent quadriplegic, participated in a home-based employment program. A former college computer science student, Ryan desired to work in a field allowing him to use his computer abilities. The occupational therapist contacted various companies to ascertain job openings based on Ryan's skills. It was arranged with a desktop publishing company that with a modem connected to his Macintosh home computer, Ryan would be able to receive assignments from a desktop publishing company. He received a salary of $15 per hour. Assignments included creating brochures and preparing artwork for the company using his computer.

REFERENCES

1. Castro, J. Staying Home Is Paying Off. *Time*, October 26, 1987.
2. Commonwealth of Massachusetts Department of Labor and Industries. Industrial Bulletin Number 20 Containing the Laws Relative to the Control of Industrial Homework and Revised Rules and Regulations Concerning Homework.
3. First Efroymson, S. The Great Office Escape: Telecommuting. *Working Mother*, February, 1990.
4. Hopkins, H. L. and Smith, H. D. *Willard and Spackman's Occupational Therapy (6th ed.)*. Philadelphia: Lippincott, 1983.
5. Internal Revenue Service, Department of the Treasury. *Jobs and Research Credits*. Publication 906 (Rev. November, 1986).
6. Knowlton, J. Smile for the Camera: Job Seekers Make More Use of Video Resumes. *Wall Street Journal*, June 22, 1987.
7. Krucoff, C. Futurists Taking Stock of Coming Age. *The Washington Post*, Friday, August 12, 1983.
8. Kuhlman, G. A. Follow Up of a W. P. Training and Employment Program for Home-bound Persons with Disabilities. *J. Rehab.* 54:2, 1988.
9. MacNeice, J. Home Jobs: Still a Long Way to Go. *USA Today*, April 14, 1986.
10. Melnik, M. Home Movement Analysis.
11. Sidler, M. Occupational Therapy Questionnaire.
12. Staff. Home Is Where the Work Is. *Industry*, November, 1989.

11

Educational Curricula on Work Practice

Today's occupational therapy curricula must be adapted to the changing needs of today's consumers [1].

It is only through updating and revising our educational curricula that we will be able to produce therapists with the knowledge and skills to keep pace with the changing health care environment. Although the area of work practice has greatly expanded in the 1980s, a trend that is predicted to continue into the 21st century, this trend is not yet reflected in our curriculum content.

In *Work Hardening: State of the Art*, Niemeyer and Jacobs predict that "educational programs for occupational therapists will need to provide curriculum to keep pace with work program practice" [2]. I support this suggestion and would like to propose that a course on work become incorporated into the occupational therapy curriculum and scheduled in the last semester of academic training. In this sequence, the course would be able to build upon the principles and knowledge acquired in foundation courses, such as physical disabilities, psychosocial dysfunction, and human development [4, 5]. Also this sequencing would allow the course to introduce selected skills and techniques of work practice that could build upon core knowledge. The development of clinical reasoning skills should be reinforced through use of case study analyses and fieldwork experiences in a variety of work practice settings, including supported employment settings, schools, industry, and work hardening programs. Creativity should be fostered.

An interdisciplinary focus of practice should be reinforced through exposure to vocational rehabilitation counselors and evaluators, social workers, physical therapists, rehabilitation nurses, and other work practice–related practitioners in the community. These individuals might be contacted to lecture on selected topics. For example, an attorney who specializes in work injuries could lecture about providing expert witness testimony, the litigation process, giving a deposition, and the importance of documentation.

WORK ASSESSMENT AND PROGRAMS: A MODEL COURSE

In 1986, a course entitled "Work Assessments and Programs" was developed as a four-credit elective through the Department of Occupational Therapy at Boston University. The course was funded by a three-year RSA grant. Curriculum content was based, in part, on information gathered from a needs assessment survey to occupational therapists working in a variety of work programs. These individuals were asked to identify knowledge, principles, skills, and techniques that they found valuable in their respective programs. From this information, in addition to reviewing future environmental trends that might affect practice, a curriculum for the course was devised.

The following common understandings were the basic framework for the course:

1. Work is an occupational performance area.
2. Work occurs over the life span.
3. Assessment and programming should be age appropriate.
4. Programming is most effectively delivered using an interdisciplinary approach.
5. Wellness and prevention are important.
6. Early intervention is critical to effective programming.

The course included the following content areas:

1. Anatomy and physiology of the back
2. Body mechanics
3. Lifting techniques
4. Anatomy and physiology of the hand
5. Cumulative trauma disorders
6. Ergonomics and job modification
7. Use of work references by the U.S. Department of Labor, e.g., *Dictionary of Occupational Titles*, *Guide to Occupational Exploration*, *Occupational Outlook Handbook*, and *Classification of Jobs*
8. Uniform terminology based on AOTA's *Uniform Terminology—2nd Edition* (Figure 2-1), Workers' Compensation Laws, Commission on Accreditation of Rehabilitation Facilities (CARF) Work Hardening Guidelines (Appendix 1-1)
9. Career theories
10. Regulatory guidelines, e.g., CARF Work Hardening Guidelines, Public Laws, Workers' Compensation Laws
11. Work evaluations, e.g., work samples, job analysis
12. Programming in a variety of settings, e.g., schools, industry, rehabilitation centers, private practice
13. Transitioning and the job coach
14. Retirement and the older worker
15. Prevention and wellness, including stress management
16. Marketing
17. Reimbursement
18. Keeping outcome data for efficacy studies
19. Litigation process, deposition, and expert witness testimony
20. Work practice legislation, e.g., Americans with Disabilities Act (ADA) [3].

Course requirements have included:

1. A three-part job site:
   a. an analysis by the student of the worker performing the job tasks, b. an analysis by the worker describing job task requirements, and c. supervisor's description of the worker's job. The student would write up a comparison of the three analyses.
2. Evaluation of individuals of various ages using work assessments and/or evaluations, such as the Jacobs Prevocational Skills Assessment (Chapter 4), the Skills Assessment Module (Chapter 3), the Perceptual-Motor Test for Children (Chapter 3), and the WEST 7—Bus Bench (Chapter 3).
3. Student presentations to the class on selected work topics such as job coaching and interest inventories.
4. Case study analyses, which included developing a treatment plan, and a proposal for adaptation of the work site.
5. Development of normative data on various work evaluations, such as the WEST 7—Bus Bench.
6. Development of a work sample.

Concurrent fieldwork placement in work practice sites is the ideal method to allow students to apply the knowledge and principles acquired in academic programming. Joint collaboration between these sites should be encouraged. In fact, the professor and students could provide assistance to the work sites by collecting outcome data to document the efficacy of work intervention.

CONCLUSION

The preceding content was provided only as a guide for curriculum development. Since work practice is an expanding area, course content should be periodically revised to incorporate information on emerging issues. It is hoped that providing students with both academic and fieldwork experiences in work practice will better prepare them to enter this highly competitive and challenging practice arena.

---

*Case Study 1**
Name: Alex O.
Age: 30
Sex: M
Job: Grounds Keeper
Type of Industry: School District
Job Description: Responsible for landscape maintenance, including mowing and hedge trimming, and maintenance of irrigation equipment.
Circumstances of Injury: Lifted a trash can into a truck bed and experienced sharp pain in his back and down his left leg.
Primary Diagnosis(es), Industrial: Severe lumbosacral sprain/strain with associated left sciatic neuritis. Herniated nucleus pulposus, L5–S1.
Pertinent History: Initial treatment consisted of heat, muscle relaxants, and pain medication. Has been undergoing chiropractic treatments three times weekly

*Courtesy of Linda Ogden Niemeyer, OTR.

since injury; treatments included cryotherapy, ultrasound, support belt, therapeutic exercise, moist heat, and chiropractic manipulation. His condition was evaluated by an orthopedic surgeon, who recommended surgical intervention. The client declined surgery and elected to continue chiropractic care.

Pertinent Physical Findings: Mild left lumbosacral tenderness and pain on flexion and rotation with extension. Paresthesia to left lateral thigh. Lumbar and left gluteal muscle spasms and myofascitis.

Pertinent Psychosocial Factors: Lives with his wife and two children in a small, well-kept home which he is purchasing from his parents.

Prior Participation in Vocational Evaluation and/or Pain Program: None.

Physician's Restrictions: No heavy lifting or repeated bending and stooping.

Intake Interview
Height: 70"
Weight: 190#
Dominance: R
Language: English
Medications: Calcium supplements and Tylenol
Assistive/Supportive Devices: None
Work Since Injury: Attempted to return to modified employment with same employer six weeks after injury, but experienced a recurrence of severe back and leg pain after two to three weeks. He has not returned to work since.
Description of Function: Loves to cook and has continued to cook for his family despite his injury. Is no longer able to participate in hobbies/interests of skiing and doing carpentry, painting, and wallpapering in his home. He is unable to do yard work, wash his car, or perform home maintenance activities. His back pain is aggravated by almost any activity, and he finds bending particularly stressful.
Description of Limiting Symptoms: Sharp pain in the low back extending to the left buttocks, thigh, and calf, causing a weakness in the left leg and numbness in the side of the thigh.
Goals: Wants to "get well" and return to work. Interested in possible employment as a landscape draftsman, or possibly in getting his contractor's license. Wants to use skills developed through extensive experience in landscape maintenance and construction.

Interview Observations
Weight: Slightly overweight
Posture/Gait: Sat with good posture, but gait was uneven, unbalanced, and antalgic.
Dress/Grooming: Neat, casual clothing and good grooming.
Affect: Presented himself as a pleasant individual and communicated easily.
Other Behavior: Arrived early for the interview. During interview, changed positions in chair frequently and moved in a somewhat stiff and guarded manner. Got up and stretched after 20 minutes sitting.

Case Study 2*
Name: Phyllis M.
Age: 53
Sex: F
Job: Waitress
Type of Industry: Restaurant
Job Description: Her job as a waitress required her to do light lifting, heavy lifting, frequent bending, stooping, prolonged walking, prolonged standing, and working with the arms overhead.
Circumstances of Injury: The client was carrying a tray of food to the dining area when she slipped on some spilled sour cream. She did not fall, but the tray, weighing 25–30 pounds, struck her in the left neck and shoulder area. She

*Courtesy of Linda Ogden Niemeyer, OTR.

experienced swelling shortly afterward and felt immediate shoulder and neck pain, which was accompanied by upper back pain.

Primary Diagnosis(es), Industrial: Soft tissue trauma of the neck, left trapezius, and shoulder. Severe myofascial sprain of the cervical spine. Suspect C6–7 herniated pulposus of the cervical spine. Possible rupture of the left trapezius. Adhesive capsulitis of the left shoulder. One physician diagnosed "anxiety hysteria" and stated, "As far as rehabilitation potential is concerned, this will depend on the patient's motivation, which I feel is a big factor."

Pertinent History: The client was hospitalized for diagnostic tests, and was placed in cervical traction. She received physical therapy for one month, including transcutaneous neural stimulation, heat, ultrasound, and massage. The treatments did not help. She was seen by a chiropractor on two occasions, and this caused her to have increased pain. She was provided with cervical traction, which she continued to use at home. She improved and then markedly deteriorated.

Pertinent Physical Findings: Slight to moderate muscle spasm and pain to palpation of the paraspinal muscles at C6–7 is noted. Range of motion of the cervical spine approximately 60% normal range of motion. No vein distension is noted. There is tenderness to palpation throughout the entire left trapezius from the base of the skull to below the scapula. Deep tendon reflexes are bilaterally equal and active. An electronic infrared thermogram was performed 3/20/89, with equivocal findings indicating possible underlying musculoligamentous spasm or myofascitis in the left scapular area of the back, and possible C6–7 sensory fiber tract irritation patterns/autonomic dysfunction. CT scan, myelogram, and EMG were normal.

Pertinent Psychosocial Factors: Has been widowed for several years. She has brother that lives with her and helps out and two daughters who live nearby. She has lived in the same home for six years; the home has been paid for. She was very energetic and industrious before her injury and was involved with sport fishing, various handicrafts, and home maintenance/improvement activities. She has an excellent work record, including 30 years of performing duties as a waitress.

Prior Participation in Vocational Evaluation and/or Pain Program: None.

Physician's Restrictions: Avoid very heavy lifting and activities that require the left upper extremity to function above the level of the shoulder.

Intake Interview

Height: 63″

Weight: 145#

Dominance: R

Language: English

Medications: Valium, Darvocet, and Tylenol. She takes 8–10 Tylenol per day and 1–2 Darvocet.

Assistive/Supportive Devices: Initially stated that she uses no assistive or supportive devices. She later remarked that she kept her left arm in a sling most of the time until a doctor told her to discontinue using the sling.

Work Since Injury: Has not worked since injury.

Description of Function: The client is able to drive her automatic transmission car using her right hand only. She stated that she does some light housework at a slow pace, and that her brother does most of the housecleaning, cooking, and shopping. Customary hobby activities, including silverwork and lapidary, fashioning of elaborately costumed china dolls, and home building projects, have been discontinued due to pain.

Description of Limiting Symptoms: The client describes intense burning pain "like scalding water" in the upper left scapular area and the back of the left shoulder. She reports intense stabbing, throbbing, and aching pain along the medial border of the left scapula extending into the left side of the neck, as well as in the left upper arm and forearm. She reports a sensation of swelling in the left upper back and hypersensitivity to even minimal pressure. She reports that left shoulder flexion and external rotation cause immediate pain, and that the pain is tolerable only when the left arm is immobilized against her body with a sling. *Goals*: She exhibited a real willingness to consider vocational alternatives, yet expressed concern that her condition appeared to be getting worse. She expressed a desire to receive appropriate medical treatment for her condition before she starts efforts to return to work.

Interview Observations
Weight: Slightly overweight
Posture/Gait: Sitting posture is poor; gait is even, comfortable, and balanced.
Dress/Grooming: Clothes are clean and casual, grooming of hair is plain, and she wears no makeup.
Affect: The client answers questions willingly and openly, yet her appearance and demeanor suggest that she is depressed.
Other Behavior: She keeps her left arm against her body, often tucked into her blouse, and does not spontaneously use it.

REFERENCES

1. Marshall, E. and Anzai, D. Work evaluation in the entry level curriculum. *Work Programs SIS Newsletter* 3:1–3, 1989.
2. Ogden Niemeyer, L., and Jacobs, K. *Work Hardening: State of the Art*. Thorofare, NJ: SLACK, Inc., 1989.
3. Taylor, S. E. Occupational therapy in industrial rehabilitation. In H. L. Hopkins and H. D. Smith (Eds.), *Willard and Spackman's Occupational Therapy* (7th ed.). Philadelphia: Lippincott, pp. 299–307.
4. Tomlin, G. From exposure to practice: Vocational skills hierarchy in an occupational therapy curriculum. *Work Programs SIS Newsletter* 4:1–2, 1990.
5. West, W. L. Nationally speaking perspectives on the past and future, part 2. *AJOT* 44:9–10, 1990.

Future Outlook

Let's ponder the implications of the following environmental trends on work practice:

The average worker today is a middle-aged white male. The new worker in the 1990s will be a young woman. By the year 2000, minorities will account for 55% of labor force growth.
Source: *American Demographics*, Nov., 1989.

The relative education and skill level of new workers is declining. The entire labor force is shrinking.
Source: *Workforce 2000: Work and Workers for the 21st Century*, 1987.

By the year 2030, 18% of the American population will be 65 or over.
Source: *Braintree Council on Aging News*, 4:2, Sept., 1982.

There is a shortage of occupational therapy personnel.
Source: AOTA.

The future holds only nominal growth in inpatient hospital care. Growth will be in outpatient alternatives to illness prevention, diagnosis, and treatment.
Source: *Modern Healthcare*, Feb. 26, 1990.

Almost half of all hospitals have implemented occupational health or industrial medicine programs. Only 4% had them in 1978.
Source: *AHA News*, Nov. 30, 1989.

In 1988, about 13.4 million working age Americans believed they had a disability that blocked or interfered with work.
Source: US Census Bureau.

Injury is "the principal health problem in America today."
Source: National Academy of Sciences.

The estimated yearly cost of low back pain is $16–$20 billion. This results in Workers' Compensation costs of approximately $6 billion annually.
Source: R. Sutherland & W. Counihan. Functional restoration for the back-injured worker: A sports medicine approach. *OTP* 1:2, March 1990.

Occupational therapists are emerging as consultants to industry and multi-state organizations on issues of ergonomics, prevention of work injuries, and job redesign.
Source: Melanie Ellexson, Chairperson, AOTA's Work Programs Special Interest Section, 1987–1990.

Occupational therapists are increasingly involved in work place adaptation for injury prevention.

Source: Melanie Ellexson, Chairperson, AOTA's Work Programs Special Interest Section, 1987–1990.

By 1991, there will be approximately 150 programs accredited by CARF in work hardening. Kentucky, Florida, and Ohio have adopted these guidelines as mandatory for reimbursement.

Source: A. Toppel, AOTA Work Programs Special Interest Section Annual Business Meeting, April, 1990.

In *Work Hardening: State of the Art*, Niemeyer and Jacobs proposed some predictions for work hardening [1]. Since the publication of that text in 1989, some of these predictions have become realities while others are evolving. They are:

1. There will be a movement toward multidisciplinary involvement.
2. There will evolve a balance between high-tech and high-touch styles of practice.
3. Work hardening will be provided in large centers, while evaluation will be available in both small and large centers.
4. Early intervention, total continuity of care, and prevention will be the next logical steps in industrial rehabilitation.
5. Insurance industry support needs to be actively pursued.
6. There will be a shift from a clinic-based medical model to an industrial-based wellness model.
7. There will be a need to use uniform terminology.
8. There will be a need to collect outcome data for efficacy information and quality assurance.
9. There will be a need to develop and apply business skills, particularly marketing. (Author's note: Gather support from satisfied customers!)
10. Occupational therapy curricula need to keep pace with work practice.

Occupational therapists need to respond to these environmental trends proactively. We are challenged to examine our knowledge, principles, skills, and techniques in the area of work practice and ascertain whether we are prepared to deliver services. Do we need additional training to better prepare us to meet these environmental trends? Specialized training may be needed in areas such as ergonomics, rehabilitation engineering, gerontology, law, and marketing. Do we need to modify our present academic curricula to better prepare our future therapists? I strongly believe so, and have offered suggestions in Chapter 11.

We need to clearly define the contributions we can make in work practice. Many opportunities await us in the future. These may include:

Working more actively with older workers, e.g., dealing with the physical changes that come with the normal aging process

Positioning ourselves as the primary providers of work practice, particularly in industry, utilizing a wellness/prevention model

Rigorously developing work programs with elementary school-aged children. For example, prevention of back injuries could begin early by teaching children proper body mechanics.

Reestablishing our role in the transition process for students completing high school education.

Working collaboratively with political and regulatory agencies and the insurance industry

Working as advocates for individuals with disabilities in the pursuit of work, e.g., becoming experts and assisting in the implementation of the Americans with Disabilities Act (ADA).

The key is anticipation of change, so that we and our clients will be ready to meet the demands of the future.

REFERENCE

1. Ogden Niemeyer, L., and Jacobs, K. Work Hardening: State of the Art. Thorofare, NJ: SLACK, Inc., 1989.

Index